Biochemistry of Nutrition I

Publisher's Note

The *International Review of Biochemistry* remains a major force in the education of established scientists and advanced students of biochemistry throughout the world. It continues to present accurate, timely, and thorough reviews of key topics by distinguished authors charged with the responsibility of selecting and critically analyzing new facts and concepts important to the progress of biochemistry from the mass of information in their respective fields.

Following the successful format established by the earlier volumes in this series, new volumes of the *International Review of Biochemistry* will concentrate on current developments in the major areas of biochemical research and study. New volumes on a given subject generally appear at two-year intervals, or according to the demand created by new developments in the field. The scope of the series is flexible, however, so that future volumes may cover areas not included earlier.

University Park Press is honored to continue publication of the *International Review of Biochemistry* under its sole sponsorship beginning with Volume 13. The following is a list of volumes published and currently in preparation for the series:

Volume 1: **CHEMISTRY OF MACROMOLECULES** (H. Gutfreund)
Volume 2: **BIOCHEMISTRY OF CELL WALLS AND MEMBRANES** (C. F. Fox)
Volume 3: **ENERGY TRANSDUCING MECHANISMS** (E. Racker)
Volume 4: **BIOCHEMISTRY OF LIPIDS** (T. W. Goodwin)
Volume 5: **BIOCHEMISTRY OF CARBOHYDRATES** (W. J. Whelan)
Volume 6: **BIOCHEMISTRY OF NUCLEIC ACIDS** (K. Burton)
Volume 7: **SYNTHESIS OF AMINO ACIDS AND PROTEINS** (H. R. V. Arnstein)
Volume 8: **BIOCHEMISTRY OF HORMONES** (H. V. Rickenberg)
Volume 9: **BIOCHEMISTRY OF CELL DIFFERENTIATION** (J. Paul)
Volume 10: **DEFENSE AND RECOGNITION** (R. R. Porter)
Volume 11: **PLANT BIOCHEMISTRY** (D. H. Northcote)
Volume 12: **PHYSIOLOGICAL AND PHARMACOLOGICAL BIOCHEMISTRY** (H. Blaschko)
Volume 13: **PLANT BIOCHEMISTRY II** (D. H. Northcote)
Volume 14: **BIOCHEMISTRY OF LIPIDS II** (T. W. Goodwin)
Volume 15: **BIOCHEMISTRY OF CELL DIFFERENTIATION II** (J. Paul)
Volume 16: **BIOCHEMISTRY OF CARBOHYDRATES II** (D. J. Manners)
Volume 17: **BIOCHEMISTRY OF NUCLEIC ACIDS II** (B. F. C. Clark)
Volume 18: **AMINO ACID AND PROTEIN BIOSYNTHESIS II** (H. R. V. Arnstein)
Volume 19: **BIOCHEMISTRY OF CELL WALLS AND MEMBRANES II** (J. C. Metcalfe)
Volume 20: **BIOCHEMISTRY AND MODE OF ACTION OF HORMONES II** (H. V. Rickenberg)
Volume 21: **MICROBIAL BIOCHEMISTRY** (J. R. Quayle)
Volume 22: **DEFENSE AND RECOGNITION IIA — CELLULAR ASPECTS** (E. S. Lennox)
Volume 23: **DEFENSE AND RECOGNITION IIB — STRUCTURAL ASPECTS** (E. S. Lennox)
Volume 24: **CHEMISTRY OF MACROMOLECULES IIA — SIMPLE MACROMOLECULES** (R. E. Offord)
Volume 25: **CHEMISTRY OF MACROMOLECULES IIB — MACROMOLECULAR COMPLEXES** (R. E. Offord)
Volume 26: **NEUROCHEMISTRY AND BIOCHEMICAL PHARMACOLOGY** (K. F. Tipton)
Volume 27: **BIOCHEMISTRY OF NUTRITION I** (A. Neuberger and T. H. Jukes)

Consultant Editors: H. L. Kornberg, Sc.D., F.R.S., Department of Biochemistry, University of Cambridge; and D. C. Phillips, Ph.D., F.R.S., Laboratory of Molecular Biophysics, Department of Zoology, University of Oxford.

INTERNATIONAL REVIEW OF BIOCHEMISTRY

Volume 27

Biochemistry of Nutrition I

Edited by

A. Neuberger

Lister Institute of Preventive Medicine and
Charing Cross Hospital Medical School
London, England

and

T. H. Jukes

Space Sciences Laboratory
University of California, Berkeley

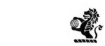

UNIVERSITY PARK PRESS

Baltimore

UNIVERSITY PARK PRESS
International Publishers in Science, Medicine, and Education
233 East Redwood Street
Baltimore, Maryland 21202

Copyright © 1979 by University Park Press

Composed by University Park Press, Typesetting Division.

Manufactured in the United States of America by
Universal Lithographers, Inc.,
and The Optic Bindery Incorporated.

Library of Congress Cataloging in Publication Data

Main entry under title:

Biochemistry of nutrition I.

   (International review of biochemistry; v. 27)
   Bibliography: p.
   Includes index.
   1. Nutrition. 2. Diet in disease.
   3. Biological chemistry. I. Neuberger, Albert. II. Jukes, Thomas Hughes,
1906–   III. Series QP501.B527 vol. 27 [QP141]   547.1'92'08s [547.1'3]
ISBN 0-8391-1083-9 (v. 1).   79-12429

Consultant Editors' Note

The *International Review of Biochemistry* was launched to provide a critical and continuing survey of progress in biochemical research. In order to embrace even barely adequately so vast a subject as "progress in biochemical research," twelve volumes were prepared. They range in subject matter from the classical preserves of biochemistry — the structure and function of macromolecules and energy transduction — through topics such as defense and recognition and cell differentiation, in which biochemical work is still a relatively new factor, to those territories that are shared by physiology and biochemistry. In dividing up so pervasive a discipline, we realized that biochemistry cannot be confined to twelve neat slices of biology, even if those slices are cut generously: every scientist who attempts to discern the molecular events that underlie the phenomena of life can legitimately parody the cry of *Le Bourgeois Gentilhomme,* "Par ma foi! Il y a plus de quarante ans que je dis de la Biochimie sans que j'en susse rien!" We therefore make no apologies for encroaching even further, in this second series, on areas in which the biochemical component has, until recently, not predominated.

However, we repeat our apology for being forced to omit again in the present collection of articles many important matters, and we also echo our hope that the authority and distinction of the contributions will compensate for our shortcomings of thematic selection. We certainly welcome criticism — we thank the many readers and reviewers who have so helpfully criticized our first series of volumes — and we solicit suggestions for future reviews.

It is a particular pleasure to thank the volume editors, the chapter authors, and the publishers for their ready cooperation in this venture. If it succeeds, the credit must go to them.

H. L. Kornberg
D. C. Phillips

Contents

Preface

In this volume, we have assembled several articles that describe recent developments in biochemical topics that are related to nutrition. Historically, the science of nutrition has developed through discoveries, such as the identification of vitamins, essential amino acids, and essential minerals, that are followed by biochemical explanation of their metabolic functions. This trend continues, with growing emphasis on pharmacology and toxicology of overdosage of nutrients and on non-nutrients that are present in the food supply.

As nutrition has grown more complex, interest in it has mounted, together with a demand that information be excessively simplified for the benefit of members of the public. This book does not present such oversimplification, but it is hoped that it will be useful for scientists who are involved in what is often termed "nutrition education."

There is great interest in the relation of nutrition to good health. It is an everyday topic of conversation, but too often such discussions are subjective and anecdotal. Dr. W. R. Beisel corrects this by reviewing findings on the immune response under conditions of malnutrition. Dr. Eric Conn's chapter on cyanogenic glycosides draws on his wide experience in research on these compounds, and is of great value as a source of corrective data in the face of the propaganda for "laetrile." Dr. Leon Ellenbogen presents a detailed account of findings with intrinsic factor and *trans*-cobalamin that will be of special interest to those who have followed the history of pernicious anemia. The chapter on protease inhibitors and lectins by Irving Liener has an important bearing on the study of actual utilization of vegetable proteins, a topic that is of great interest now.

An important topic — the vitamin C requirements of man and the effect of large dosages of this vitamin — is critically discussed by Dr. G. N. Schrauzer. Another field that gives rise to considerable public discussion is the importance of fiber in the diet. Its role in diseases of the intestinal tract and vascular system is carefully and comprehensively assessed by Jon Story and David Kritchevsky. Elizabeth and James Miller were both elected to the National Academy of Sciences (U.S.) during the period they were writing their review on naturally occurring carcinogens, a topic that is in the forefront of public discussion today. G. A. Rose and H. D. Tunstall Pedoe bravely tackle a subject that has been debated endlessly for at least 30 years: can we stave off heart disease by stern adherence to a restricted diet? Eric Underwood is a well-known authority on trace minerals, and his textbook, the standard reference on the subject, is updated in his chapter. Finally, R. G. Whitehead writes on the daily needs for energy and nutrients, a topic of world-wide interest whose importance increases year by year.

A second volume on nutrition is now underway, and we hope that it will be equally timely.

A. Neuberger
Thomas H. Jukes

Biochemistry of Nutrition I

International Review of Biochemistry
Biochemistry of Nutrition IA, Volume 27
Edited by A. Neuberger and T. H. Jukes
Copyright 1979 University Park Press Baltimore

1
Malnutrition and Immune Response

W. R. BEISEL

United States Army Medical Research Institute of Infectious Diseases,
Fort Detrick, Frederick, Maryland

The adverse effects of malnutrition on host resistance against infection have been widely documented (1). Although this relationship appears to be increasing in its clinical importance among adults who become malnourished as a secondary consequence of severe disease or trauma, the combination of malnutrition and infection is encountered most frequently in the infants and young children of impoverished societies. Not only do malnourished children have a higher frequency of diarrheal and respiratory infections, but the infections they develop tend to be more severe and prolonged (2).

The mechanisms used by a normal host to resist infection seem to be impaired to some degree by severe nutritional deficits. Although malnutrition can reduce the effectiveness of nonspecific defensive mechanisms and lead to structural defects in anatomical barriers, such as epithelial and mucosal surfaces, the most important causes for an impairment of host resistance can be found within the areas of immunological function.

The effects of protein-energy malnutrition on immunological competence were not widely recognized until recently, despite the long-standing availability of published data describing the consistent presence of anatomical defects in lymphoid organs and tissues in malnourished children and laboratory animals (3-5). However, in concert with recent technological and conceptual advances in the field of immunology, systematic immunological studies have been carried out in pediatric malnutrition clinics in Africa (6-12), Thailand (13-17), India (18-24), and the Americas (22, 25-28). Similar investigations have also begun in malnourished adult patients. These types of studies are already providing direct clinical benefits for patients with serious and chronic illness. Surgical teams, for example, are finding it of value to survey their patients with a variety of nutritional and immunological tests, and to use vigorous supportive nutritional therapy to improve or correct host defenses, including immunological functions (29-31).

Thus, most of the information available for this chapter has come from clinical studies performed in man. The potential usefulness of experimentation in animals, on the other hand, has not as yet been fully used to determine mechanistic details concerning the interrelationships between malnutrition and specific immunological dysfunctions. As of the present time there are no completely satisfactory animal models available for studies of these interactions. Nevertheless, it is possible, through nutritional manipulations under controlled conditions, to influence both the function and numbers of T- and B-lymphocytes in laboratory animals and change the serological and cell-mediated responses to standardized antigens (32). Interpretation of animal data and their applicability to man will have to take into account the differences in immunological response that can be attributed to the type of nutritional deficit and its speed of onset and duration, as well as the differences caused by the species of animal used for a study (32).

The complex interrelationships between malnutrition and immunocompetence were evaluated in detail during a 1976 Kroc Foundation Workshop, the proceedings of which were published as a monograph edited by R. M. Suskind (33). Other recent reviews have also been stimulated by the importance of the problem (4, 34–38).

CHANGES IN LYMPHOID TISSUES

The widespread anatomical changes in lymphoid organs that accompany various generalized forms of malnutrition provide evidence of immunological cell dysfunction that is relatively easy to identify and quantitate.

Atrophy of the thymus gland in malnourished children was described as early as 1845 by Simon (5), who taught that the thymus was a very delicate barometer of malnutrition. Although thymus involution has consistently been viewed as a key indicator for the severity of malnutrition, the spleen, lymph nodes, tonsils, appendix, Peyer's patches, and other lymphoid tissues may also become atrophic. Clinical examinations of severely malnourished children revealed a prevalence of 36–65% in whom the tonsils could not be visualized or were only "trace" in size (9). Such atrophic changes can generally be reversed by refeeding, although the rate of recovery of individual thymolymphatic tissues is variable in different species.

During generalized malnutrition, thymic involution can advance to a point at which virtually all lymphoid elements and Hassal's corpuscles are replaced by fibrous stroma. The anatomical changes in other lymphoid organs involve primarily the thymic-dependent areas. The depletion of T-lymphocytes in the paracortical areas depends to some degree upon the severity of malnutrition. Studies in guinea pigs show the paracortical lymphocytes to have slowed turnover and mitotic rates (39). Reduction in the size and number of germinal centers is also noted. B-cells in perifollicular areas may be fewer, but plasma cell numbers in medullary areas are usually maintained. Variable reductions have been reported in the number of lymphocytes circulating in peripheral blood during malnutrition, with the greatest reduction occurring in spontaneously rosetting, thymus-dependent T-cells (3, 9, 17, 18, 34, 40–43).

The combination of anatomical findings and changes in peripheral blood lymphocyte counts is compatible with the view that malnutrition has a greater impact on the function of T-cells and cell-mediated immunity than it does on B-cell function and antibody-synthesizing mechanisms.

CELL-MEDIATED IMMUNITY

Generalized nutritional deficits appear to have a clearly adverse effect upon cell-mediated immunity (CMI). This arm of the immunological system includes the many immune phenomena that depend on T-cell function for their induction and expression. Subpopulations of T-lymphocytes include killer, suppressor, and helper cells. The adverse effects of malnutrition on CMI have only been recognized during the past decade, but appear to affect lymphoid tissue anatomy, allograft rejection, delayed dermal hypersensitivity, T-cell numbers, and in vitro tests of lymphocyte function. Since the T-cell functions appear to be essential components for host defense against many viruses, fungi, and facultative intracellular mycobacteria, it is not surprising that infections such as tuberculosis, measles, herpes simplex, vaccinia, and pneumocystis pneumonia all exhibit a more virulent course when they occur in malnourished children. Furthermore, a variety of tests conducted in vivo or in vitro combine to show that, in human beings, T-lymphocyte function and CMI are compromised by malnutrition (3, 4, 7–12, 17, 18, 22, 25, 27–38). Similar findings have also been obtained in laboratory animals (7, 23, 32, 44–52).

Many of the tests used clinically for assessing T-cell functions or other parameters of immunological competence are altered by the presence (or recent occurrence) of an infection. Since infections are commonly present in malnourished patients, published data are often difficult to interpret because no information is given concerning the presence or absence of infectious diseases in the patient population under study.

Circulating T-Lymphocyte Numbers

Actual counts of lymphocyte subpopulations consistently indicate that the number of T-cells, identified by their ability to form rosettes with sheep red blood cells, is diminished in patients with marasmus or kwashiorkor (3, 8, 9, 17, 28, 36, 37, 41–43). A similar depression in numbers has also been noted during malnutrition in several animal species (51). In the presence of normal or slightly depressed total lymphocyte counts in peripheral blood, the depression in T-lymphocyte numbers appears to be made up primarily by lymphocytes lacking T- or B-cell surface markers (null cells). The T-cell percentages fall to about one-fourth to one-half of their normal values in patients with severe protein-energy malnutrition.

Delayed Dermal Hypersensitivity

Delayed dermal hypersensitivity to various common antigens is one of the most widely used in vivo tests for evaluating CMI. A positive response requires prior sensitization to the antigen and is manifest by the delayed development of localized dermal infiltration by mononuclear cells and the accumulation of protein-rich fluid. The magnitude of the response is best evaluated by measuring the diameter of palpable dermal thickening at 48 hr. Strongly positive responses may progress to the point of dermal necrosis.

The ability of a previously sensitized patient to develop a positive response is commonly lost during generalized malnutrition (3, 6, 9, 11, 12, 24, 27, 29, 42, 49) if the patient is tested by an intradermal injection with one or more of the ubiquitous antigens such as tuberculin, *Monilia,* trichophyton, *Candida,* mumps, streptokinase-streptodornase (SK-SD), or phytohemagglutinin (PHA). Neumann and her colleagues (9) found that the incidence of delayed dermal hypersensitivity to PHA was reduced to 44–45% in a group of severely malnourished Ghanaian children, in marked contrast to an almost 100% positive response in normal American children. The inability to manifest delayed dermal hypersensitivity may be partial, or it may be dose dependent, requiring larger quantities of antigen to elicit a positive response. Dermal hypersensitivity responsiveness is generally restored progressively as nutritional deficits are corrected.

Attempts to use delayed dermal hypersensitivity responses as clinical indicators of CMI are influenced by a lack of knowledge concerning the prior immunological experience of the patient (i.e., does he have the prior sensitization required for a test to be positive?), by the dose of the antigen being used, and by the possible presence of a concomitant infection. In emphasis of this latter point, Schlesinger et al. (27) found that only 1 of 12 marasmic children had a positive tuberculin skin test despite the fact that all had received a BCG vaccination at birth. This anergic response of marasmic children contrasted to the development of a positive dermal response in 46 of 52 healthy, similarly vaccinated control children. However, only two positive tuberculin skin tests occurred among eight other normally nourished, vaccinated children who were experiencing an incidental, intercurrent infection at the time of testing (27). Since infections are quite common in marasmic children, their lack of a delayed dermal hypersensitivity response could be associated with intercurrent infection, nutritional deficiency, or a combination of both insults.

A positive delayed dermal hypersensitivity reaction requires a functional response by each of three independent component portions of the basic response mechanism (3). These include sensitization, recognition (elicitation or recall), and inflammation. All three components may be disrupted, singly or in combination, in the presence of malnutrition (3).

Patients with severe protein-energy malnutrition may not become sensitized by an antigen to which they would normally respond. The sensitization component can be tested in vivo by administering an unusual or unfamiliar antigen (such as keyhole limpet hemocyanin) to a patient or experimental animal and determining whether dermal hypersensitivity develops within a 2–3-week period. Using such a test sequence, Smith et al. (11) found that 12% of a group of 17 severely malnourished children failed to become sensitized, whereas all control subjects developed positive tests. A deficient ability to become sensitized generally responds rapidly to successful dietary therapy despite the initial severity of the malnutrition (9).

Malnourished patients who were previously sensitized to an antigen may fail to respond to it because their immunological recognition mechanism is faulty. This type of deficit can generally be detected clinically by skin-testing patients with one or more of the ubiquitous antigens in a range of doses.

Even if both the sensitization and recognition limbs of a delayed dermal hypersensitivity response were intact, a positive reaction would not occur if the functional mechanisms for generating a localized area of inflammation were impaired. An inflammatory response is initiated in large measure because of the localized release from injured cells and activated lymphocytes of chemotactic factors and other chemical mediators. Children with severe protein-energy malnutrition may fail to develop a localized inflammatory response (3) on dermal testing with nonspecific irritant doses of chemicals such as 2,4-dinitrofluorobenzene (DNFB) or 2,4-dinitrochlorobenzene (DNCB). Monocytes of malnourished children infiltrate only sluggishly into areas of inflammation (3), and their release of (or response to) endogenous mediators of inflammation seems to be abnormal.

The possibility that delayed dermal hypersensitivity responsiveness can be transferred passively to a severely malnourished person remains an unsettled question. Brown and Katz (6) inoculated 12 African children suffering from either kwashiorkor or marasmus and five healthy controls with transfer factor extracted from the peripheral lymphocytes of a tuberculin-positive subject; all recipients developed a positive tuberculin skin test. This study has been criticized, however, on several grounds, including the ambiguous nature of transfer factor per se, a possible transient booster effect caused by closely repeated skin tests, and the fact that the malnourished children under study were receiving nutritional therapy during the course of the studies (3). In a subsequent randomized double-blind clinical trial that compared transfer factor injections with saline injections in 32 Guatemalan children who were recovering from protein-energy malnutrition, Walker et al. (53) failed to find a demonstrable effect of transfer factor on the recovery of delayed dermal hypersensitivity responses.

Lymphocyte Transformation Studies

Lymphocyte blastogenic transformation studies, performed in vitro, are of value for measuring the responsiveness of T-lymphocytes to familiar specific antigens or certain nonspecific mitogens. Normal lymphocytes respond in vitro to the presence of nonspecific mitogens, such as phytohemagglutinin, by undergoing blastogenic transformation. This response can be quantitated by measuring the increased cellular uptake of [³H]thymidine in PHA-stimulated cultures in comparison to responses of identical control cultures not exposed to the mitogen. Cells from a healthy subject, previously sensitized to an antigen, also respond in vitro to the presence of that antigen by blastogenic transformation. T-cells also respond in mixed leukocyte cultures to surface alloantigens on cells of another person or individual of the same species, or to xenogenic cells in animal studies. All three types of T-cell mitogenic responses may be lost or impaired in patients or animals with severe generalized nutritional deficits (31).

When tested by these in vitro methods, the T-lymphocytes from malnourished patients are generally found to exhibit depressed blastogenic responses to mitogens (3, 4, 8–10, 17, 18, 24, 29, 30, 34, 36, 42). This lymphocytic impairment correlates well in individual patients with depressed dermal hypersensitivity reactions and can be corrected by appropriate nutrient replacement therapy. Mixed leukocyte cultures can also be used to assess the blastogenic responsiveness of T-cells. Use of this recently introduced technique in patients with marasmus provided additional evidence for T-cell deficiency (31).

While many animal data appear to confirm the depression in mitogenic responsiveness observed in lymphocytes from malnourished patients (3, 4, 32, 47, 48), some dietary manipulations that produce deficiencies in single amino acids or protein (3, 32) appear to inhibit B-cell function without inhibiting cellular immunity. In fact, a depression of serum-blocking antibodies in mice with protein deficiency appeared to enhance the effectiveness of cytotoxic lymphocyte actions against mouse tumors (32).

Transplantation Immunity

The ability of a host to reject allografted tissue depends on CMI functions, primarily through the actions of killer T-lymphocytes. This CMI function may also be depressed in malnourished animals, in which the grafted allogenic tissues remain viable for longer periods of time (46, 51).

In a series of investigations concerning killer T-lymphocyte functions, Good et al. (32) found that allograft survival and killer cell function could be manipulated through dietary changes toward either an enhanced or a depressed apparent level of killer cell function. A chronic deprivation of dietary protein caused mice to reject either allogenic spleen cells or skin grafts at an accelerated rate. The accelerated response could be abrogated by prior thymectomy. In contrast, killer cell functions were reduced by short-term protein restrictions followed by high protein feedings, or by diets with a chronic limitation in their essential amino acid content (32). These paradoxical findings suggested that the several types or durations of nutrient deficiencies may be having a different effect on the production of blocking antibodies or cytotoxic antibodies versus the function of cytotoxic cell-mediated immunity (32).

Lymphokine and Interferon Production

A large variety of diverse non-antibody substances is released by lymphocytes into the surrounding body fluids or tissue culture media. These substances, collectively termed lymphokines, include macrophage migration inhibitory factor, mitogenic factor, and other biologically active products. The lymphokines serve an important function in activating macrophages and are also believed to play a role in modulating other body defense and immunological functions. However, little is known about the molecular structure or function of lymphokines. The production or release of interferon from lymphocytes and other cells may be suppressed in malnourished patients (27) or animals (3, 54).

Nutritional Deficiencies Associated with Impaired Cell-mediated Immunity

Although most clinical studies reporting cell-mediated immunosuppression have focused on patients with generalized forms of malnutrition, there is also evidence, derived especially from animal studies, that single-nutrient deficiencies can diminish immunological responsiveness. Pyridoxine deficiency in experimental animals produces thymic and lymph node atrophy, prolonged skin graft rejection times, impairment of both sensitization and recognition mechanisms for mycobacterial antigens, and impairment of in vitro lymphocyte responses to test antigens (44–46). Deficiencies of other B complex vitamins, including thiamine or pantothenic acid, produce less clearly defined changes. Axelrod (46) suggested that pyridoxine deficiency has its principal effect on nucleic acid synthesis, whereas pantothenic acid deficiency could interfere with the release of immunoglobulins from lymphoid cells into the surrounding fluids. No consensus has been reached on the role of vitamins A or C on CMI competence (3).

Since zinc plays a role in nucleic acid synthesis and is also an essential component of many metalloenzymes, it is not surprising that a deficiency of body zinc could lead to impaired immunological functions. Balb/C mice fed a zinc-deficient diet developed a selective exaggerated decrease in the weight of all lymphoid organs in comparison with those of other organs of the deficient mice as well as in comparison with organs of control mice pair-fed a zinc-sufficient diet (55). The zinc-deficient mice showed a delayed response in the number of splenic plaque-forming cells after immunization with sheep red blood cells, an antigen that requires T-cell helpers in addition to a B-cell response (55).

The familial disease acrodermatitis enteropathica is now known to be due to an inherited disorder in zinc absorption from the intestine. The disease is manifested by chronic dermal lesions, diarrhea, alopecia, and eye lesions, with frequent superimposed yeast and bacterial infections, all of which can be dramatically reversed by correcting the zinc deficiency (56). Although defective cell-mediated and humoral immune functions may contribute to the disease picture, recent case studies suggest that the immunological defects are not due to the zinc deficiency, per se, but to the generalized malnutrition that typically accompanies severe forms of the disease (56, 57).

Considerable evidence obtained in man suggests that deficiencies of iron or folic acid or both produce an impairment of lymphocyte function (7, 15). While the individual roles for each nutrient and their interactions have yet to be clarified with respect to CMI functions, there is evidence that severe iron deficiency impairs the ability of lymphocytes to respond, in vitro, to mitogens or antigens or to produce macrophage migration-inhibitory factor. Folic acid deficiencies are also said to impair delayed dermal hypersensitivity reactions in in vitro lymphocyte transformation responses (7, 58). Furthermore, studies in rats with experimental deficiencies of lipotropic factors (choline, methionine, B_{12}, and folic acid) showed impairments in cell-mediated functions as assessed by atrophy of lymphoid tissues, diminished response to sheep RBC antigens, and impaired [^{3}H]thymidine incorporation by PHA-stimulated thymic and splenic cells (58). This effect of lipotropic factors suggests that methyl group metabolism is intimately involved in the maintenance of adequate CMI.

These data, in combination, make it seem likely that some portion of the immunological incompetence ascribed to generalized deficiencies of protein or energy could well be due to coexisting deficiencies of specific nutrients.

HUMORAL IMMUNITY

Humoral immunity depends on the ability of lymphocytes in the presence of macrophages to recognize foreign antigens and then to initiate the production of specific antibodies against them. In the course of their normal circulation via the blood stream, T- and B-lymphocytes enter lymphoid tissues, remain for about 1 day, leave via the lymph, and recirculate. If the highly individualized cell surface receptors of an individual lymphocyte match up with an antigen, allowing it to impinge upon the exterior lymphocyte surface membrane, the cell begins to replicate, producing large numbers of clonal daughter cells, which in turn undergo differentiation and transformation into immunoregulatory T-cells and mature, immunoglobulin-secreting plasma cells.

Humoral immunity can be assessed by a variety of methods. Conventional serological tests such as the complement fixation, neutralization, and hemagglutination reactions are most widely used to detect the presence of specific antibody that can interact with specific antigens. A different kind of information about heterologous antibody classes is obtained through quantitation of the several types of immunoglobulins in serum, i.e., IgG, IgA, IgM, IgD, and IgE. The ability of the host to initiate a serological response can be evaluated by in vivo tests with the use of specific antigens administered as vaccines or toxoids. B-lymphocytes can be identified by the immunoglobulins on their surface and counted. By using more sophisticated tissue culture methods (i.e., the Jerne plaque assay), the actively secreting plasma cells in tissue homogenates from some species can be identified and counted on the basis of the type of specific antibody they produce.

The impact of various forms of malnutrition upon humoral immunity has been difficult to determine with certainty (59). Some studies appear to suggest that humoral immune functions are actually enhanced by malnutrition. The possible presence of coexisting infectious or parasitic diseases may account for some of the increase in immunoglobulin production. In any event, data compiled from all available human and animal studies allow for important differences in their possible interpretations.

Evidence for Normal (or Enhanced) Humoral Immunity

Total B-lymphocyte counts in peripheral blood generally remain near normal values during severe protein-energy malnutrition (4, 9, 35, 36, 38). B-cell populations in lymphoid tissues show far less depletion than do the T-cell populations, whereas total plasma cell numbers seem to be maintained. Plasmacytoid cells have been observed in the peripheral blood of malnourished children (27, 28).

The total gammaglobulin concentrations in plasma may remain normal or be increased (14, 59, 60); rarely are they said to decline. IgM values tend to be increased in some newborn infants with fetal malnutrition (25), and they may also be high in older children, although low or normal values have been reported (14, 59, 60). The IgG values of malnourished infants are often increased (14, 59, 60) and may approach adult levels by 1 or 2 years of age (34). IgA values in plasma often increase, but they may remain in the normal range or decrease (14, 59, 60). Relatively few studies have been reported and published on IgD or IgE values, but these suggest that concentrations of both are increased (14, 59, 60).

In addition to the increase in serum concentration of several classes of immunoglobulins during malnutrition, some data describe increases in the titer of antibodies with a specific function. Good and his collaborators (32) have described a series of experiments in laboratory animals in which they could manipulate the type, magnitude, and duration of a dietary deficit in a manner that would increase the production rate and titer of blocking antibodies or cytotoxic antibodies. Chandra (19) has reported an increased incidence in malnourished children of antibodies against various foods. He suggested that these antibodies resulted as a secondary consequence of gut mucosa atrophy and impaired production of secretory IgA, which in combination permitted the passage of whole or partially degraded food protein molecules into the blood stream.

These several types of data can be interpreted to imply that humoral immunity may be enhanced and that B-cell functions remain intact despite generalized protein-energy malnutrition, or, at the very least, that humoral immunity is sustained more effectively than CMI. On the other hand, it may be argued that serum IgG values tend to be low in malnourished children kept free of infection (18). Greater-than-normal IgG concentrations could result from an extraordinarily severe and continuing exposure of the child to the multiple antigens associated with heavy parasitic infestations, repeated bacterial and viral infections, and an unfavorable social environment (2, 25).

Evidence for Suppressed Humoral Immunity

Absent, delayed, or inadequate developments of serological titers have been reported in studies after inoculation of malnourished individuals with standardized doses of well-characterized antigens. A variety of vaccines may fail to generate the expected serological titer values when given to malnourished patients (14, 20, 21, 24, 30, 32, 37, 60, 62). These findings include impaired antibody responses to influenza, typhoid, and live measles, polio, and smallpox vaccines. Comparable impairments in humoral response have been reported in malnourished animals immunized with antigens such as flagellin, tobacco mosaic virus, and allogeneic red blood cells (32, 46, 47, 50–52, 60–62). McFarlane and Hamid (51) found a marked decrease in both the primary and secondary immunological responses of malnourished rats given initial and booster inoculations of sheep red blood cells. The impairment in splenic T-cell numbers was greater than the suppression of antibody-producing cells after the primary inoculation, whereas the reverse was true after the second inoculation. Other indices of CMI suggested a greater degree of T-cell depression than exhibited by B-cell functions. Other studies in mice (50) suggested that, although all aspects of antibody responses to new antigens were depressed by protein-deficient diets, the capacity to produce IgG was more vulnerable than the capacity to produce IgM.

These types of studies have focused upon primary responses to a "new" antigen (62). Little is known about the responsiveness of malnourished persons to secondary or booster stimuli with familiar antigens, but some malnourished patients with nondetectable antibody titers against an antigen may show an anamnestic type of booster response if administered an antigen (60). This suggests that "memory" had been present because of some prior experience with the antigen.

Studies of humoral responsiveness are also confounded by differences in the molecular composition of nonviable antigens, the route of their administration, their physical state (soluble versus particulate), or the presence and effectiveness of adjuvants. Live vaccines are especially hard to evaluate (62) since they introduce multiple antigenic combinations, undergo "processing" by a variety of host cells, and achieve an ultimate antigenic mass that depends primarily on organism multiplication within the host rather than on the initial dose of inoculated organisms. Some malnourished patients have been found to generate an apparently normal serological response to one live attenuated viral vaccine while at the same time failing to show any response to another (62).

Nutritional Deficiencies Associated with Impaired Humoral Immunity

Although some studies reveal normal humoral responses after an antigenic stimulus, depressed responses are common in both human and animal studies in which the malnutrition may be generalized. A similar depression of response has sometimes been associated with an induced deficiency in a single nutrient. Impaired humoral responsiveness has been demonstrated in animals during induced deficiencies of pyridoxine or pantothenic acid but not vitamins A or C (44–46).

In a series of papers published in the early 1960s, Hodges and his co-workers (63–66) described impairments in the serological responses to several vaccines administered to adult volunteers who had been rendered deficient in one or more specific nutrients. Antibody responses to tetanus and typhoid vaccines were poor in a volunteer eating a protein-deficient diet (63). Men receiving a pantothenic acid-deficient diet, with or without an added pantothenic acid antagonist, showed depressed responses to influenza and tetanus vaccines, but had normal responses to typhoid antigens and normal skin allograft rejection (64). Only minimal impairments to tetanus and typhoid vaccines were seen during pyridoxine deficiency (65), but volunteers with combined pyridoxine-pantothenic acid deficiencies developed depressed serum IgG concentrations and responded poorly to tetanus and typhoid O antigens, minimally to typhoid H, and excellently to live polio vaccine (66). The defective responses were all corrected by restoring the two missing vitamins.

SURFACE IMMUNITY

The secretory antibody system must be considered as separate from the serum antibodies. It provides antibodies for body surfaces such as the respiratory system and gastrointestinal and genitourinary tracts, and in body secretions, including saliva and milk. Secretory IgA is manufactured locally by plasma cells situated near the point of secretion. The secreted molecule consists of two IgA molecules linked by a J-chain (also produced by the plasma cell) and a secretory component that is synthesized by epithelial cells and attached to the combined 5,000,000 MW molecule prior to its secretion into a glandular duct. IgA from the serum is not incorporated into the secretory IgA molecule. Small amounts of IgG and IgE may also be synthesized locally and secreted via exocrine glands. The localized application of an unfamiliar antigen onto a mucosal surface can stimulate the induction of secretory IgA without the initiation of a humoral antibody response.

Relatively few studies are available to document changes in surface immunity in malnutrition, but these indicate deficiencies in the system (13, 20, 60, 67–69). Nasopharyngeal, lacrimal, and salivary gland secretions show a selective reduction in secretory IgA relative to their content of total protein and albumin (13, 20, 60, 69). The most severely malnourished of a group of Colombian children had depressed secretory IgA values in tears, in contrast to IgG values, which were high (69). The responses of secretory IgA were poor in malnourished children immunized with live attenuated measles or polio vaccines; in addition, serum antibodies failed to appear or were delayed and of low titer (60). The concentration of secretory IgA in the nasal washings demonstrated a modest but significant depression in Thai children (13) who had either generalized protein-energy malnutrition or vitamin A deficiency. Low values persisted throughout the period of nutritional repletion. The deficient secretory IgA values could not be correlated with serum IgA values, which were high (13, 69), or with the presence or absence of upper respiratory infections (13).

AGE-RELATED CHANGES

Although the majority of studies that describe the effects of malnutrition on the immune response have been performed in weanling infants, nutritional immunodeficiencies may develop at any age.

Fetal Malnutrition

Mata et al. (2) have reviewed the evidence from underdeveloped societies that fetal malnutrition often begins during gestation as a direct consequence of deficient maternal diets during pregnancy, continuous exposure to unsanitary conditions, and recurrent clinical or subclinical maternal infections that sometimes involve the placenta and fetus as well. These effects can combine to cause premature births or intrauterine growth retardation. Infants with a birth weight of less than 2,500 g are at special risk and suffer the highest neonatal mortality rates. Many of these small babies already exhibit an increase in their serum IgM concentrations at the time of birth. This finding may be attributed to antenatal antigenic stimulation by maternal or intrauterine fetal infections.

Chandra (21, 34) found that low birth weight newborn infants could respond normally to tetanus and typhoid immunizations, but their antibody response to live poliomyelitis vaccine was impaired. Reduction in both B- and T-lymphocyte numbers may be evident at birth (11, 40), and in vitro lymphocyte responses to PHA may be impaired. Undernourished or undersized newborn infants may also fail to become sensitized if tested with DNCB. Subsequently the rate of physiologic decrease in their serum IgG concentrations may be exaggerated between the ages of 3–5 months (21, 34).

Experimental evidence in rats suggests that the effects of maternal malnutrition may be manifested in later generations. Prolonged partial restriction of caloric intake in rats resulted in slowed growth, lymphopenia, involution of lymphoid tissues, and an impaired response to primary immunization (61). Both the first and second generation offspring from these starved mothers subsequently showed an impaired response to immunization with sheep red blood cells manifested by a reduced appearance of serum hemolysin titers and a smaller number of antibody-forming cells in the spleen (61).

Childhood Malnutrition

The breast-fed periods of infancy are usually free of severe malnutrition or serious infection in the underdeveloped societies. Breast-fed infants initially tend to grow rapidly, remaining in the growth tracks for body weight, height, and head circumference predicted from their weight at birth. Until weaning, the nursing infant is protected by the nutrients in maternal milk, by the presence of viable phagocytic cells and immunoreactive lymphocytes (70), by the passive immunity afforded by secretory IgA and other antibodies, and by other substances such as complement, interferon, lactoferrin, and bifidus factor (68). Reddy et al. (71) found the concentration of immunoglobulins and lactoferrin to be highest in colostrum, while lysozyme values increased throughout the period of lactation. There appeared to be no differences in the milk from well-nourished or undernourished Indian women (71). Severe malnutrition and the immunodeficiencies described in earlier sections of this chapter begin to appear in the postweaning years as a result of both dietary deficiencies and the nutrient-wasting effects of repeated infections that often combine to produce a vicious cycle and high rates of childhood mortality (1).

Adult Malnutrition

Nutritional deficiencies that occur during later life can also lead to impaired immunological functions. The important studies of Law et al. (29) in surgical patients with secondary malnutrition showed deficiencies in both humoral and cell-mediated immune functions. Failure to manifest delayed dermal hypersensitivity and impaired in vitro lymphocyte responses to phytohemagglutinin gave evidence for T-cell dysfunction. Although total serum immunoglobulin concentrations were in the normal range, the patients failed to produce an early serum IgM response after immunization with keyhole limpet hemocyanin and thus showed evidence of B-cell dysfunction as well. These combined system impairments responded promptly to nutritional repletion (29, 31, 47).

Most studies performed in man suggest that nutritional immunosuppression can be reversed by the appropriate repletion of existing deficiencies. Several studies in experimental animals, however, suggest that long-term effects of postweaning malnutrition may be observed, including some that paradoxically seem beneficial. Good et al. (32) found that a simple reduction in caloric intake could double the life-span of $(NZB \times NZW)_{F1}$ strain mice that regularly die as the result of antigen-antibody complex deposition within the renal glomerular tufts. Similarly, a normally long-lived (C57BL/6J) strain of mice studied by Gerbase-DeLima et al. (48) had their life-span prolonged even further by restricting their caloric intake after weaning. The mice that were fed a fully nutritious, normal diet, but only on alternate days, showed a generalized immunosuppression throughout the first half of their life-span. This was manifested by impaired lymphocyte blastogenic responses to B- and T-cell mitogens, by poor serologic responses to sheep red blood cell antigens, and by delayed skin allograft rejection times. These deficiencies gradually corrected themselves late in life in the undernourished mice, while at the same time the normally fed control mice developed an immunosuppressed state as they aged. The control mice died earlier than the undernourished ones.

INTEGRATION OF THE IMMUNE SYSTEMS

Much recent research has been aimed at identifying and quantitating individual mechanistic aspects of T-cell and B-cell functions. Major progress has also been made in defining the structure of immunoglobulins, their interaction with antigens, and the nature of cell surface receptors. As these important revelations emerge, they must be fitted individually into their appropriate niche in our overall understanding of the complex interrelationships that exist within the immune systems and their integration with other mechanisms of host defense.

Specific Immunity

Immunological defensive mechanisms are unique in their ability to recognize and respond to the specific molecular configurations in the structure of individual antigens. The process of generating and maintaining an immune response to a specific antigen is a complex one, complete with innate modulating systems of checks and balances analogous to those that help regulate the hormonal and neurotransmission systems. The cellular processing of antigens and their trapping within lymph nodes involve the interaction of various phagocytes, macrophages, and lymphocytes and the differentiation, maturation, and proliferation of B-lymphocytes in the presence of helper and suppressor T-cells and their secretory products. Virtually nothing is known about the primary impact of malnutrition on these regulatory mechanisms when considered at the molecular or biochemical level.

Nonspecific Defense Mechanisms

The immune system functions of a malnourished subject are undoubtedly influenced by the occurrence of concomitant changes in nonspecific host defense mechanisms (68, 72). Malnutrition-induced changes in neutrophil functions include delayed chemotaxis and defective microbicidal activities (26, 68, 72), although neutrophil recognition and endocytosis functions remain normal. Electrolyte transport across leukocytic membranes is impaired in protein-energy malnutrition (26). Resting activity of the hexosemonophosphate shunt may be increased in neutrophils, while the burst of activity that accompanies phagocytosis may be diminished. The release of acid phosphatases from intracellular neutrophilic lysosomes may also be impaired

(73). The mononuclear cells of malnourished children contain diminished activities of the enzymes phosphoglycerate kinase and pyruvate kinase (74). A decrease in the migration of macrophages into areas of inflammation can also contribute to delays in antigen processing (16).

Several groups have described a reduction in total hemolytic complement activity during generalized malnutrition (3, 13). This defect is a reflection of the diminished concentrations in plasma of all individual components of the complement system except C_4 in children with severe protein-energy malnutrition (3).

Concentrations of other proteins with known antimicrobial functions may be depressed in the serum of patients with severe protein-energy malnutrition. These include depressions of serum transferrin, lactoferrin, and lysozyme and an impaired release of interferon from cells (27, 54, 68, 72). On the other hand, the increased hepatic production of acute-phase reactant proteins such as orosomucoid, α-antitrypsin, haptoglobin, C-reactive protein, and ceruloplasmin that normally occurs in response to infection or an inflammatory stimulus continues to occur in children or experimental animals despite the severity of coexisting generalized protein-energy malnutrition (72). Some of these acute-phase reactants, such as C-reactive protein, are now being recognized as modulators of immune functions. α-Fetoprotein of hepatic origin may similarly be increased in malnourished infants (23). Other nonspecific factors that could influence the immune systems include a malnutrition-induced increase in plasma glucocorticoid values, an inhibition of febrile and inflammatory responses, an altered integrity of such mechanical barriers to infection as body secretions and epithelial surfaces, and an altered composition of microorganisms that constitute the normal body flora (68, 72).

Since endocrine changes are known to accompany malnutrition, it is also possible that some of the observed immunodeficiencies could result, in part, as a secondary consequence of hormonal actions. An increase in plasma concentrations of total and free cortisol known to occur during severe protein-energy malnutrition could exert antilymphocyte effects. In support of this concept, McFarlane (8) has reported an increase in the uptake of [^{3}H]corticosteroid by the spleen and thymus of underfed growth-retarded rats.

SUMMARY

There can be no doubt that malnutrition has an adverse impact on immunological functions and can serve to suppress cell-mediated, humoral, and secretory immune competence. While most clinical studies have been performed in patients with generalized forms of malnutrition, immunosuppression has been found to occur with deficiencies of essential single nutrients.

Rarely does even a severely malnourished child exhibit the degrees of impairment in any immune function comparable to those experienced in congenital, primary immunodeficiency states. Furthermore, nutritional immunodeficiencies in human beings appear to respond well to dietary therapy, with improvement in some functions becoming evident within a few days of initiating a refeeding program.

No entirely satisfactory animal model has yet been developed to replicate human forms of malnutrition. Nevertheless, animal models have considerable potential usefulness for probing the mechanisms of nutritional immunosuppression at the molecular level.

REFERENCES

1. Beisel, W. R., Blackburn, G. L., Feigin, R. D., Keusch, G. T., Long, C. L., and Nichols, B. L. (1977). Am. J. Clin. Nutr. 30:1203.
2. Mata, L. J., Kromal, R. A., Urrutia, J. J., and Garcia, B. (1977). Am. J. Clin. Nutr. 30:1215.
3. Edelman, R. (1977). In R. M. Suskind (ed.), Malnutrition and the Immune Response, p. 47. Raven Press, New York.
4. Faulk, W. P., Mata, L. J., and Edsall, G. (1975). Trop. Dis. Bull. 72:89.
5. Simon, J. (1845). A Physiological Essay on the Thymus Gland. Henry Renshaw, London.
6. Brown, R. E., and Katz, M. (1967). J. Pediatr. 70:126.
7. Gross, R. L., and Newberne, P. M. (1976). Adv. Exp. Med. Biol. 73(B):179.
8. McFarlane, H. (1977). In R. M. Suskind (ed.), Malnutrition and the Immune Response, p. 127. Raven Press, New York.
9. Neumann, C. G., Stiehm, E. R., Swenseid, M., Ferguson, A. C., and Lawlor, G. (1977). In R. M. Suskind (ed.), Malnutrition and the Immune Response, p. 77. Raven Press, New York.
10. Schopfer, K., and Douglas, S. D. (1977). In R. M. Suskind (ed.), Malnutrition and the Immune Response, p. 123. Raven Press, New York.
11. Smith, N. J., Khadroui, S., Lopez, V., and Hamza, B. (1977). In R. M. Suskind (ed.), Malnutrition and the Immune Response, p. 105. Raven Press, New York.
12. Heyworth, B. (1977). Trans. R. Soc. Trop. Med. Hyg. 71:251.
13. Sirisinha, S., Suskind, R. M., Edelman, R., Asvapaka, C., and Olson, R. E. (1977). In R. M. Suskind (ed.), Malnutrition and the Immune Response, p. 195. Raven Press, New York.
14. Suskind, R. M., Sirisinha, S., Edelman, R., Vithayasai, V., Damrongsak, D., Charupatana, C., and Olson, R. E. (1977). In R. M. Suskind (ed.), Malnutrition and the Immune Response, p. 185. Raven Press, New York.
15. Suskind, R. M., Kulapongs, P., Vithayasai, V., and Olson, R. E. (1977). In R. M. Suskind (ed.), Malnutrition and the Immune Response, p. 387. Raven Press, New York.
16. Kulapongs, P., Edelman, R., Suskind, R., and Olson, R. E. (1977). Am. J. Clin. Nutr. 30:367.
17. Kulapongs, P., Suskind, R. M., Vithayasai, V., and Olson, R. E. (1977). In R. M. Suskind (ed.), Malnutrition and the Immune Response, p. 99. Raven Press, New York.
18. Chandra, R. K. (1972). J. Pediatr. 81:1194.

19. Chandra, R. K. (1975). Arch. Dis. Child. 50:532.
20. Chandra, R. K. (1975). Br. Med. J. 32:583.
21. Chandra, R. K. (1975). Am. J. Dis. Child. 129:450.
22. Chandra, R. K. (1977). In R. M. Suskind (ed.), Malnutrition and the Immune Response, p. 111. Raven Press, New York.
23. Chandra, R. K., and Bhujwala, R. A. (1977). Int. Arch. Allergy Appl. Immunol. 53:180.
24. Kielmann, A. A. (1977). In R. M. Suskind (ed.), Malnutrition and the Immune Response, p. 429. Raven Press, New York.
25. Mata, L. J., and Faulk, W. P. (1974). Bol. Of. Sanit. Panam. 77:410.
26. Patrick, J., and Golden, M. (1977). Am. J. Clin. Nutr. 30:1478.
27. Schlesinger, L., Ohlbaum, A., Grez, L., and Stekel, A. (1977). In R. M. Suskind (ed.), Malnutrition and the Immune Response, p. 91. Raven Press, New York.
28. Keusch, G. T., Urrutia, J. J., Guerrero, O., Casteneda, G., and Douglas, S. D. (1977). In R. M. Suskind (ed.), Malnutrition and the Immune Response, p. 117. Raven Press, New York.
29. Law, D. K., Dudrick, S. J., and Abdou, N. I. (1973). Ann. Intern. Med. 79:545.
30. Carpentier, Y., Delespesse, G., Janne, P., Mendès da Costa, P., and Collet, H. (1976). Acta Chir. Scand. 466(suppl.):122.
31. Kahan, B. E. In P. L. White (ed.), Metabolic Aspects of Critically Ill Patients. A. M. A. Publications, Chicago. In press.
32. Good, R. A. Jose, D., Cooper, W. C., Fernandes, G., Kramer, T., and Yunis, E. (1977). In R. M. Suskind (ed.), Malnutrition and the Immune Response, p. 169. Raven Press, New York.
33. Suskind, R. M. (ed.) (1977). Malnutrition and the Immune Response. Raven Press, New York.
34. Chandra, R. K., and Newberne, P. M. (1978). Nutrition, Immunity, and Infection: Mechanisms of Interaction. Plenum Publishing Corp., New York.
35. Douglas, S. D., and Schopfer, K. (1976). Clin. Immunol. Immunopathol. 5:1.
36. Faulk, W. P., Paes, R. P., and Marigo, C. (1976). Proc. Nutr. Soc. 35:253.
37. McFarlane, H. (1976). Proc. Nutr. Soc. 35:263.
38. Katz, M., and Stiehm, E. R. (1977). Pediatrics 59:490.
39. Bhuyan, U. N., and Ramalingaswami, V. (1974). Am. J. Pathol. 75:315.
40. Moscatelli, P., Bricarelli, F. D., Piccinini, A., Tomatis, C., and Dufour, M. A. (1976). Helv. Paediatr. Acta 31:241.
41. Chandra, R. K. (1977). Pediatrics 59:423.
42. Rafii, M., Hashemi, S., Nahani, J., and Mohagheghpour, N. (1977). Clin. Immunol. Immunopathol. 8:1.
43. Gleason, W. A., Jr., and Roodman, S. T. (1977). J. Pediatr. 90:1032.
44. Axelrod, A. E., Hopper, S., and Long, D. A. (1961). J. Nutr. 74:58.
45. Axelrod, A. E., Trakatellis, A. C., Bloch, H., and Stinebring, W. R. (1963). J. Nutr. 79:161.
46. Axelrod, A. E. (1971). Am. J. Clin. Nutr. 24:265.
47. Dionigi, R., Zonta, A., Dominioni, L., Gnes, F., and Ballabio, A. (1977). Ann. Surg. 185:467.
48. Gerbase-DeLima, M., Liu, R. K., Cheney, K. E., and Walford, R. L. (1975). Gerontologia 21:184.
49. Ghavami, N. A., and Mohagheghpour, N. (1975). Nutr. Metab. 19:158.
50. Malavé, I., and Layrisse, M. (1976). Cell. Immunol. 21:337.
51. McFarlane, H., and Hamid J. (1973). Clin. Exp. Immunol. 13:153.
52. Rao, V. G., and Padma, M. C. (1975). Indian J. Exp. Biol. 13:168.

53. Walker, A. M., García, R., Pate, P., Mata, L. J., and David, J. R. (1975). Cell. Immunol. 15:372.
54. Younger, J. S., and Salvin, S. B. (1973). J. Immunol. 111:1914.
55. Frost, P., Chen, J. C., Rabbani, I., Smith, J., and Prasad, A. S. (1977). In G. J. Brewer and A. S. Prasad (eds.), Zinc Metabolism: Current Aspects in Health and Disease, p. 143. Alan R. Liss, Inc., New York.
56. Hambidge, K. M., Walravens, P. A., and Neldner, K. H. (1977). In G. J. Brewer and A. S. Prasad (eds.), Zinc Metabolism: Current Aspects in Health and Disease, p. 329. Alan R. Liss, Inc., New York.
57. Van Gool, J. D., Went, K., and Zegers, B. J. M. (1976). Lancet 1:1085.
58. Newberne, P. M. (1977). In R. M. Suskind (ed.), Malnutrition and the Immune Response, p. 375. Raven Press, New York.
59. Neumann, C. G., Stiehm, E. R., and Swendseid, M. (1977). In R. M. Suskind (ed.), Malnutrition and the Immune Response, p. 191. Raven Press, New York.
60. Chandra, R. K. (1977). In R. M. Suskind (ed.), Malnutrition and the Immune Response, p. 155. Raven Press, New York.
61. Chandra, R. K. (1975). Science 190:289.
62. Katz, M. (1977). In R. M. Suskind (ed.), Malnutrition and the Immune Response, p. 421. Raven Press, New York.
63. Hodges, R. E., Bean, W. B., Ohlson, M. A., and Bleiler, R. E. (1962). Am. J. Clin. Nutr. 10:500.
64. Hodges, R. E., Bean, W. B., Ohlson, M. A., and Bleiler, R. E. (1962). Am. J. Clin. Nutr. 11:85.
65. Hodges, R. E., Bean, W. B., Ohlson, M. A., and Bleiler, R. E. (1962). Am. J. Clin. Nutr. 11:180.
66. Hodges, R. E., Bean, W. B., Ohlson, M. A., and Bleiler, R. E. (1962). Am. J. Clin. Nutr. 11:187.
67. Michalek, S. M., Rahman, A. F. R., and McGhee, J. R. (1975). Proc. Soc. Exp. Biol. Med. 148:1114.
68. Neumann, C. G. (1977). In R. M. Suskind (ed.), Malnutrition and the Immune Response, p. 355. Raven Press, New York.
69. McMurray, D. N., Rey, H., Casazza, L. J., and Watson, R. R. (1977). Am. J. Clin. Nutr. 30:1944.
70. Schlesinger, J. J., and Covelli, H. D. (1977). Lancet 2:529.
71. Reddy, V., Bhaskaram, C., Raghuramulu, N., and Jagadeesan, V. (1977). Acta Paediatr. Scand. 66:229.
72. Beisel, W. R. (1977). In R. M. Suskind (ed.), Malnutrition and the Immune Response, p. 341. Raven Press, New York.
73. Felsenfeld, O., and Gyr, K. (1977). Am. J. Clin. Nutr. 30:1393.
74. Das, M., Stiehm, E. R., Borut, T., and Feig, S. A. (1977). Am. J. Clin. Nutr. 30:1949.

International Review of Biochemistry
Biochemistry of Nutrition IA, Volume 27
Edited by A. Neuberger and T. H. Jukes
Copyright 1979   University Park Press   Baltimore

2
Cyanogenic Glycosides

E. E. CONN

University of California, Davis, California

The author's research in cyanogenic glycosides described in this chapter has been supported in part by continuing grant GM-05301 from the National Institute of General Medical Sciences, United States Public Health Service, and by National Science Foundation Grants GB-30319 and BMS 74-11997.

The ability of a wide variety of plants to produce toxic levels of hydrocyanic acid (HCN) has been known for more than a century. HCN, a gas, does not exist in the free state to any extent in the plant. Instead it is produced by enzymes acting on one or more compounds that serve as precursors. These compounds are usually O-β-glycosides of α-hydroxynitriles and are known as cyanogenic glycosides.

Plant tissues or preparations commonly consumed by man or animals that are produced by cyanogenic species include cassava tubers, sorghum seed and foliage, white clover foliage, linseed presscake, lima beans, bamboo shoots, and nuts of the almond and macadamia trees. Other cyanogenic plants that are not normally used for food but have caused accidental poisoning of animals include acacia (leaves), apricot (seeds) and other rosaceous species (foliage of wild cherry, chokecherry, and mountain mahogany), and arrow grass (foliage). The conditions under which these plant materials may be toxic vary greatly. This chapter describes the phenomenon of cyanogenesis, lists some of the plants and compounds involved, and discusses the conditions that may render cyanogenic plants unsafe for eating. Discussion of this subject is appropriate at this time for several reasons. There is an international effort directed toward increasing the potential of cassava (*Manihot esculenta* Crantz), a well-known cyanogenic species, as a food for man and other animals. There is an increased interest in using plants, especially legumes, to meet the protein needs of less developed countries (cyanogenesis is a frequent occurrence in the Leguminosae). Also one cyanogenic glycoside, amygdalin, is actively promoted in the United States and elsewhere as a treatment for cancer without scientific basis for such claims.

THE PHENOMENON OF CYANOGENESIS

Enzymic Hydrolysis of Cyanogenic Glycosides

The production of HCN by a biological organism is called cyanogenesis. The process is usually enzymatic and in higher plants depends on the co-occurrence of the HCN precursor and catabolic enzymes in the cyanogenic species. The process is represented in Figure 1 for the cyanogenic glucoside prunasin that occurs in many rosaceous species. Initially the β-glucosidic bond linking a sugar, usually D-glucose, to an α-hydroxynitrile (cyanohydrin) is hydrolyzed by a β-glucosidase. The α-hydroxynitrile, being unstable, then dissociates to produce HCN and benzaldehyde in the case of prunasin. While the dissociation of the α-hydroxynitrile can and does occur nonenzymatically, enzymes (hydroxynitrile lyases) that catalyze this type of reaction are known and have been studied in the Rosaceae (1) and in *Sorghum bicolor* (2). The presence of this enzyme in other cyanogenic plants such as cassava and white clover may therefore be predicted.

The enzymatic hydrolysis of prunasin yields an equimolar mixture of HCN, benzaldehyde, and glucose, and the reaction can be monitored by

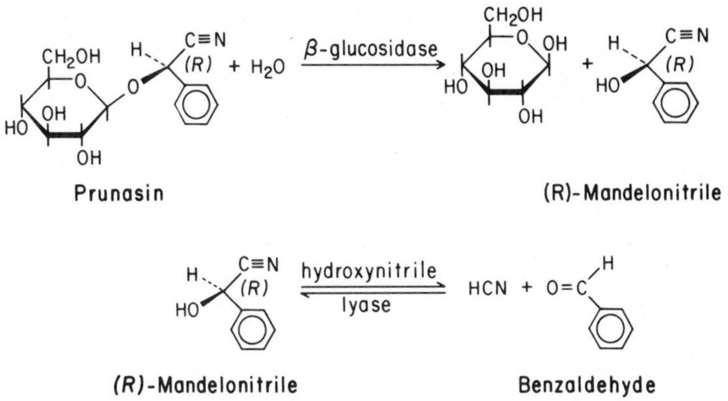

Figure 1.   Enzymatic hydrolysis of prunasin and dissociation of *(R)*-mandelonitrile.

following the formation of any one of these products. Other cyanogenic glycosides (see under "Chemical Nature") yield other aldehydes or ketones, and analytical procedures can be based on the colorimetric or spectrophotometric determination of the carbonyl compound that is formed (3). The action of β-glucosidase can be followed independent of the hydroxynitrile lyase reaction by using specific chemical reagents or, in the case of D-glucose, glucose oxidase to measure the sugar released (4). Generally, however, it is the production of HCN that is followed, especially if the chemical nature of the cyanogenic precursor is not known. Sensitive colorimetric methods for HCN analysis are available (5, 6), and procedures for measuring the release of HCN from cyanogenic plant tissues have been described (7, 8).

The hydrolysis of a cyanogenic glycoside as represented in Figure 1 occurs at a significant rate only after the tissue of the cyanogenic plant has been macerated and the glycoside is brought into contact with its catabolic enzymes. This assumes a spatial (intercellular or intracellular) separation of the enzymes from the glycoside in the intact plant. Evidence supporting this assumption is discussed elsewhere (9). If either the cyanogenic substrate or the enzymes are lacking, the production of HCN does not occur on maceration. These conditions do occur in some plants because of the polymorphic nature of cyanogenesis and are discussed under "Genetics of Cyanogenesis." If only the cyanogenic substrate is present in a plant but there is an agent, enzymatic or chemical, that can subsequently bring about its hydrolysis, the plant material obviously maintains its potential for toxicity. Conditions under which this situation exists do occur and are discussed under "Chemical Nature and Occurrence of Cyanogenic Glycosides in Food Plants."

The first cyanogenic glycoside to be described was amygdalin (10), and its discovery was soon followed by the report of its enzymic hydrolysis (11). Amygdalin, found primarily in seeds of members of the Rosaceae, is atypical among the cyanogenic glycosides in that it is a diglucoside (Figure 2). Studies on the enzymatic hydrolysis of amygdalin were reviewed by Haisman and

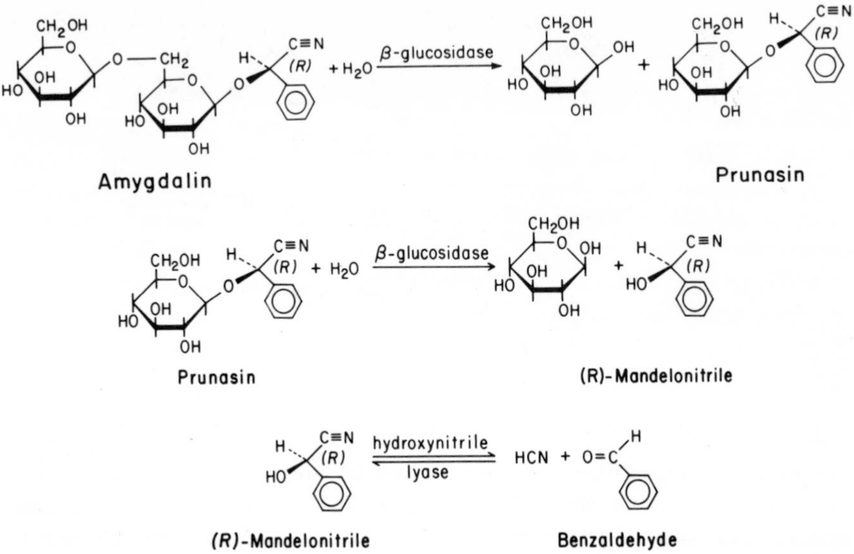

Figure 2.   Stepwise hydrolysis of amygdalin forming prunasin, *(R)*-mandelonitrile, benzaldehyde, and HCN.

Knight (12), who showed that the enzyme preparation called almond emulsin (11) contains three separate enzymes. One of these is amygdalin hydrolase, a β-glucosidase that catalyzes the removal of the terminal glucose residue to form prunasin, the *O*-β-glucoside of *(R)*-mandelonitrile. A second β-glucosidase in almond emulsin, prunasin hydrolase, then catalyzes the hydrolysis of prunasin to form *(R)*-mandelonitrile. The third enzyme, an α-hydroxynitrile lyase, then catalyzes the dissociation of the cyanohydrin, forming HCN and benzaldehyde.

The enzymes in almonds that exhibit β-glucosidase activity have been the subject of several investigations in recent years (see ref. 13 for review). These studies are of some interest in that they have demonstrated the existence of isozymic forms, some of which hydrolyze β-D-galactopyranosides as well as β-D-glucopyranosides. However, one should question their relationship, if any, to the enzymes in almond that catalyze the hydrolysis of amygdalin and prunasin. These recent studies and others cited therein have used synthetic, chromogenic substrates such as *p*-nitrophenyl-β-D-glucopyranoside instead of the natural substrates that occur in almonds and other members of the stone fruits. There has been no attempt in these recent studies to correlate the actions of these highly purified proteins on amygdalin.

Mao and Anderson (4) have shown that vegetative tissue of sorghum contains an enzyme (glucosidase I) that hydrolyzes *p*-nitrophenyl-β-D-glucopyranoside ($K_m = 0.31$ mM) but is inactive toward dhurrin, the cyanogenic glucoside found in sorghum. On the other hand, sorghum seed contains a second enzyme (glucosidase II) that uses dhurrin as a substrate, with a K_m of 0.55 mM. The seed enzyme also hydrolyzes the chromogenic substrate, but that activity may have been due to the presence of glucosidase I in the seed preparation.

The work of Mao and Anderson suggests that cyanogenic plants may contain β-glucosidases possessing great specificity for the cyanogenic glucosides found in those plants. This view is supported by the discovery and characterization (14) of a β-glucosidase in *Alocasia macrorrhiza* that is highly specific for triglochinin, the cyanogenic glucoside found in this species. The K_m for triglochinin is 3×10^{-4} (15). The enzyme is essentially inactive toward eight other cyanogenic glycosides that were tested (14). The V_{max} for p-nitrophenyl-β-glucoside is one-tenth that for triglochinin, whereas the K_m is 10 times that of triglochinin. Further support for this view is the observation by Heuser (16) that an enzyme preparation from stems of a hybrid plum, "marianna," hydrolyzed prunasin but not amygdalin.

Enzymes that catalyze the hydrolysis of the cyanogenic glucoside linamarin (see under "Chemical Nature") have been partially purified from flax seed *(Linum usitatissimum)* (17) and cassava parenchymal tissue (18). Studies on the substrate specificity of the flax enzyme demonstrated that it hydrolyzed glycosides having both aliphatic (linamarin) and aromatic (prunasin, taxiphyllin, and dhurrin) aglycones. It did not, however, hydrolyze amygdalin, which has a disaccharide as its sugar component. The substrate specificity of the cassava enzyme toward cyanogenic glycosides other than linamarin ($K_m = 1.45$ mM) was not examined, but the enzyme was active toward p-nitrophenyl-β-D-glucopyranoside ($K_m = 0.46$ mM). The specific activities of crude extracts from cassava peel were much higher than those from parenchymal tissue, but the peel enzyme was not stable.

Chemical Hydrolysis of Cyanogenic Glycosides

The β-glycosidic bonds of the cyanogenic glycosides are predictably labile to acid and are cleaved in dilute acid at elevated temperatures, yielding sugar components and characteristic α-hydroxynitriles. The latter, being labile, dissociate to HCN and the corresponding carbonyl compound. The products of hydrolysis by dilute acids, therefore, are similar to those of enzymatic hydrolysis.

Early studies on the chemistry of cyanogenic glycosides were centered on amygdalin because of its history and availability and are summarized by Viehoever and Mack (19). These workers reported that the hydrolysis of amygdalin proceeds in 1 N HCl at a detectable rate only at 60°C or higher. Hydrolysis by hot concentrated HCl yields mandelic acid and NH_3 instead of HCN and benzaldehyde. These products would be expected if the rate constant for acid hydrolysis of the nitrile group in amygdalin were greater than that for hydrolysis of the β-glycosidic bonds.

Hydrolysis under mild alkaline conditions hydrolyzes the nitrile group in several cyanogenic glycosides to a carboxylic function and NH_3 without cleavage of any other bonds. The product formed is the glycosidic acid. The alkaline hydrolysis of amygdalin to amygdalinic acid, studied by Liebig and Wöhler (11), proceeds through the amide intermediate, amygdalinamide.

Dhurrin and its epimer taxiphyllin (see under "Chemical Nature"), in contrast to amygdalin and prunasin, are labile to dilute alkali and decompose rapidly at room temperature to glucose, HCN, and p-hydroxybenzaldehyde. Dilute alkaline conditions facilitate epimerization at the carbinol carbon atom of cyanogenic glycosides having electron-withdrawing groups (e.g., an aromatic ring) adjacent to that carbon atom (20). This lability erroneously led to the report of a naturally occurring epimeric mixture of (R,S)-mandelonitrile glucoside in cherry laurel (21). Nahrstedt (20) has shown that epimerization of amygdalin occurs even at neutrality at elevated temperatures. Such findings require that care be taken in isolation procedures involving boiling aqueous solutions in order to avoid epimerization.

Other Chemical Properties

A listing of all recorded properties of cyanogenic glycosides is beyond the scope of this chapter. A recent review by Seigler (3) describes many of the chemical and physical properties of the cyanogenic glycosides as well as those of the cyanolipids and pseudocyanogenic glycosides. A renewed interest in the alleged therapeutic value of amygdalin in the treatment of cancer has resulted in the application of newer analytical methods to amygdalin. Recent studies record the application of high performance liquid chromatography (22, 23), carbon-13 nuclear magnetic resonance (22), chemical ionization mass spectrometry (22), gas chromagraphy (22, 24), and high field nuclear magnetic resonance spectrometry (25) to amygdalin or related compounds.

CHEMICAL NATURE AND OCCURRENCE
OF CYANOGENIC GLYCOSIDES IN FOOD PLANTS

Chemical Nature

Although 23 different cyanogenic glycosides have been isolated from higher plants, this chapter treats only those that occur in plants intentionally used by animals for food. The conditions that determine the release of HCN from such compounds, and therefore the toxicity, can be amply illustrated and discussed with these examples. Reviews concerned with the chemical nature and properties (3, 26) of all 23 compounds, their distribution (26) and metabolism (27, 28) are available.

The structures of linamarin (2-hydroxyisobutyronitrile-β-D-glucopyranoside) and (R)-lotaustralin (2-hydroxy-2-methylbutyronitrile-β-D-glucopy-

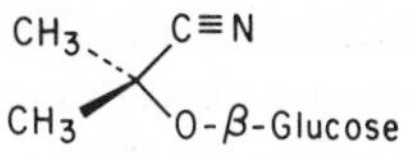

CH₃ — C≡N
CH₃ — O-β-Glucose

Linamarin

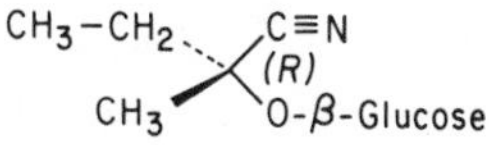

CH₃—CH₂ — C≡N
(R)
CH₃ — O-β-Glucose

(R)-Lotaustralin

Figure 3.   Structures of linamarin and *(R)*-lotaustralin.

ranoside) are presented in Figure 3. These two compounds, without apparent exception, always occur in the same plant, although not necessarily in the same ratio. Thus, Butler (29) found that linamarin predominated over lotaustralin by the ratio of 19:1 in seed of *Phaseolus lunatus,* whereas the reverse ratio of 1:19 was observed in seed of *Lotus tenuis.* The co-occurrence of these two cyanogenic glycosides in linen flax, the only species in which biosynthesis has been investigated in detail, is ascribed to the existence of a single set of biosynthetic enzymes that can act on either valine or isoleucine and produce linamarin or lotaustralin, respectively (27).

Figure 3 emphasizes the chiral (asymmetric) nature of the carbinol carbon atom (i.e., the carbon atom bearing the glucose moiety) in *(R)*-lotaustralin. In lotaustralin and most of the other cyanogenic glycosides, this chiral center means that two epimers differing only in the configuration at that carbon atom can exist. Such epimers do occur, although never in the same species, with apparently one exception (30).

Figure 4 shows the structures of two such epimers, dhurrin and taxiphyllin. Both glycosides contain the sugar D-glucose, linked in an *O-β*-glyco-

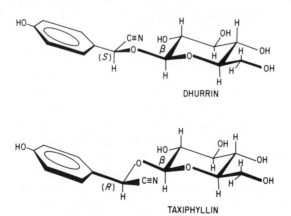

DHURRIN

TAXIPHYLLIN

Figure 4.   Structures of dhurrin and taxiphyllin.

side bond to an α-hydroxynitrile (cyanohydrin). Since the carbon in the α-hydroxynitrile is chiral, the α-hydroxynitrile can occur in two forms called the *(R)* and *(S)* enantiomers that are mirror image isomers. When the hydroxyl group in these two enantiomers is linked to D-glucopyranose, two stereoisomers are formed that differ only in configuration at that single carbon atom. The two compounds, therefore, are epimeric. Dhurrin, first isolated from sorghum, is the trivial name that was assigned to the *(S)* epimer (4-hydroxy-*S*-mandelonitrile-β-D-glucopyranoside) (31). Taxiphyllin is the trivial name of the *(R)* epimer (4-hydroxy-*R*-mandelonitrile-β-D-glucopyranoside) (32). Their natural occurrence is discussed in the next section.

The structures of amygdalin and prunasin (Figure 2) illustrate another relationship. As is evident, prunasin and amygdalin are glycosidic derivatives of the same aglycone, *(R)*-mandelonitrile. In prunasin the sugar is D-glucopyranose, while in amygdalin the sugar is the disaccharide D-gentiobiose. Amygdalin is one of the three cyanogenic glycosides having disaccharides as the sugar moiety. Vicianin (33) is the vicianoside of *(R)*-mandelonitrile and lucumin (34) is the primaveroside of *(R)*-mandelonitrile.

To complete the list of cyanogenic glycosides found in food plants, proteacin has been isolated from bitter nuts of *Macadamia ternifolia* (35). Proteacin is related to dhurrin (Figure 4) in that a second glucose moiety is bound in glycosidic linkage to the aromatic hydroxyl group of dhurrin. Proteacin, therefore, is a diglucoside (and not a disaccharide) derivative of *p*-hydroxy-*(S)*-mandelonitrile. Dhurrin also is present in *M. ternifolia* (36).

Occurrence

Table I lists some typical values for the amounts of HCN released from various parts of cyanogenic plants. In studies of this sort it is important to specify which tissue was analyzed because it may or may not be identical with the plant part that is used as food. An informative example is the sorghum plant, whose starchy seed has served as human food for centuries and whose foliage is often consumed by animals as ensilage. The leaves of sorghum species were first shown to be cyanogenic by Dunstan and Henry (31), who isolated and characterized dhurrin from "the great millet" of Egypt, known also as dhurra shirshabi. The young green leaves of sorghum [*S. bicolor* (Linn.) Moench] and the dark-grown shoots have been extensively used in biosynthetic studies (27); the coleoptile and first leaf of 3-day-old dark-grown seedlings can contain up to 25% (dry weight) of dhurrin. However, the dry seed that is used for food contains no detectable cyanogenic compound (37), which means that the dry, unsoaked seed can be eaten with impunity, although the young green tissue of plants growing in a field must be avoided. The poisoning of transport animals of Kitchener's army in the Sudan by sorghum species growing wild in the Upper Nile Valley provided the impetus for identifying the toxic agent in the green herbage. Accidental poisoning of livestock occurs when they are introduced into a field of im-

Table 1.   HCN released from various plant tissues

Plant	HCN yield (mg/100 g)	Reference
Sorghum		
mature seed	0	(37)
etiolated shoot tips	240	(77)
young green leaves	60	(77)
Almond		
bitter seed	290	(77)
young leaves	20	(77)
Apricot, seed	60	(77)
Peach		
leaves	125	(77)
seed	160	(39)
Wild cherry, leaves	90–360	(39)
Lima bean, mature seed		
Puerto Rico, small black	400	(47)
Puerto Rico, black	300	(43)
Arizona, colored	17	(46)
America, white	10	(46)
Linen flax		
seedling tops	910	(29)
linseed cake	50	
White clover, young leaves	3–352	(29)
Cassava		
less toxic clones		(95)
bark of tuber	69	
inner part of tuber	7	
leaves	77	
very toxic clones		
bark of tuber	84	
inner part of tuber	33	
leaves	104	

mature green sorghum (38). Sorghum leaves may be used as silage, but fermentation in the silo is required to decompose the cyanogenic glycoside.

Another example in which some tissues of a plant are cyanogenic and others are not is the stone fruits of the edible Rosaceae. The fruits of domesticated apple, pear, peach, apricot, and cherry have been enjoyed by man through the ages. The seeds of these species, on the other hand, are well known to be cyanogenic, probably containing amygdalin. What is less well known or appreciated is that the leaves of the domesticated stone fruits are variably cyanogenic, and animals should not have access to their foliage. Kingsbury (39) reports that leaves of several species of wild cherry have been responsible for poisoning of livestock in the eastern United States.

If, as indicated, the pits (seeds) of the stone fruits are cyanogenic, it would seem a simple matter to avoid their consumption. However, the literature (40) contains a report of four cases of poisoning of children by western chokecherries because the children ate the fruit whole, broke up the seed in the mouth, and swallowed indiscriminately. In another case, a small child is reported (41) to have dipped kalabey apricot seeds, which are bitter, in sugar before eating a quantity that poisoned him. To these can be added reports on poisonings, some fatal, after the ingestion of peach seeds, apricot seeds, and bitter almonds (see ref. 42 for review).

The promotion of Laetrile (amygdalin or vitamin B_{17}) in the treatment of cancer has also indirectly resulted in some cases of poisoning due to the ingestion of apricot seeds (42). Knowing that apricot seeds contain amygdalin, people have consumed an excess of the bitter kernels in one form or other. Within an hour or two such symptoms as abdominal discomfort, tachycardia, vomiting, flushing, dizziness, or faintness were noted and, where treatment was sought, a diagnosis of cyanide poisoning was made.

The almond *(Prunus amygdalus)* is an important example of a cyanogenic stone fruit that has been selectively bred to produce a nut that is sweet, edible, and commercially valuable. Although the nut is sweet, leaves of such commercial trees are strongly cyanogenic, the HCN arising from prunasin. The amygdalin concentration of sweet almonds is low but still detectable with qualitative tests for HCN. Bitter almonds, on the other hand, contain approximately 100 μmol/g. It apparently is amygdalin that imparts the bitter flavor, because crystalline amygdalin is bitter to the human taste. Apricot seeds, which contain approximately 20–80 μmol/g of amygdalin, are also noticeably bitter. The commercial oil of almond, which contains benzaldehyde, glucose, and HCN, is obtained from bitter almonds or alternatively from apricot and peach seeds.

Beans of the lima type *(P. lunatus)* represent one of the most important edible legumes. This American species, already in many varietal forms, was known to Spanish explorers of the 15th century and together with cassava was introduced both into the Old World and the Far East for cultivation. Viehoever (43), who has reviewed the botanical and chemical characteristics of the bean in a thorough study, collected and determined the cyanogenic potentials of varieties collected from around the world. This study and others reviewed elsewhere (44, 45) permit the following general conclusions. All parts of the growing plant, including the developing seed pods, can be cyanogenic. The cyanogenic potential of the mature bean, on the other hand, varies with the color, shape, and size of the bean. The small, black or dark-colored wild lima of Central America in general has the highest content of cyanogenic glycoside, predominately linamarin. Such beans can contain 70–140 μmol/g, equal to 190–380 mg of HCN/100 g of air-dried seed. (The HCN that could be released from 25 g of seed could easily be fatal to a 70-kg man.) Limas cultivated for large size and white color (butter beans) have only a fraction (1–2%) of the linamarin found in the wild type (43). Beans intermediate in size and color might be expected to have intermediate levels of cyanogenic glycoside, and to some extent this is indicated by the literature. Such beans are readily available in the public markets of tropical countries, where they are favored for their flavor over the common noncyanogenic bean, *Phaseolus vulgaris*. This author, however, is unaware of any data on the cyanogenic content of such market beans.

Cyanogenic beans contain linamarase, the β-glucosidase that hydrolyzes linamarin to form HCN, acetone, and glucose (43, 46). It therefore is undesirable to soak colored beans without an additional step to remove the HCN that is released on soaking. Boiling of dry beans should inactivate the β-glucosidase and therefore decrease the release of HCN from linamarin. However, people have been poisoned by colored lima beans after boiling and draining, as well as under other conditions. At the turn of the 20th century the matter attracted sufficient attention and concern so that the importation of beans with significant levels of cyanogen into the United States and Britain was carefully regulated (43).

Viehoever (43) reports that leaves and stems of bean plants are cyanogenic and that HCN is released from the pods of lima beans. These observations would seem to call for caution in using green leaves and pods as food. However, Burkill (48) cites the human consumption of young seedlings and pods as well as the use of dried vines as hay.

Cassava (*M. esculenta* Crantz) contains linamarin and lotaustralin, the same cyanogenic glycosides that are found in the lima bean, with linamarin again predominating (95%). The potential toxicity of the plant presumably was known to its users in pre-Columbian times (48). The fact of its toxicity was first recorded in 1605 (49), and the production of HCN by the plant was reported by Henry and Boutron-Charland in 1836 (50). Dunstan et al., in 1906 (51), showed that the principal cyanogenic glycoside of cassava was identical with the glycoside linamarin known from studies on *Phaseolus* and *Linum*.

Cassava provides the basic calorie intake for approximately 200–300 million people. Although it is one of the world's major crops (52, 53), its potential as a carbohydrate source for human and domestic animals is largely undeveloped. For this reason there is a major international effort directed at developing this potential (52). Connected with this effort is a concern for its cyanogenic nature and the fact that chronic cyanide toxicity may be associated with consumption of cassava food products that contain low levels of cyanogenic glycosides (see under "Pathological Conditions Possibly Associated with Prolonged Ingestion of Cyanogenic Glycosides").

The cyanogenic glycosides are found in all parts of the cassava plant, and the concentrations in the edible tuber vary not only with the plant variety but also with climatic and cultural conditions. Coursey (54), who reviews the literature on this subject, states that the amount of HCN that can be produced from the tuber ranges generally between 30 mg and 150 mg of HCN/kg of fresh tuber. The literature refers to "sweet" and "bitter" varieties, and there is a tendency to associate the bitter variety with higher levels of cyanogenic glycoside (54). However, there is much overlap in the actual values of HCN produced, and there are instances of the bitter variety being preferred because of the generally bland, starchy taste of the sweet form.

As in other cyanogenic plants, HCN is released when the cassava tuber is processed for eating. The tuber contains linamarase, which is brought in contact with its substrate when the cellular structure of the plant is disrupted by a variety of traditional processing methods (54). Grinding or grating procedures presumably accomplish a more thorough enzymic hydrolysis; the HCN, which is released together with any unhydrolyzed glucoside, can then be removed by soaking in static or running water. Drying in the sun or over a fire probably would cause extensive cellular disruption and enzymatic hydrolysis, but not as much as grinding. The HCN released could then escape as a gas, but some unhydrolyzed glucoside would undoubtedly remain in such preparations. Simple cooking techniques, as with beans, would tend to inactivate the endogenous hydrolytic enzymes but would not destroy the relatively stable glucoside. The wide variety of processing techniques for cassava, together with the variation in the amount of cyanogenic glucoside in different varieties eaten, makes it impossible to generalize as to the amount of intact cyanogenic glucoside that might be consumed. However, values are available for certain processed cassava foods that are consumed in Africa (54). The linamarin content of a product called gari, together with its large intake (0.8 kg/day) by some populations, means that such individuals are potentially exposed to approximately 20 mg of HCN daily (see under "Pathological Conditions Possibly Associated with Prolonged Ingestion of Cyanogenic Glycosides").

White clover *(Trifolium repens)* is a cyanogenic species that is also a major herbage crop. Those varieties that are most productive and long lived are also those having a higher content of the cyanogenic glucosides lotaustralin and linamarin (ratio of 4:1). Because the plant is used extensively in New Zealand and Australia, its potential toxicity to sheep has been examined. These studies, carried out largely in the 1940s, have been reviewed by Tapper and Reay (55). Of particular interest is the fact that cyanogenic glycosides, often present in clover in amounts insufficient to show acute toxicity, can have a goitrogenic action in sheep. This results from the fact that HCN released from the ingested cyanogenic clover is detoxified by conversion to thiocyanate by the action of rhodanase. Butler et al. (56) found elevated levels of serum thiocyanate and evidence of goiter formation in sheep.

Young bamboo shoots, a delicacy in many countries, have been responsible for some cases of human cyanide poisoning (57). The cyanogenic material in *Banbusa vulgaris* has been identified as taxiphyllin (Figure 4), and its unusual thermolability studied (58). At pH 5.5 (0.2 M phosphate), the compound has a half-life of 5 min at 100°C, decomposing to HCN, glucose, and *p*-hydroxybenzaldehyde. This means that boiling bamboo shoots in water for 35–40 min should destroy the cyanogenic glycoside. If the HCN released is then removed in the cooking procedure, the bamboo should be safe to eat.

Other members of the Gramineae and Leguminosae are well established food plants. Since cyanogenesis is fairly common in these two families, members have been examined for their ability to produce HCN. Clark (59) has cited maize, sugar cane, various millets, oat, rye, wheat, and barley as being cyanogenic plants, but no figures are given for their cyanogenic capacity. Petrie (60), examining over 100 species of grasses for cyanogenesis, found 20 that were cyanogenic. He also refers to older reports of cyanogenic grasses, but gives no quantitative data. In our work dark-grown seedlings of commercial varieties of wheat, rice, and barley were found to contain 0.3, 0.5, and 1.9 mg of HCN/100g of tissue, respectively. However, maize, millet, and rye were negative in the preliminary surveys. Montgomery (44) has reported the following legume seeds to be cyanogenic: black-eyed pea (*Vigna sinensis,* 2.1 mg/100 g); common pea (*Pisum sativum,* 2.3 mg/100 g); kidney or navy bean (*P. vulgaris,* 2.0 mg/100 g); chick pea (*Cicer arietinum,* 0.8 mg/100 g), and common vetch (*Vicia sativa,* 52 mg/100 g). With the exception of vetch, the values reported indicate little possibility of these species being acutely toxic. Vetch, on the other hand, has a significant history as a toxic plant because it contains the lathyrism factor β-cyanoalanine (61). The nitrile group of β-cyanoalanine arises in the plant from HCN released from the cyanogenic glycoside vicianin that it contains (62). The HCN is then converted to β-cyanoalanine by reaction with cysteine in the presence of β-cyanoalanine synthase (63).

Genetics of Cyanogenesis

The polymorphic nature of cyanogenesis has been alluded to by references in the preceding sections to sweet and bitter almonds or sweet and bitter cassava, i.e., plants of the same species that differ in their content of cyanogenic glycosides. The polymorphism is indicated by the existence of both cyanogenic and noncyanogenic plants in a population of a single species, and has been extensively studied in *T. repens* and *Lotus corniculatus* (64). *S. bicolor, P. amygdalus, M. esculenta,* and *M. ternifolia* undoubtedly are also polymorphic since there are individual plants within these species that are either strongly cyanogenic or only weakly so (65).

The genetic relationship for *T. repens* is indicated in equation 1, in which the synthesis of the cyanogenic glycosides is determined by alleles of the gene *(Ac).*

$$\text{Precursors} \xrightarrow{\ Ac\ } \begin{array}{c}\text{cyanogenic}\\\text{glycosides}\end{array} \xrightarrow{\ Li\ } \begin{array}{c}\text{ketone,}\\\text{HCN,}\\\text{glucose}\end{array} \qquad (1)$$

The hydrolysis of the glycosides is determined by alleles of another independently inherited gene, *Li*, which regulates the presence of the catabolic β-glucosidase. Only plants that possess one dominant allele of both genes are cyanogenic (i.e., can release HCN). By selective breeding it is possible to obtain the four homozygous genotypes of white clover: *AcAcLiLi, AcAclili, acacLiLi, acaclili.* Only the first of these genotypes is independently cyanogenic, i.e., can release HCN from the glucosides that it contains. The second genotype contains the cyanogenic substrate and, therefore, has the potential to be cyanogenic. However, it requires a source of the β-glucosidase before it can release HCN.

Plant breeders have made extensive practical use of this genetic information in the case of cyanogenic plants. Strains of white clover having a low cyanoglucoside content are the varieties used commercially in New Zealand and Australia. Although the genetic relationship for cyanogenesis in *S. bicolor* is not as simple as indicated in equation 1, high- and low-cyanide strains of *S. bicolor* are known and have been used in preparing commercial hybrids. Pomologists have used the information on genetic polymorphism in breeding the sweet almonds produced commercially. It presumably is genetic polymorphism in *P. lunatus* that made it possible to obtain the low-cyanide white butter beans of commerce from the tiny black lima native to much of tropical America. The phenomenon of polymorphism is sufficiently common that it must be expected in any cyanogenic population.

TOXICITY OF HCN

Acute Toxicity

Cyanide as HCN or NaCN is rapidly absorbed from the upper digestive tract. Once in the circulation, HCN exhibits its toxic action since it has a strong affinity for enzymes associated with cellular respiration, notably cytochrome oxidase (66). When that enzyme is combined with cyanide it cannot react with O_2, and consequently aerobic cellular respiration ceases. Death ensues from a generalized anoxia, the central nervous system being the most susceptible tissue.

The lethal dose of HCN for humans is given as 0.5–3.5 mg/kg of body weight taken orally (45). This corresponds to 1.0–7.0 mg of KCN/kg and refers to a single dose taken at one time. The heart, brain, and nervous system are rapidly affected and, if the dose is relatively large, death ensues within a few minutes. If the dose encountered produces acute toxicity but not death, the condition must be quickly recognized and treatment rapidly initiated. The treatment is based on the fact that ferrihemoglobin (methemoglobin) forms a strong but dissociable complex with cyanide. Therefore, oxidizing agents such as $NaNO_2$ or aminophenols (67) are injected to increase the relative amounts of ferrihemoglobin. Care must be taken not to oxidize too much of the hemoglobin to ferrihemoglobin; otherwise the O_2-carrying capacity of the blood is reduced and death from hypoxia still occurs (68). After the injection of $NaNO_2$, sodium thiosulfate ($Na_2S_2O_3$) is administered to provide an adequate supply of sulfur as a substrate for rhodanese (see below) to react with cyanide produced on dissociation of the cyanoferrihemoglobin.

Chronic Toxicity

Man is exposed to small doses of HCN continually in polluted atmospheres, through cigarette smoke, and through his diet. These small doses of HCN are converted to thiocyanate by the rhodanese (sulfur transferase) system described in the next section, and the exposure can be monitored to some extent by measuring the thiocyanate excreted in the urine. Thiocyanate is also a metabolic product derived from the metabolism of mustard oil glycosides (glucosinolates) in the diet. Therefore, reliance on urinary thiocyanate values must take into account the intake of any dietary glucosinates, usually acquired by eating plants of the Crucifereae family.

Workers in certain occupations are exposed to HCN over and above those sources encountered by the general public. These individuals have been studied to ascertain whether or not chronic cyanide poisoning is a clinical entity, and there appears to be some disagreement on this question (69). Symptoms that such workers exhibit include headache, vertigo, tinnitus, nausea, vomiting, and tremor. Although these symptoms are sufficiently documented and characteristic, they are transitory in that exposure to fresh air causes their disappearance. Whether or not the repeated exposure causes irreversible lesions is not clearly established. If there are irreversible changes, they do not seem to produce the outward symptoms of tropical ataxic neuropathy (TAN), a pathological condition that has been attributed in part to exposure to cyanide or cyanogenic glycosides in certain preparations (see under "Pathological Conditions Possibly Associated with Prolonged Ingestion of Cyanogenic Glycosides").

Detoxification of Cyanide by Rhodanese

It is difficult to estimate the degree or intensity of cyanide poisoning by measuring the levels of free HCN in body fluids. HCN is a highly reactive chemical that undergoes reaction with other functional groups as well as binding to proteins. In addition, HCN is rapidly converted to thiocyanate by the enzyme rhodanese (thiosulfate sulfur transferase EC 2.8.1.1), which catalyzes the reaction (70).

$$CN^- + S_2O_3^{2-} \xrightarrow{\text{rhodanese}} SCN^- + SO_3^{2-}$$

Rhodanese occurs in several animal tissues, with highest concentrations in liver, and apparently is responsible for the observation that dietary cyanide is largely converted to thiocyanate and excreted in the urine. The effectiveness of this process depends on a supply of $Na_2S_2O_3$, and, as stated above, acutely poisoned animals are often given an injection of $Na_2S_2O_3$. Animal tissues can also catalyze the transfer of the sulfur atom of cysteine to cyanide and form thiocyanate. The immediate sulfur donor is mercaptopyruvate, which is obtained by transamination of cysteine.

The production of thiocyanate in this detoxification process is of concern because thiocyanate is an established goitrogen. Thiocyanate exerts its goitrogenic action by inhibiting the uptake of iodine by the thyroid gland. The glucosinolate compounds found in members of the Crucifereae have long been recognized for their goitrogenic properties because of their metabolic conversion in part to thiocyanate. If thiocyanate is formed in significant quantities by detoxification of dietary cyanide, goiter might be observed as an indication of chronic cyanide poisoning occurring over a period of time. Such a situation has been described for human populations in the Congo and in Nigeria (see under "Pathological Conditions Possibly Associated with Prolonged Ingestion of Cyanogenic Glycosides").

TOXICOLOGY OF CYANOGENIC GLYCOSIDES

The potential toxicity of a cyanogenic plant depends primarily on its capacity to produce a concentration of HCN that is toxic to the animal being exposed. However, other factors should be considered. For example, little attention has been paid to the other noncarbohydrate compounds produced on hydrolysis of a cyanogenic glycoside. While aliphatic ketones such as acetone or 2-butanone may be of little concern, the production of aromatic aldehydes may well be harmful. At the very least, energy must be expended in their detoxification and excretion.

Other factors that influence the toxicity of a plant include the size and kind of animal that may eat the plant, the type of food consumed at the same time, the rate of ingestion, the possibility of the plant's hydrolytic enzymes remaining active in the digestive tract of the animal, the possibility of intracellular enzymes in the animal hydrolyzing any glycoside that is absorbed into the blood stream, and the ability of the animal to detoxify any HCN that it encounters. With the exception of this last factor, which has been discussed, there are few detailed studies on any of these topics. Nevertheless, certain interrelationships can be stated that might provide some insight into the poisoning process.

Autohydrolysis

If ingestion of a cyanogenic plant produces acute symptoms indicative of HCN poisoning, this indicates that the plant has provided both the cyanogenic substrate and the enzymes necessary for release of the HCN. Moreover, enough of the plant material must have been ingested in a sufficiently short period of time to produce a quantity of HCN that is toxic. The amount of HCN required obviously depends on the size of the animal; the minimum amount of plant material to be ingested is determined by the concentration of cyanogenic glycoside in the plant.

The release of HCN requires that the degradative enzymes in the plant be sufficiently active to produce the required quantity of HCN in the short time interval between mastication of the plant material and its arrival in the stomach. This condition seems necessary at least in man and other monogastric animals in which the high acidity (pH 2) of the stomach presumably would inhibit the action of the plant enzymes, which have an optimum pH of 5–6. Whether the inactive enzymes are also irreversibly denatured by the acid medium is not known. If they are not, they could regain their catalytic activity in the duodenum after the stomach contents have mixed with the alkaline bile juice and the pH has been raised to neutrality.

In ruminants the ingested food materials are not exposed to acid, and the neutral pH of the rumen strongly favors the continued action by the plant's hydrolytic enzymes. It is also possible that rumen bacteria, with their ability to hydrolyze the β-glycosidic linkages of cellulose, may also act on the β-glycosidic bonds of the cyanogenic glycosides. Coop and Blakley (71) reported that the rumen flora in sheep can hydrolyze lotaustralin, and Moran (72) has indicated that ruminants are more susceptible to poisoning by cyanogenic plants than are nonruminants.

If an animal eats a plant that contains a cyanogenic glycoside but not the hydrolytic enzymes, the situation is less clear. This obviously raises the question of the existence in the animal of other enzymes or conditions that can hydrolyze the glycoside (see next section). Seddon and King (73) pointed out the hazards in simultaneous ingestion of other plants that have β-glucosidase activity but not a cyanogenic glycoside, and performed some model experiments using sweet almonds to release HCN from foliage of *Acacia glaucescens* and *Eremophilia maculata,* which contained a cyanogenic glycoside but no enzyme. Only a little work has been done on the ability of noncyanogenic plants to hydrolyze cyanogenic glycosides, but edible plants such as lettuce, celery, and mushrooms have the ability to hydrolyze amygdalin (74). Clearly this calls for some caution in consuming these plants and a source of cyanogenic glycoside simultaneously.

Cooking to inactivate the degradative enzymes is not a procedure normally employed with domestic animals, but it is commonly used by man in the preparation of food products derived from the cassava tuber and some other cyanogenic plants (e.g., beans and bamboo). If cooking serves only to inactivate the degradative enzymes and not to destroy the glycoside, then there remains the question of whether the glycoside itself can be toxic or be degraded by intracellular enzymes (see next section). Heat presumably destroys only taxiphyllin, since thermolability has not been observed for the other glycosides.

The foregoing discussion of various factors that may influence the acute poisoning of an animal must not obscure the basic fact that cyanogenic plants can be toxic if ingested. Reference has already been made under "Occurrence" to specific cases of poisoning. The literature on poisonous and medicinal plants contains many additional references to poisoning of animals, including man (39, 75, 76).

Hydrolysis in Animals

Several mechanisms have been proposed for hydrolysis of cyanogenic glycosides after they have been ingested. For example, there are references to the possible hydrolysis of these compounds by the acid contents of the stomach. However, incubation of amygdalin and linamarin at 37°C for 18 h in 0.1 N H_2SO_4 failed to hydrolyze either of these compounds (77). While these conditions do not mimic the acid contents of monogastric animals, they do show that these two cyanogenic glucosides are stable to acid. These observations confirm the report by Caldwell and Courtauld (78) that amygdalin is not hydrolyzed at a significant rate in 1 N HCl at temperatures below 60°C.

It has sometimes been inferred that the digestive juices of the mammalian digestive tract hydrolyze cyanogenic glycosides. However, the glycosidases in the gastrointestinal tract are α-glycosidases and would not be expected to hydrolyze the β-glycosidic link found in the cyanogenic glycosides. Studies on the hydrolysis of amygdalin or other cyanogens by purified intestinal carbohydrases have apparently not been carried out.

There is the general impression that the bacteria of the digestive tract can hydrolyze cyanogenic glycosides. However, the literature is not clear on this point. Winkler (79) refers to the hydrolysis of amygdalin by *Escherichia coli,* but gives no quantitative data. The rumen flora are apparently capable of hydrolysis (71), but Jansz et al. (80) report that coliform bacteria did not hydrolyze linamarin.

Barrett et al. (81) have carried out an important study showing that linamarin administered orally to rats is both absorbed and metabolized to yield thiocyanate, which is then excreted in the urine. These workers found that 19% of single doses of linamarin administered orally appeared as the intact glucoside in the urine in the first 24 h. Another 24% was excreted as urinary thiocyanate, but no linamarin was found in the feces. The formation of urinary thiocyanate was attributed to hydrolysis of the linamarin in the body of the rat and its conversion to thiocyanate by intracellular rhodanese. Whether hydrolysis occurred in the digestive tract or the linamarin was first absorbed and then hydrolyzed by intracellular enzymes cannot be answered by these experiments. If hydrolysis did occur in the digestive tract, the HCN released obviously was absorbed and converted to thiocyanate. Clearly, linamarin also was absorbed into the circulatory system of the rat, where it might be acted upon by intracellular β-glycosidases. Such enzymes are known in mammalian tissue, but their activity against amygdalin or other cyanogens was not examined (82).

In a recent study Ng (83) measured the activity of a partially purified steroid β-D-glucosidase preparation from rabbit liver against several cyanogenic glycosides. These studies showed that the rabbit liver preparation, which had as its preferred substrate a steroid glucoside, could also hydrolyze prunasin, amygdalin, dhurrin, taxiphyllin, and linamarin. However, the K_m values for these substrates were large and the rates of hydrolysis low in contrast to those values reported for the preferred substrate.

Relevant to the foregoing discussion are two recent reports on human fatalities associated with the oral ingestion of Laetrile (amygdalin). In one case (84), an 11-month-old child accidentally consumed up to five 500-mg tablets of amygdalin that belonged to her father. The child exhibited signs of cyanide poisoning within 1 h and had a significant concentration of cyanide in her blood. Treatment with $NaNO_2$ and $Na_2S_2O_3$ occurred 3½ h after ingestion with no success, and the patient died in 72 h. In the other case (85) a 17-year-old girl swallowed 3½ ampules of Laetrile stated to contain a total of 10.5 g of amygdalin. Within 10 min she exhibited signs of poisoning and shortly became comatose. Although her stomach was lavaged and she received other assistance, she died 24 h after ingestion of the cyanogenic glycoside. Analysis performed 1 month later on samples of blood and urine taken at 36 h showed the cyanide levels to be normal.

These cases indicate that amygdalin taken orally can be rapidly hydrolyzed in humans to produce HCN. It is unlikely that hydrolysis resulted from the action of microorganisms in the gastrointestinal tract, because the rapid onset of symptoms (within 1 h) occurred before the material would have moved into the portion of the tract inhabited by bacteria. The presumably normal acidic pH of the stomach of the patients involved would not have caused hydrolysis. Although there are no reports on the ability of human gastric contents to hydrolyze amygdalin, the known enzymes in saliva and gastric juice should not act on cyanogenic glycosides. These observations permit the tentative conclusion that amygdalin can be absorbed into the circulatory system of man and that sufficient hydrolysis by intracellular enzymes released sufficient HCN to produce the fatality. In support of this conclusion are the studies by Barrett et al. (81) showing the uptake of linamarin from the intestinal tract of the rat.

Pathological Conditions Possibly
Associated with Prolonged Ingestion of Cyanogenic Glycosides

Osuntokun (86, 87) has described a chronic degenerative disease known as tropical ataxic neuropathy (TAN) that occurs in several parts of Africa in communities with a low standard of nutrition. TAN is characterized by myelopathy, bilateral optical atrophy, and perceptive deafness. In Nigeria the disease is associated with long-standing consumption of large amounts of certain foods prepared from cassava. Individuals suffering from TAN exhibit high levels of plasma and urinary thiocyanate. The levels fall when patients are hospitalized and fed a low-cassava diet, and the levels rise again when patients return to cassava meals. The sulfur amino acids are low or absent in the plasma of TAN patients. This is attributed to poor nutrition, cyanide-induced deficiency, or both because the sulfur for detoxification of cyanide by rhodanese can come from these amino acids.

Osuntokun (88), who has collected and evaluated most of the epidemiological data on TAN in Nigeria, has concluded that chronic cyanide intoxication is an important etiological factor for the disease in West Africa. Moreover, he identifies cyanogenic glucosides in cassava as the main source of the cyanide. Montgomery (45) has commented on the possibility that both TAN and amblyopia in West Africa may be the result of chronic cyanide poisoning by cassava or certain cyanogenic legumes (pulses) commonly taken as a source of protein.

Studies on endemic goiter in Africa have identified iodine deficiency and an antithyroid activity of cassava diets as major etiological factors of the disease (89, 90, 91). The antithyroid action of cassava is due to thiocyanate, a well-established goitrogen, which is produced on detoxification of HCN released from the daily consumption of foods prepared from cassava. These conclusions are supported by experiments showing that the uptake of radioactive ^{131}I into the thyroid gland was significantly less in humans on cassava diets as compared with control subjects on rice, banana, or peanut diets (91). These effects on the uptake of ^{131}I were observed only with foods grown in goitrous regions of Idjwi Island in Zaire, where endemic goiter has been extensively studied. When individuals on cassava and rice diets in the nongoitrous regions of Idjwi were compared, there was no significant difference in ^{131}I uptake. Such results indicate that there are multifactorial causes of goiter that may be associated with sources of dietary cyanide and call for experiments with laboratory animals to identify these factors. Recent studies with neonatal iodine-deficient rats support the proposition that cyanogenic glycosides and thiocyanate derived therefrom may affect thyroid function (92). A further complication in this field is the association of endemic goiter with endemic cretinism of the myxedematous type (93). The widespread occurrence of endemic goiter, which may affect as many as 200 million people in tropical areas of the world (94), urgently calls for studies establishing how much cassava and other cyanogenic species as staple foods contribute to these conditions.

As noted above, cassava is believed to have a significant potential for increased food production in developing countries in the tropics. However, unless efforts emphasizing increased production and usage of cassava are coupled with research designed to eliminate or minimize the health problems apparently associated with its consumption under some conditions, the future of this plant as a major food crop cannot be taken for granted.

REFERENCES

1. Becker, W., and Pfeil, E. (1966). Biochem. Z. 346:301.

2. Seely, M. K., Criddle, R. S., and Conn, E. E. (1966). J. Biol. Chem. 241:4457.
3. Seigler, D. S. (1977). In L. Reinhold, J. B. Harborne, and T. Swain (eds.), Progress in Phytochemistry, Vol. 4, p. 83. Pergamon Press, Inc., New York.
4. Mao, C.-H., and Anderson, L. (1967). Phytochemistry 6:473.
5. Epstein, J. (1947). Anal. Chem. 19:272.
6. Lambert, J. L., Ramasamy, J., and Pankstelis, J. V. (1975). Anal. Chem. 47:916.
7. Hahlbrock, K., and Conn, E. E. (1971). Phytochemistry 10:1019.
8. Reay, P. F., and Conn, E. E. (1970). Phytochemistry 9:1825.
9. Conn, E. E. (1979). In G. A. Rosenthal and D. H. Janzen (eds.), Herbivores: Their Interaction with Secondary Plant Metabolites. Academic Press, Inc., New York. In press.
10. Robiquet, P. J., and Boutron-Charland, A. F. (1830). Ann. Chim. Physique Ser. 2 44:352.
11. Wöhler, F., and Liebig, J. (1837). Justus Liebigs Annalen. Pharm. 22:1.
12. Haisman, D. R., and Knight, D. J. (1967). Biochem. J. 103:528.
13. Grover, A. K., MacMurchie, D. D., and Cushley, R. J. (1977). Biochim. Biophys. Acta 482:98.
14. Hösel, W., and Nahrstedt, A. (1975). Hoppe Seylers Z. Physiol. Chem. 356:1265.
15. Hösel, W., and Nahrstedt, A. (1976). Hoppe Seylers Z. Physiol. Chem. 357:1681.
16. Heuser, C. W. (1972). Phytochemistry 11:2455.
17. Butler, G. W., Bailey, R. W., and Kennedy, L. D. (1965). Phytochemistry 4:369.
18. Cooke, R. D., Blake, G. G., and Battershill, J. M. (1978). Phytochemistry 17:381.
19. Viehoever, A., and Mack, H. (1935). Am. J. Pharmacol. 107:397.
20. Nahrstedt, A. (1975). Arch. Pharm. 308:903.
21. Plouvier, V. (1935). C. R. Acad. Sci. (Paris) 200:1985.
22. Cairns, T., Froberg, J. E., Gonzales, S., Langham, W. S., Stamp, J. J., Howie, J. K., and Sawyer, D. T. (1978). Anal. Chem. 50:317.
23. Nahrstedt, A. (1978). J. Chromatogr. 152:265.
24. Nahrstedt, A. (1970). J. Chromatogr. 50:518.
25. Turczan, J. W., Medwick, T., and Plank, W. M. (1978). J. Assoc. Off. Anal. Chem. 61:192.
26. Eyjolfsson, R. (1970). Fortschr. Chem. Org. Naturst. 28:74.
27. Conn, E. E. (1973). Biochem. Soc. Symp. 38:277.
28. Conn, E. E., and Butler, G. W. (1969). In J. B. Harborne and T. Swain (eds.), Perspectives in Phytochemistry, p. 47. Academic Press, Inc., New York.
29. Butler, G. W. (1965). Phytochemistry 4:127.
30. Jensen, S. R., and Nielsen, B. J. (1973). Acta Chem. Scand. 27:2661.
31. Dunstan, W. R., and Henry, T. A. (1902). Phil. Trans. R. Soc. Lond., Ser. A, 199:399.
32. Towers, G. H. N., McInnes, A. G., and Neish, A. C. (1964). Tetrahedron 20:71.
33. Kofod, H., and Eyjolfsson, R. (1969). Phytochemistry 8:1509.
34. Eyjolfsson, R. (1971). Acta Chem. Scand. 25:1888.
35. Young, R. L., and Hamilton, R. A. (1966–1967). Proc. Hawaii Macadamia Soc. 6:27.
36. Plouvier, V. (1974). C. R. Acad. Sci. (Paris) 279:1689.
37. Akazawa, T., Miljanich, P., and Conn, E. E. (1960). Plant Physiol. 35:535.
38. Gibb, M. C., Carbery, J. T., Carter, R. G., and Catalinac, S. (1974). N. Zl. Vet. J. 22:127.

39. Kingsbury, J. M. (1964). Poisonous Plants of the U.S. and Canada. Prentice-Hall Inc., Englewood Cliffs, New Jersey.
40. Pijoan, M. (1942). Am. J. Med. Sci. 204:550.
41. McTaggart, C. M. (1936). Br. Med. J. 2:100.
42. Lewis, J. P. (1977). West. J. Med. 127:55.
43. Viehoever, A. (1940). Thai. Sci. Bull. 2:1.
44. Montgomery, R. D. (1965). Am. J. Clin. Nutr. 17:103.
45. Montgomery, R. D. (1969). In I. E. Liener (ed.), Toxic Constituents of Plant Foodstuffs, p. 143. Academic Press, Inc., New York.
46. Montgomery, R. D. (1964). West. Indian Med. J. 13:1.
47. Clegg, D. O., Conn, E. E., and Janzen, D. H. (1979). Nature. (In press).
48. Burkill, I. H. (1966). A Dictionary of the Economic Products of the Malay Peninsula, Ministry of Agriculture and Co-Operatives, Kuala Lumpur.
49. Clusius, C. (1605). Exoticorum, libri decem.
50. Henry, O., and Boutron-Charland, A. F. (1836). Mem. Acad. Med. (Paris) 5:212.
51. Dunstan, W. R., Henry, T. A., and Auld, S. J. M. (1906). Proc. R. Soc. Lond. (Biol.) 78:152.
52. Nestel, B. (1973). In B. Nestel and R. MacIntyre (eds.), Chronic Cassava Toxicity, p. 11. International Development Research Center Monograph-010e, Ottawa, Canada.
53. Yeoh, H. H., and Chew, M. Y. (1974). Malay. Agric. J. 49:332.
54. Coursey, D. G. (1973). In B. Nestel and R. MacIntyre (eds.), Chronic Cassava Toxicity, p. 27. International Development Research Center Monograph-010e, Ottawa, Canada.
55. Tapper, B. A., and Reay, P. F. (1973). In G. W. Butler and R. W. Bailey (eds.), Chemistry and Biochemistry of Herbage, Vol. II, p. 447. Academic Press, Inc., New York.
56. Butler, G. W., Flux, D. S., Petersen, G. B., Wright, E. W., Glenday, A. C., and Johnson, J. M. (1957). N. Z. J. Sci. Technol. 38A:793.
57. Bagchi, K. N., and Ganguli, H. D. (1943). Indian Med. Gazette 78:40.
58. Schwarzmaier, U. (1976). Chem. Ber. 109:3379.
59. Clark, A. (1936). J. Trop. Med. Hyg. 39:269.
60. Petrie, J. M. (1913). Proc. Linnean Soc. N. S. Wales 38:624.
61. Ressler, C. (1962). J. Biol. Chem. 237:733.
62. Tschiersch, B. (1966). Flora (Abt. A) 157:43.
63. Hendrickson, H. R., and Conn, E. E. (1969). J. Biol. Chem. 244:2632.
64. Nass, H. G. (1972). Crop Sci. 12:503.
65. Jones, D. A. (1972). In J. B. Harborne (ed.), Phytochemical Ecology, p. 213. Academic Press, Inc., New York.
66. Warburg, O. (1927). Biochem. Z. 189:354.
67. Kiese, M., and Weger, N. (1969). Eur. J. Pharmacol. 7:97.
68. Lorcher, W., and Weger, N. (1971). Arch. Pharm. 270:R88.
69. National Institute for Occupational Safety and Health Criteria Document (1976). Occupational Exposure to Hydrogen Cyanide and Cyanide Salts, Publication No. 77-108.
70. Westley, J. (1973). Advan. Enzymol. 39:327.
71. Coop, I. E., and Blakley, R. L. (1949). N. Z. J. Sci. Technol.30A:277.
72. Moran, E. A. (1954). Am. J. Vet. Res. 15:171.
73. Seddon, H. R., and King, R. O. C. (1930). J. Aust. Coun. Sci. Ind. Res. 3:14.
74. Stone, M., and Conn, E. E. Unpublished results.
75. Everist, S. L. (1974). Poisonous Plants of Australia. Angus and Robertson, Pty. Ltd., Sydney.

76. Watt, J. M., and Breyer-Brandwijk, M. F. (1962). The Medicinal and Poisonous Plants of Southern and East Africa, Ed. 2. E. & S. Livingstone, Ltd., London.
77. Dunn, J. E., and Conn, E. E. Unpublished results.
78. Caldwell, R. J., and Courtauld, S. L. (1907). J. Chem. Soc. 91:666.
79. Winkler, W. O. (1951). J. Assoc. Off. Anal. Chem. 34:541.
80. Jansz, E. R., JeyaRaj, E. E., Pieris, N., and Abeyratne, D. J. (1974). J. Natl. Sci. Coun. Sri Lanka 2:57.
81. Barrett, M. D., Hill, D. C., Alexander, J. C., and Zitnak, A. (1977). Can. J. Physiol. Pharmacol. 55:134.
82. Cohen, R. B., Rutenberg, S. H., Tsou, K., Woodbury, M. A., and Seligman, A. M. (1952). J. Biol. Chem. 195:607.
83. Ng, S.-C. J. (1975). M. S. thesis, University of California, Davis.
84. Humbert, J. R., Tress, J. H., and Braico, K. T. (1977). JAMA 238:482.
85. Sadoff, L., Fuchs, K., and Hollander, J. (1978). JAMA 239:1532.
86. Osuntokun, B. O. (1973). In B. Nestel and R. MacIntyre (eds.), Chronic Cassava Toxicity, p. 127. International Development Research Center Monograph 010e, Ottawa, Canada.
87. Osuntokun, B. O. (1975). Bull. Schweiz. Akad. Med. Wiss. 31:353.
88. Osuntokun, B. O. (1971). Trans. R. Soc. Trop. Med. Hyg. 65:454.
89. Delange, F., and Ermans, A. M. (1971). Am. J. Clin. Nutr. 24:1354.
90. Ekpechi, O. L. (1973). In B. Nestel and R. MacIntyre (eds.), Chronic Cassava Toxicity, p. 139. International Development Research Center Monograph 010e, Ottawa, Canada.
91. Delange, F., van der Velden, M., and Ermans, A. M. (1973). In B. Nestel and R. MacIntyre (eds.), Chronic Cassava Toxicity, p. 147. International Development Research Center Monograph 010e, Ottawa, Canada.
92. Kreutler, P. A., Varbanov, V., Goodman, W., Olaya, G., and Stanbury, J. B. (1978). Am. J. Clin. Nutr. 31:282.
93. Ermans, A. M., Delange, F., van der Velden, M., and Kinthaert, J. (1972). In J. B. Stanbury and R. L. Kroc (eds.), Human Development and the Thyroid Gland, p. 456. Plenum Publishing Corp., New York.
94. Dorozynski, A. (1978). Nature 272:121.
95. de Bruijn, G. H. (1973). In B. Nestel and R. MacIntyre (eds.), Chronic Cassava Toxicity, p. 43. International Development Research Center Monograph 010e, Ottawa, Canada.

International Review of Biochemistry
Biochemistry of Nutrition IA, Volume 27
Edited by A. Neuberger and T. H. Jukes
Copyright 1979   University Park Press   Baltimore

3
Uptake and Transport of Cobalamins

L. ELLENBOGEN

Lederle Laboratories, Medical Research Division, American Cyanamid Company,
Pearl River, New York

The human body contains three classes of vitamin B_{12} (cobalamin)-binding proteins with different functional, structural, and immunological properties. These are 1) intrinsic factor, which facilitates the gastrointestinal absorption of cobalamin, 2) transcobalamin II, which mediates the transport of cobalamin from blood to tissues, and 3) R-type cobalamin-binding proteins (also called cobalophilin), which include transcobalamin I and III and whose functions are not unequivocally known.

In discussing the relationship of intrinsic factor, cobalamin absorption, and pernicious anemia, Castle (1) said: "Thus this disease would not develop if the patient could effect daily the transfer of a millionth of a gram of vitamin B_{12} the distance of a small fraction of a millimeter across the intestine and into the blood stream. This he cannot do, principally as a result of failure of his stomach to secrete into its lumen some essential but still unknown substance." The existence of this essential substance, now known as intrinsic factor, was postulated by Castle and his associates (2, 3) about 50 years ago. However, it is only in the past decade that much progress has been made in understanding the mechanism by which ingested cobalamin is transported across the intestinal wall, mediated by intrinsic factor, and enters the blood bound to the specific carrier proteins, transcobalamins, from which the cobalamin is discharged to needed tissues. This chapter is concerned with this problem. The role of these proteins in the absorption and transport can be better appreciated if, in addition, their properties, site of secretion, purification, and so on, are also discussed. There has been major progress in some of these areas recently.

THE ANION IN COBALAMINS

The isolation of vitamin B_{12} was reported by Rickes et al. (3a) and by Smith (3b). Smith noted that more than one pink, clinically active pigment was present in liver extract. Two crystalline "vitamin B_{12}" preparations were obtained from cultures of *Streptomyces aureofaciens* (3c). The first of these had an absorption spectrum identical with that reported for vitamin B_{12} (3d, 3e), but the second had a different spectrum and was termed vitamin B_{12b}. Unlike vitamin B_{12} (3f), B_{12b} did not contain cyanide, and it was named hydroxocobalamin (3g). Vitamin B_{12b} was indistinguishable from cyanocobalamin in biological activity, including effectiveness for pernicious anemia (3h). The cyanide in cyanocobalamin apparently originated from charcoal used in the concentration process.

Studies by Barker et al. (4, 5), who isolated the coenzyme forms of vitamin B_{12}, led to the further recognition that cyanocobalamin (vitamin B_{12}) is not the naturally occurring form of the vitamin, but is rather an artifact that arises from the original isolation procedure. In clinical practice cyanocobalamin, however, is the most widely used form of the cobalamin because of its availability. Most of the studies in gastrointestinal absorption and transport have used cyanocobalamin. However, as is discussed in the relevant portions of this chapter, there is no evidence that the mechanism of absorption and transport is different from that observed with the naturally occurring cobalamins. Additional information on selected aspects of the subject can be found in recent reviews (6–14).

ABSORPTION

Site of Intrinsic Factor Secretion

The basic and pioneering work of Castle established the concept of the gastric origin of intrinsic factor in humans. He was the first to show that the ingestion of normal human gastric juice mixed with beef muscle protein caused an erythropoietic response in pernicious anemia (2). Castle's description of his early studies — "Intrinsic factor is secreted by the active normal gastric mucosa and not present in detectable amounts in the gastrointestinal tract of patients with pernicious anemia or in normal saliva or duodenal contents free of gastric juice" — showed that saliva and normal duodenal juice were also devoid of intrinsic factor (3). This was confirmed by Landboe-Christensen and Bohn (15). Further studies from Landboe-Christensen et al. (16) showed that desiccated preparations of normal human duodenum, but not jejunum, contained a small amount of intrinsic factor activity. This was undoubtedly due to contamination of the tissue by gastric juice, because patients who have undergone total gastric resection cannot absorb cobalamin, and intestinal juices of most patients are devoid of intrinsic factor activity (17–20).

The fundic (corpus) and cardiac regions of the normal human stomach have been identified as the sites of intrinsic factor formation (21–23). These results are in agreement with histological findings that atrophy of the stomach, characteristically seen in pernicious anemia, occurs in the fundic area but not in the pyloric region (24–26). Additional evidence for the belief that the fundic part of the human stomach is responsible for intrinsic factor production comes from the report of impaired cobalamin absorption in patients who underwent a selective resection of this portion of the stomach (27). The stomach seems to be the only site of intrinsic factor, as indicated by numerous reports on the development of pernicious anemia several years after total gastrectomy (19, 28–32). After partial gastrectomy, in which the fundus is left intact, megaloblastic anemia or malabsorption of vitamin B_{12} does not develop (33).

With the use of autoradiographic and immunological procedures, it has been shown that intrinsic factor is elaborated by the hydrochloric acid-secreting parietal cells (34, 35). Studies using the immunofluorescence method have confirmed the fact that, in man, intrinsic factor is derived from parietal cells (36, 37). Fractionation studies of human gastric mucosal extracts indicate that intrinsic factor activity is present in both mitochondria and particle-free supernatant fluid (38).

Since the nutrition of the fetus takes place through capillaries in the placenta, there appears to be no reason to believe that the fetus could make use of gastric intrinsic factor. By means of radioimmunoassays, however, Schwartz and Weber (39) have recently shown that intrinsic factor is produced in the fetal stomach from about the 11th to the 13th week. While intrinsic factor is found mostly in the fundus of the neonate, a considerable amount of intrinsic factor was found in the pyloric part of the stomach of the fetus. It therefore appears that the production of intrinsic factor begins several months before the substance can be presumed to be of any value to the individual, and intrinsic factor may be one of the first important substances to appear in gastric juice.

Purification and Properties of Intrinsic Factor

Since hog intrinsic factor is active in facilitating cobalamin absorption in humans, investigators have been concerned with the isolation of hog as well as human intrinsic factor. Various laboratories have recently succeeded in isolating human and hog intrinsic factor in homogenous or nearly homogenous form (40–43). The methods used were laborious and only small amounts of material were isolated. Despite these difficulties, material active at a dose of 40–50 μg was obtained, which represented a purification of about a million-fold.

The development of affinity chromatography proved to be an attractive method for the isolation of significant amounts of intrinsic factor and other cobalamin-binding proteins; the isolation of cobalamin-binding proteins by affinity chromatography has recently been described (44–49). In the studies by Allen's group the affinity ligand was prepared by partial acid hydrolysis of an amide group of the unsubstituted propionamide side chains of the corrin ring of cyanocobalamin. The resulting mixture of mono-, di-, and tricarboxylic cobalamin derivatives was separated by chromatography, and the monocarboxylic derivatives of cyanocobalamin were coupled covalently to the free amino group of 3,3′-diaminodipropylamine-substituted Sepharose, thereby regenerating native cyanocobalamin stably coupled to Sepharose. The cobalamin-Sepharose proved to be an effective absorbent and was used to isolate human granulocyte cobalamin-binding protein, human transcobalamin II, human intrinsic factor, and hog intrinsic factor.

The groups of Gräsbeck, Holdsworth, and Ellenbogen were able to separate the cobalamin-binding protein of hog gastric mucosa into two fractions by ion-exchange chromatography. Only one fraction contained intrinsic factor activity. The fraction without intrinsic factor, called nonintrinsic factor (i.e., unable to promote intestinal absorption), is one of a number of related cobalamin-binding proteins collectively called "R" binders or cobalophilin. These are discussed further under "Transport." In Allen's laboratory, the two cobalamin-binding proteins were separated by a method of selective affinity chromatography with an affinity absorbent containing covalently bound derivatives of cobalamin that lack the nucleotide portion of the native vitamin. The active fraction was not adsorbed to the substituted Sepharose on the column.

Ellenbogen's group reported a molecular weight of about 50,000 for both of their protein fractions in the absence of cobalamin, whereas formation of an oligomer of molecular weight about 100,000 was observed in the presence of cyanocobalamin (50). Similar observations were made by Allen and Mehlman with hog intrinsic factor, but no oligomer formation was observed with the nonintrinsic factor binder by these workers (48). Cyanocobalamin and intrinsic factor react in approximately equimolar amounts. Both groups of workers have shown that hog intrinsic factor has a lower affinity for pseudovitamin B_{12} relative to cyanocobalamin than does the hog nonintrinsic factor preparation. The differences in the carbohydrate and amino acid composition between these two proteins were much more marked in the studies by Allen and Mehlman (48) than in those of Ellenbogen and Highley (42).

Hog intrinsic and nonintrinsic factor are probably separate proteins, and such properties as facilitation of absorption and cobalamin binding by guinea pig ileal mucosal homogenates and blockade of cobalamin binding by anti-intrinsic factor antibody are not shared by the hog nonintrinsic factor fraction. The function of hog nonintrinsic factor is not known. Since it has been obtained in three different laboratories with different techniques, it would appear that it is not an artifact of isolation.

Isolation of human intrinsic factor from normal human gastric juice has been accomplished by Gräsbeck's laboratory (41, 43), Allen's laboratory (47), and by Christensen et al. (49). A molecular weight of 119,000 has been obtained for the intrinsic factor–cobalamin complex in Gräsbeck's early work, and these investigators suggested that this complex is a dimer (41). A molecular weight of 60,000–73,000 (monomeric form) was obtained in their later work (43). The elegant work on the isolation of human intrinsic factor by Allen's laboratory by affinity chromatography also suggests a monomer-to-oligomer formation, but these investigators obtained a molecular weight of 44,000 for their monomer (47). A nonintrinsic factor binder was not obtained by Allen and Mehlman, whereas Gräsbeck's group isolated a nonintrinsic factor binder from human gastric juice.

As was observed with the homogenous hog preparation, the homogenous human preparation obtained by Allen's group facilitated binding to homogenates of guinea pig and human distal ileum (47). Preparations of both pure hog and human intrinsic factor have single cobalamin-binding sites, and both bind about 30 μg of cyanocobalamin per mg of protein. The spectral maximum of 361 nm for unbound cyanocobalamin shifts to 362 nm when the vitamin is bound to either protein, suggesting that determination of cobalamin content by using the extinction coefficient at 361 nm would result in falsely elevated values.

Preparations of homogenous hog and human intrinsic factor display certain differences in properties. Anti-intrinsic factor antibody from the serum of a pernicious anemia patient has a lower affinity for hog intrinsic factor than for human intrinsic factor. Both human and hog intrinsic factor contain relatively large amounts of carbohydrate, as was suspected from the early fractionation studies. Human intrinsic factor has a molecular weight of 44,000, whereas an approximate value of 55,000 was obtained for hog intrinsic factor. Hog intrinsic factor was isolated from stomach mucosa and human intrinsic factor from gastric juice. The isolation of human intrinsic factor from gastric mucosa would be of interest in order to determine whether the differences in their properties represent a species difference.

Christensen et al. (49) also isolated intrinsic factor from human gastric juice by affinity chromatography. Hydroxocobalamin was made insoluble by covalent coupling to albumin, which in turn was coupled to bromoacetyl-activated cellulose. This allowed specific absorption of cobalamin-binding proteins from the human gastric juice. The cobalamin-binding proteins were eluted by increase of temperature and addition of cyanocobalamin instead of guanidine. [Weiss et al. (51) have criticized the use of guanidine to dissociate intrinsic factor from the cobalamin-Sepharose complex because it is claimed that this resulted in decreased affinity for the intestinal receptors.] The molecular weight of the isolated human intrinsic factor obtained by Christensen et al. was about 60,000, and the amino acid composition was similar to that of hog intrinsic factor isolated by Ellenbogen's group.

Recently Francis et al. (51a) isolated 99% pure hog intrinsic factor by affinity chromatography with the monocarboxylic acid derivative of vitamin B_{12} covalently coupled to 1,6-hexanediamine–substituted Sepharose. Intrinsic factor was separated from nonintrinsic factor in one step with a selective linear gradient of guanidine-HCl. Their technique resulted in a 1033-fold purification of intrinsic factor with a 40% recovery of that present in the original sample.

In addition, Gräsbeck's laboratory recently described a simple combined immuno- and affinity chromatographic system for the isolation of single proteins from preparations containing various kinds of cobalamin-binding proteins (52). The isolated proteins were identical in properties with the corresponding protein not subjected to affinity chromatography.

Binding of Cobalamins to Intrinsic Factor

One of the most important properties of intrinsic factor is its binding by cobalamins, first observed by Ternberg and Eakin (53). The ability to bind cobalamin is an essential property of intrinsic factor. The isolation of hog and human intrinsic factor not only confirmed the hypothesis regarding the binding properties of intrinsic factor, but also helped to clarify some of the confusion about the correlation between intrinsic factor activity and binding (41, 42, 47–49). These investigators were able to purify two fractions from hog pylorus and human gastric juice. Both fractions combined with cyanocobalamin, but only one possessed intrinsic factor activity.

It is important to emphasize that cobalamin binding is only one of the properties of intrinsic factor. There may be several sites on the intrinsic factor molecule necessary for its activity. Intrinsic factor probably contains a site for cobalamin binding and at least one site concerned with absorption or attachment to ileal receptors in the intestine (54–59). Both groups would be necessary for activity. If the "absorption site" were absent or destroyed, the material would be inactive but would retain its ability to bind cobalamin.

Structural Specificity of Binding Cyanocobalamin, aquocobalamin, adenosylcobalamin, and methylcobalamin each have the same binding constant to intrinsic factor, which indicates that the substituent at the fifth coordination position is not important in the formation of the cobalamin–intrinsic factor complex (60–65). Intrinsic factor does not bind pseudovitamin B_{12} to any significant extent, whereas pseudovitamin B_{12} competes with cyanocobalamin for nonintrinsic factor binders (48, 54, 66). Any observed pseudovitamin binding by human gastric juice or hog gastric mucosa concentrates is a result of their nonintrinsic factor content (42, 54).

Intrinsic factor does not appear to bind to other cobalamin analogs in which the nucleotide is modified. From these observations, Gräsbeck inferred that the nucleotide of the vitamin faces inward in the complex and the cyanide side of its planar structure faces outward (67). Chemical and immunological findings also suggest that cyanocobalamin fits into a "pit" in the molecule and that intrinsic factor has an open structure that closes around the cobalamin after it is bound (68, 69).

Physical and Chemical Nature of Cobalamin Binding The rate of binding of cyanocobalamin to intrinsic factor is rapid (50, 70). The reaction is complete in less than 1 min. Hippe and Olesen (61) determined certain thermodynamic parameters for binding of cyanocobalamin to a purified preparation of human intrinsic factor, transcobalamin I, and transcobalamin II. Equilibrium constants in the order of $10^9 M^{-1}$ were obtained and are similar to those reported by other investigators (47, 65, 71, 72). The reaction between cyanocobalamin and intrinsic factor is exothermic, DH^0 being -22.7 kcal/mol (61).

The binding of cyanocobalamin to intrinsic factor causes certain physical changes in the intrinsic factor molecule (40, 41, 50). Bromer and Davisson (40) reported an increase in sedimentation constant from 3.1 to 4.4 Svedberg units after the addition of cyanocobalamin to their purified hog intrinsic factor and speculated that association had occurred or that the complex was "unusually dense." Highley et al. (50, 68) demonstrated very clearly that, after cyanocobalamin binding, hog intrinsic factor undergoes a slow dimerization, although the rate of binding is instantaneous. Similar findings have been reported by Gräsbeck et al. (41). Hippe (73, 74) found a decrease in the Stokes radius of human intrinsic factor and transcobalamin II, indicating a conformational charge after binding by cyanocobalamin. After binding to cyanocobalamin, the behavior of the complex in gel filtration is slightly different from that of free intrinsic factor. Since the complex is resistant to various enzymes, through some conformational change the cobalamin protects the peptide bonds from enzymatic attack (55, 75-77).

Circular dichroism studies on the methylcobalamin-intrinsic factor complex, together with studies on the carbethoxylation of histidine residues in this complex, indicate that 5,6-dimethylbenzimidazole is probably displaced by a histidine residue of intrinsic factor that coordinates with the cobalt atom at the sixth coordination site. In addition, the stability of the Co-C bond for methylcobalamin bound to intrinsic factor is identical with that of the free methylcobinamide-histidine complex, but differs considerably from the stability of this bond in free methylcobalamin (78, 79).

When cyanocobalamin binds human intrinsic factor, the spectral maximum shifts from 361 nm to 362 nm and the absolute absorbance at 361 nm increases by approximately 30% (47). The bond between cyanocobalamin and hog intrinsic factor or human gastric juice is quite strong, particularly at lower temperatures (54, 80-82). There is appreciable exchange, however, at 37°C between free cobalamin and gastric juice-bound cobalamin (83).

Comparatively little has been published on attempts to detach cobalamin from intrinsic factor or transcobalamins. At pH 12.3, no dissociation occurs, but at pH 12.6 there is almost complete dissociation (84). The complex can also be dissociated slowly by 5M guanidinium chloride (50), undoubtedly due to unfolding of the protein molecule. The rate constant for dissociation at pH 7.4 and 30°C is very low (72).

Inhibition of Cobamide Coenzyme Activity Intrinsic factor preparations have been found to inhibit several cobamide coenzyme-dependent reactions, presumably by combining with the added coenzyme to decrease the effective concentration. Good correlation between the clinical activity of intrinsic factor preparations and their specific activity as inhibitors of the coenzyme-dependent glutamate isomerase reaction has been found (85).

The inhibition of cobamide coenzyme activity by intrinsic factor is the basis for its usefulness in the study of the role and mechanisms of action of the cobalamin coenzymes in several metabolic reactions. Thus, intrinsic factor has been helpful in providing additional evidence that the cobamide structure is involved in specific enzymic reactions. In certain instances in which separation of the coenzyme from the apoenzyme is difficult, specific inhibition of the coenzyme such as that obtained with intrinsic factor may be the only means of providing proof of a cobamide coenzyme requirement (86, 87).

Immunological Properties

The findings by Taylor (88) and Schwartz (89, 90) that the sera from pernicious anemia patients inhibited the gastrointestinal absorption of cobalamin and the demonstration that these sera contain antibodies to intrinsic factor (91, 92) provided the impetus for immunological studies with intrinsic factor. Two types of intrinsic factor antibodies are now recognized (93). These are the "blocking" antibody, which prevents the combination of cobalamin with intrinsic factor, and the "binding" antibody, which combines with cobalamin–intrinsic factor complex, thereby preventing the uptake of the complex by the intestinal mucosa (see Figure 1).

Jeffries (94) has recently summarized the evidence suggesting that immunological phenomena may be responsible for an individual's susceptibility to the development of pernicious anemia. Although the role of anti-intrinsic factor antibody in the pathogenesis of gastric mucosal atrophy is far from clear, most of the available evidence suggests that these antibodies are a consequence of rather than a cause of pernicious anemia (9). Thus, in some patients with pernicious anemia, anti-intrinsic factor antibody cannot be detected (95, 96), and such antibodies have been reported in some patients who do not have pernicious anemia (97, 98). Parietal cell antibodies frequently occur in the absence of gastric atrophy and intrinsic factor (9). A more detailed review of intrinsic factor antibodies and their role in cobalamin absorption and malabsorption has been recently presented by Donaldson (9).

Assay of Intrinsic Factor: In Vivo Techniques

The final criterion of biological activity of any intrinsic factor preparation is its ability to enhance the intestinal absorption of cobalamin. Therefore, the most unequivocal methods for measuring intrinsic factor are those techniques used to measure cobalamin absorption in man — the urinary excretion, fecal excretion, hepatic uptake, blood plasma, and total body radioactivity (see under "Methods of Determining Cobalamin Absorption in

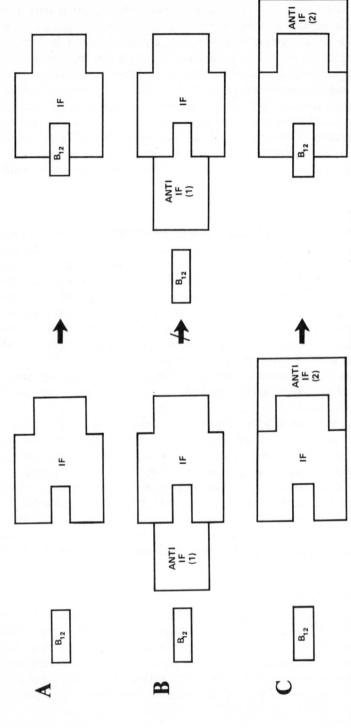

Figure 1.   Antibodies to intrinsic factor: a, normal absorption; b, blocking type of antibodies (Type 1); and c, binding type of antibodies (Type 2).

Man"). These methods are used with patients who lack intrinsic factor (as in pernicious anemia or with total gastric resection).

In the United States, the Anti-Anemia Preparations Advisory Board of the National Formulary adopted a standardized procedure and a standard intrinsic factor sample for use in the urinary excretion test for assay of commercial intrinsic factor preparations (National Formulary, 11th Edition). An outline of the procedure has been described (10). The method allows for the assay of several intrinsic factor preparations in one patient. Wider acceptance of this method recently has permitted more accurate estimation of relative activities of various preparations under investigation.

However, it would be most desirable if unequivocal in vitro techniques were available. The techniques that have been described directly and indirectly provided useful information about intrinsic factor in many respects, but have not made it possible to assay intrinsic factor quantitatively. Reviews of these in vitro assays can be found in the monographs by Glass (12) and Ellenbogen (10).

Methods of Determining Cobalamin Absorption in Man

Before the introduction of the use of labeled cyanocobalamin (99), estimates of absorption were based mostly on indirect evidence. Microbiological assays were used to measure deposition of the absorbed vitamin in tissues. Qualitatively, the degree of hematopoietic response in cobalamin-deficient patients was used as an index of absorption (100). Because of the synthesis of cobalamins by bacteria in the intestine, it has not been possible to measure microbiologically the unabsorbed cyanocobalamin from an unlabeled oral dose.

Five different methods are available for determining the absorption of an oral dose of radioactive cyanocobalamin in man. Various radioactive isotopes of cobalt have been used — ^{56}Co, ^{57}Co, ^{58}Co, and ^{60}Co. The five methods are discussed briefly here; detailed reviews of these techniques have been presented elsewhere (70, 101, 102). An excellent summary of the various methods for clinical purposes has also been given by Mollin (103).

Absorption tests have been of great value in diagnosing cobalamin deficiencies, especially in differentiating between Addisonian pernicious anemia and cobalamin malabsorption of intestinal origin (104). The administration of intrinsic factor usually corrects impaired absorption of cobalamin in patients with pernicious anemia but not in those with intestinal malabsorption.

The assimilation of cobalamins from food involves both digestive and absorptive processes (see under "Sequence of Events During Intrinsic Factor–mediated Cobalamin Absorption"). The absorption tests use labeled crystalline cyanocobalamin, which is not always physiological since it circumvents the digestive process. The importance of this digestive process is seen by the recent observations that some patients do not absorb labeled cyanocobalamin satisfactorily if it is incorporated into food, even though they absorb crystalline cyanocobalamin normally (105, 106).

Urinary Excretion Test   Introduced by Schilling, the urinary excretion method of measuring cyanocobalamin absorption is frequently called the Schilling test or UET and is the most widely used isotopic method for measuring absorption of the vitamin (107). After a small, single, oral dose of radioactive cyanocobalamin (0.5–2.0 μg), no urinary radioactivity is detected in normal or pernicious anemia subjects. However, if a parenteral injection (i.e., a "flushing dose") of 1000 μg of nonradioactive cyanocobalamin is given simultaneously or within 2 h after the oral dose, a significant amount of radioactivity is excreted by normal individuals but very little is found in pernicious anemia subjects. Excretion of substantial radioactivity in the urine of pernicious anemia patients occurs only when oral intrinsic factor is given. Not all the absorbed radioactivity is flushed into the urine by the parenteral cyanocobalamin; approximately one-third of the absorbed dose is recovered in the urine in 24 h (108–110). If a second parenteral injection of unlabeled cyanocobalamin is given 24 h after the oral test dose, an additional amount equivalent to as much as 50% of the first day's excretion may be recovered (111–113). Because of the delayed excretion of radioactivity observed in some normal and pernicious anemia subjects and in patients with renal disease, it is desirable to use two flushing doses and to collect two 24-h urine specimens after each oral dose of labeled cyanocobalamin (111, 114–116). It is absolutely necessary to use at least two flushing doses when testing intrinsic factor preparations consecutively in the same patient. The second injection also serves to eliminate further radioactivity from the body.

A shortened procedure that measures the absorption of cyanocobalamin in the presence and absence of intrinsic factor simultaneously has been proposed (117). Two different isotopes of cobalt are required, one bound to intrinsic factor and the other free. This procedure has been used successfully and was found to be acceptable to both patients and clinicians. It is extremely important to mix the intrinsic factor and labeled cyanocobalamin before administration. The administration of two separate capsules, one containing the labeled cyanocobalamin and the other a preparation of intrinsic factor, may lead to spuriously low results (118).

Many sensitive counting techniques and a large quantity of special equipment have been developed so that relatively large urine volumes may be counted with maximum precision. The advantages of the urinary excretion test are that: 1) results can be obtained in 24–48 h; 2) as much as 50% of the absorbed radioactivity can be flushed from the body; 3) the method is suitable for use with outpatients; 4) it is possible to test the greatest number of samples on the same patient in the shortest time; and 5) with the flushing dose the patient is receiving treatment during the test. The disadvantages are that it is an indirect method requiring quantitative urine collections and that increased tissue levels of cobalamins resulting from larger parenteral doses may affect the results of the test (108, 111, 119).

Fecal Excretion Test   The fecal excretion test, described by Heinle et al. (120), was the first isotopic method used for the study of cyanocobalamin absorption. The difference between the dose and the amount excreted in the feces represents the quantity of cobalamin absorbed. Normal subjects absorb from 50% to 60% of a 1.0-μg oral dose, whereas pernicious anemia subjects absorb less than 10%. When the same dose is given to pernicious anemia patients together with a fully active intrinsic factor preparation, absorption is increased to normal levels. The agreement of the results obtained with this method with those obtained by the hepatic uptake and urinary excretion tests is very good (121).

The fecal excretion technique is in theory the most accurate and quantitative means of determining absorption since it yields a direct result. Its disadvantages are that 1) 7–10 days are required to collect all unabsorbed fecal radioactivity; 2) it is the least pleasant of the methods; 3) because only a small percentage of a large dose is absorbed, it cannot be used to accurately measure absorption of doses much above 5–10 μg; and 4) fecal radioactivity does not represent exclusively unabsorbed cyanocobalamin, since it has been shown that some absorbed vitamin is excreted into the feces by the bile.

Hepatic Uptake Method   The hepatic uptake technique, described by Glass et al. (122), is concerned with the measurement of absorbed cyanocobalamin deposited in the liver. Subjects with pernicious anemia, in contrast to normal subjects, show no hepatic uptake of radioactivity after an oral dose of cyanocobalamin unless it is accompanied by the administration of intrinsic factor. By placing a directional scintillation counter over the surface projection of the liver, a semiquantitative estimate of the amount of cobalamins deposited and, indirectly, the amount absorbed can be obtained. The increase in radioactivity in the liver is slow; the peak concentration is reached 2–4 days after the oral dose. For measuring intestinal absorption by hepatic uptake, a more rapid quantitative method with the use of a double label (^{57}Co and ^{60}Co) has also been proposed (123).

Excellent correlation has been found between the hepatic uptake and the fecal and urinary excretion methods (121, 124). It is a decided advantage of the hepatic uptake method that patient cooperation is unnecessary. On the other hand, special equipment is required, and the procedure does not lend itself to consecutive assays of intrinsic factor on the patient. In addition, inhibition of uptake is observed in liver disease.

Blood Plasma Radioactivity   The blood plasma radioactivity method, introduced by Booth and Mollin (124) and Doscherholmen et al. (125), depends on the presence of a peak of radioactivity in the blood 8–12 h after giving an oral test dose. Pernicious anemia subjects, unless given intrinsic factor with the labeled dose, have very little plasma radioactivity at any time. Because in normal subjects less than 5% of the oral dose appears in the total plasma at peak concentration, this method requires the use of labeled cyanocobalamin with very high specific activity. This method shows good correlation with the urinary excretion method (126).

Whole Body Counting   Whole body counting is similar to the hepatic uptake method, but radioactivity of the whole body is measured instead of liver radioactivity (127). Whole body counting makes use of equipment that is expensive and not generally available. Typical values of the amount of radioactivity measured after a test dose of labeled cyanocobalamin with and without a potent source of intrinsic factor are given in Table 1.

Site of Cobalamin Absorption

The absorption of physiological doses of cobalamin in the human alimentary tract takes place almost exclusively in the ileum. This evidence is based on defective cobalamin absorption in diseases of the lower ileum or after resection of the ileum, measurement of intestinal radioactivity after oral administration of radioactive cyanocobalamin, and instillation of radioactive cyanocobalamin in various segments of intestine. Impaired absorption of cobalamins is found in patients who have undergone resection of the ileum, but not after resection of the duodenum or jejunum (104, 128–132). The addition of intrinsic factor or antibiotics could not correct the impaired cobalamin absorption.

Various investigators have studied the site of cobalamin absorption by following instillation of cyanocobalamin and cyanocobalamin-intrinsic factor complex. Direct instillation of cobalamins in the jejunum only (segment closed at proximal and distal ends) did not result in any significant cyanocobalamin absorption (133). Cobalamin is absorbed, whether it is instilled in the duodenum, jejunum, or ileum. The cobalamin instilled in the upper intestine probably moved down to the ileum before it was absorbed. In pernicious anemia patients, the ileum absorbed cyanocobalamin only when intrinsic factor was added. Similar experiments, conducted by Best et al. (134) and Johnson and Berger (135), implicated the ileum as the site of absorption after the use of delayed release capsules containing labeled cyanocobalamin. Using polyethylene glycol as a marker in a test meal containing labeled cyanocobalamin, samples of intestinal juice from different parts of the intestine

Table 1.   Typical values of radioactive cyanocobalamin in pernicious anemia subjects with and without intrinsic factor by five different methods

Method	Without intrinsic factor (% of oral dose)	With intrinsic factor (% of oral dose)
Urinary excretion test	0–7	10–30
Fecal excretion	80–100	30–60
Hepatic uptake	0–1	40–50
Blood radioactivity	0–1	3–5
Total body radioactivity	0–20	30–60

also lead to the conclusion that most of the absorption occurred in the terminal portion of the small intestine (136).

Various investigators have provided ample evidence that other parts of the gastrointestinal tract are of no significance in the absorption of physiological doses of cyanocobalamin (see review in ref. 12). No absorption takes place after buccal administration, and the large intestine has been shown to be incapable of absorbing small doses of cyanocobalamin (137, 138), although some absorption can take place after rectal administration of very large doses, such as 2000 μg (139). The mucosa of the large bowel, therefore, does not secrete intrinsic factor or a substance that would mediate the absorption of the vitamin.

Sequence of Events during Intrinsic Factor-Mediated Cobalamin Absorption

Cobalamin can be absorbed by two different mechanisms (125, 140, 141). The active mechanism is mediated by the intrinsic factor; absorption occurs in the ileum and is of primary importance in the absorption of physiological doses of cobalamin (approximately 2–3 μg or less). The events that take place in the intestine after the ingestion of physiological amounts of cobalamin require about 8–10 h for the completion of the absorption of the vitamin in man. The sequence of events can be classified as: 1) removal of cobalamin from combination with other dietary sources; 2) binding of cobalamin to intrinsic factor; 3) intestinal transit through the small intestine to the ileum; 4) attachment of cobalamin–intrinsic factor complex to specific receptors on the absorptive surface of the ileum; 5) transfer of cobalamin across the small intestinal epithelial absorptive cell to the portal plasma; and 6) release of the vitamin from cobalamin–intrinsic factor complex.

Removal of Cobalamins from Combination with Other Dietary Sources Essentially all dietary cobalamin is attached to protein in coenzyme form. Unless cyanocobalamin in medicinal form is ingested, the main cobalamins in food are adenosylcobalamin and hydroxocobalamin (142). Significant amounts of the coenzymes are converted to hydroxocobalamin during the preparation of the food (142, 143). Most studies concerned with cobalamin absorption have been performed with cyanocobalamin; therefore, this form is used in discussing these studies except where different analogs were specified. The absorption of cyanocobalamin, however, is essentially the same as that of hydroxocobalamin (62, 144). The cobalamins are released in vitro by heating, acid, and proteolytic enzymes (145, 146). In contrast to cobalamin–intrinsic factor complexes, pancreatic proteases readily release cobalamin from protein linkage. The release of cobalamin does not appear to be rate limiting. Because of the low dissociation constant of the R type proteins, intrinsic factor readily binds the released cobalamin (65, 71, 147, 148).

Binding of Cobalamin to Intrinsic Factor A prerequisite for the intestinal absorption of physiological amounts of cobalamin is binding to intrinsic factor. Upon release of the vitamin from food, it is bound to intrinsic factor. (The binding of cobalamins to proteins and the physical and chemical nature of binding have been discussed under "Binding of Cobalamins to Intrinsic Factor.") The intrinsic factor is secreted by the parietal cells of the stomach. There are nonintrinsic factor proteins such as salivary binding protein and the cobalamin-binding proteins of the bile, and any cobalamin attached to nonintrinsic factor proteins is transferred to intrinsic factor in the small intestine (81).

It should not be assumed that orally administered cobalamins are bound by intrinsic factor and that this complex remains intact until sometime after it becomes bound to the ileal receptor. Recent in vitro studies have shown that human salivary R protein binds cyanocobalamin with affinities that are three- and fifty-fold higher than those of human intrinsic factor at pH 8 and 2, respectively (148). Cobalamin bound to R protein was not transferred to an equal amount of intrinsic factor at either pH 8 or pH 2 (also see under "Role of the Pancreas in Cobalamin Absorption").

The intrinsic factor molecule probably has at least two functional sites, a cobalamin binding site and a receptor side that attaches to a receptor mechanism on the surface of the intestinal mucosa (54–59). There is excellent evidence that the cobalamin binding sites are protected by the bound vitamin against enzymatic digestion and heating (75–77). The presence of the vitamin also diminishes or prevents inactivation of human intrinsic factor by various means (40, 149). This stabilizing effect of cobalamin facilitates the isolation of intrinsic factor from both hog and human sources, but, more importantly, it has a useful physiological effect. It protects intrinsic factor against autodigestion during transport from the stomach to the ileum, where the intrinsic factor can then promote the uptake of the bound vitamin. Intrinsic factor also probably protects cobalamin from uptake by intestinal bacteria.

Transit through the Small Intestine   The cobalamin–intrinsic factor complex is carried to the ileum by peristalsis. The complex is resistant to enzymatic hydrolysis by various enzymes, as mentioned above. In vitro, very few enzymes can split off cobalamins from the complex or digest the complex, whereas the free intrinsic factor is more labile as well as more susceptible to enzymatic breakdown (75–77). In view of the fact that the intrinsic factor molecule dimerizes, it would appear that the polymerization causes some conformational change that prevents the enzymes from attacking susceptible bonds (41, 42, 47, 48). In addition, the dimerization must also protect the vitamin from bacterial utilization, as suggested by a large number of studies mentioned above. Callender et al. (150) have shown the importance of binding of intrinsic factor in the upper part of the intestine. Patients with esophageal occlusion whose stomachs were bypassed by a Roux-Y type of anastomosis of the esophagus to the jejunum showed decreased absorption of cobalamin in the intestine. In these patients, the intrinsic factor reached the ingested vitamin in the jejunum. Citrin et al. (133) performed intestinal intubations on normal persons and patients with pernicious anemia. A test dose of labeled cyanocobalamin delivered to the duodenum resulted in greater absorption than when the vitamin was delivered to the jejunum or the ileum. In pernicious anemia patients, administration of cyanocobalamin with intrinsic factor into the duodenum also resulted in greater absorption than when both substances were administered into the ileum. The method of Jacob and O'Brien (151), which can measure intrinsic factor bound to cobalamin, was used to study the fate of intrinsic factor–cobalamin complex during intestinal transit in two normal subjects. Approximately 50–70% of the administered radioactivity recovered from the ileum was bound to intrinsic factor, whereas 15–25% was free cobalamin and 10–30% was bound to nonintrinsic factor binders.

Attachment of Cobalamin to Ileal Receptors   Several studies indicate that the cobalamin–intrinsic factor complex is transiently attached to an ileal receptor. This is probably the first characterized process that occurs in the ileum. In vitro studies using everted sacs, whole homogenates (including human ileal homogenates), and brush border fractions demonstrated that intrinsic factor enhanced the uptake of cobalamin (59, 152–158). The proximal small intestine does not have the ability to enhance absorption of the vitamin; only the ileum has this property. Free cobalamin is attached to the ileal receptors only weakly if at all (44). This uptake is also specific for intrinsic factor. Cobalamin-binding proteins of serum, saliva, colostrum, or tears do not enhance the uptake of cobalamin (159).

Several other characteristics of this attachment to ileal receptor have been found:

1. Energy supply or a specific enzymatic step is probably not required (158). The attachment occurs in the absence of glucose or oxygen and despite poisoning with sodium azide and dinitrophenol (145).
2. Intrinsic factor enhancement of cobalamin uptake is not affected by changes in temperature from 7 °C to 37 °C (158), suggesting that the attachment of intrinsic factor–bound vitamin, although specific, results from absorption and not from a specific energy-requiring enzymatic process. The observation that increasing the time for incubation did not increase uptake of intrinsic factor–bound cobalamin supports this view (158).
3. Attachment of the complex to the receptor occurs preferentially at a pH between 6.0 and 8.0 (154, 155, 158). Lowering the pH below 5.6 impairs uptake of cobalamin by everted sacs (154), homogenates (155), and isolated brush borders (158). This pH effect is important only with the attachment of the intrinsic factor–cobalamin complex to the ileal receptor and is unimportant in the nonintrinsic factor–mediated cobalamin absorption (154). Maximal binding between human intrinsic factor–cobalamin complex and ileal mucosal homogenates has been reported to oc-

cur in the pH range of 6.5–9.5, which is in good agreement with studies in the other species (160).

4. Divalent cations are required for attachment. Removal of calcium ion from an in vitro medium or addition of a chelating agent to the medium reduces intrinsic factor uptake of cobalamin.

The precise mechanism by which calcium ions influence the attachment to the ileal receptors remains unknown. Calcium could enhance attachment of intrinsic factor–cobalamin complex to ileal receptor by directly linking anionic groups on the intrinsic factor molecule with those on ileal receptor or by forming salt bridges that alter the conformation of the intrinsic factor-cobalamin complex (161). Based on experiments with homogenous preparations of intrinsic factor–cobalamin and human ileal mucosa homogenates and unpurified human intrinsic factor and solubilized human ileal receptors, an association constant for ileal receptor of the order of $10^9 \, \text{M}^{-1}$ was obtained (160, 162). The entire human ileum contains enough receptors to bind 0.5–1.0 mg of cobalamin bound to intrinsic factor. Human intrinsic factor devoid of cobalamin does not appear to attach to human ileal receptors (160, 162, 163); large excesses of homogeneous human free intrinsic factor do not inhibit human intrinsic factor–cobalamin binding to human ileal homogenates.

Since free cobalamin or free intrinsic factor does not attach to ileal receptors, the conformational changes that occur during the formation of the intrinsic factor–cobalamin complex (see under "Purification and Properties of Intrinsic Factor") must be important with respect to the binding of the complex to the ileal receptor. A patient has been described whose intrinsic factor bound cobalamin normally but had little affinity to ileal receptors (164, 165). A schematic representation of the intrinsic factor complex on the ileal receptor as described by Herbert et al. (166) is shown in Figure 2. The complex is thought to fit into the ileal receptor by molecular complementarity in a key-in-lock fashion. This model can explain why large pharmacological doses of cobalamin are poorly absorbed and why large or excessive doses of intrinsic factor do not increase the absorption of cobalamin above a certain limit. In addition, the species specificity of the intrinsic factor can be explained by the failure of the specific receptor to bind a heterologous intrinsic factor.

To determine whether the molecular configuration of a corrinoid influences the attachment of intrinsic factor–corrin complex to ileal microvillous membrane receptor sites, Mathan et al. (65) have examined the kinetics of uptake of intrinsic factor–bound cyanocobalamin by brush borders and microvillous membranes isolated from guinea pig ileum. They have compared this uptake with that of intrinsic factor alone and with that intrinsic factor complexed with various analogs of cyanocobalamin. Attachment of intrinsic factor–bound cyanocobalamin to microvillous membranes showed satura-

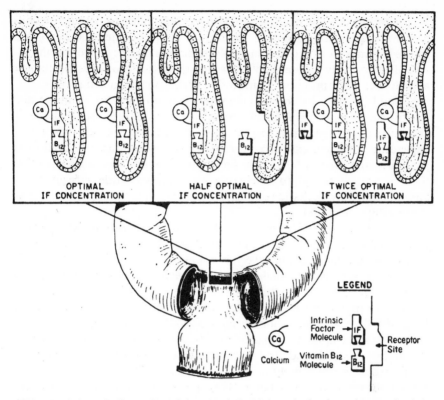

Figure 2.   Schematic illustration of the "key-in-lock" hypothesis of attachment of cobalamin–intrinsic factor complex to receptors on the brush border of the ileal-mucosa. Reproduced from Herbert et al. with permission of the Williams & Wilkins Company, Baltimore.

tion kinetics with a dissociation constant of 0.25 nM. Attachment was rapid and was 70% complete within 5 min; the second order rate constant for attachment was $1.3 \times 10^6 \ \text{M}^{-1}/\text{s}$. The half-time for dissociation of intrinsic factor–bound cyanocobalamin from the ileal receptor was approximately 35 min. Free intrinsic factor inhibited the attachment of intrinsic factor–bound cyanocobalamin. When intrinsic factor was complexed with various analogs of cyanocobalamin, the affinities of these complexes for ileal microvillous membranes were similar to that of intrinsic factor–bound cyanocobalamin. These findings suggest that the molecular configuration of the corrin is not a major determinant in the interaction between intrinsic factor–corrin complex and the ileal receptor site.

The precise nature of the ileal receptor is unknown. The receptor is probably antigenic and is specific for the distal end of the small intestine. Antisera from rabbits injected with purified microvillous membrane preparations isolated from the distal, but not proximal, hamster small intestine inhibited attachment of the intrinsic factor–cobalamin complex to the brush border of distal small intestine (167). When antibodies to the microvillous membrane are conjugated with ferritin, the ferritin-conjugated antibodies can be shown to attach to the mucopolysaccharide surface coat of the microvilli. The antibody was probably attached to the receptor in some manner and blocked absorption of the intrinsic factor–cobalamin complex.

Good progress has been made recently in attempts to solubilize and purify ileal receptors from human tissue (160, 162, 163, 168, 169). The characteristics of these purified receptors appear to be the same (temperature independence, divalent cation requirement, pH optimum near neutrality) as previously reported with less pure preparations. It has been speculated that the receptor may be a glycoprotein or a mucopolysaccharide since glycoproteins or mucopolysaccharide or both are present at the absorptive surface of the intestinal cell (158).

Transport of Cobalamin across the Intestinal Epithelial Cell   In contrast to the attachment of cobalamin to receptors on the brush borders, entry of cobalamin into the epithelial cell is a slow, endergonic process (145, 170, 171). The attachment of cobalamin to the receptors occurs within about 2–3 h after ingestion. An additional 3–4 h are required before significant amounts of the vitamin appear in the blood in humans. Peak blood levels are reached 8–12 h after ingestion in humans (172). This indicates that a slow and probably complex mechanism is involved in the transport of cobalamins across the cell membrane. Prolonged interaction between the cobalamin–intrinsic factor complex and the membrane receptor would explain the slow rate of absorption of the vitamin (173). Recent important studies with the guinea pig have shown that cobalamin accumulates in the mitochondrial fraction of the mucosal epithelium during absorption (174–176). This delay within the mitochondria is longer than the time required for attachment to the brush borders. It therefore appears that the vitamin could be concentrated in mitochondria during the period of mucosal delay.

A number of possible explanations for this localization were postulated. Latner et al. (177) have claimed, on the basis of fluoracetate inhibition studies, that conversion of cyanocobalamin to adenosylcobalamin occurs during ileal transport. The mitochondrial delay might therefore be due to the interconversion of the two forms, and the adenosyl derivative should therefore be more rapidly absorbed than cyanocobalamin. Recent detailed studies have shown that a similar period of delay within the mitochondria occurs for both of these cobalamins (178, 179). Similar delay and mitochondria localization were also observed for methylcobalamin, although the uptake of the methyl- and adenosylcobalamin by the ileum was less than that of cyanocobalamin. These studies would therefore suggest that all three cobalamins are localized in the ileal mitochondria during their absorption of the vitamin. If the mitochondria are the site of synthesis of adenosylcobalamin from cyanocobalamin, it is clearly not the sole function of the mitochondria in the transport of the vitamin. The conversion of cyanocobalamin to adenosylcobalamin is not obligatory (178, 179). Moreover, significant amounts of cyanocobalamin appear unchanged in portal plasma in man (180).

The principal form of cobalamin in guinea pig ileal mucosa is similar to that in liver — adenosylcobalamin. The localization of the adenosylcobalamin in the mitochondria is consistent with the known mitochondrial localization of methylmalonyl CoA and methyltetrahydrofolate methyltransferase (181-184). The finding of mitochondrial localization of cobalamin during its absorption does not support the hypothesis that pinocytosis is involved in cobalamin absorption (185). If pinocytosis were taking place, it would mean that intrinsic factor enters the cell. Studies by Hines et al. (171) appear to show, however, that intrinsic factor remains on the surface of the brush borders while cobalamin enters the epithelial cell. Hines et al. (171), however, used a heterologous system (hog intrinsic factor and guinea pig ileum). Peters and Hoffbrand (186), using a doubly labeled complex [^{57}Co]cyanocobalamin and [^{125}I]human intrinsic factor), could find labeled cyanocobalamin in the enterocyte, but no labeled intrinsic factor. Other investigators using similar techniques could not find any evidence of the absorption of intrinsic factor into the cell (187).

Release of Cobalamin from Cobalamin-Intrinsic Factor Complex Cobalamin is bound to intrinsic factor when it reaches the ileum, and it probably is bound to intrinsic factor when it is attached to the ileal brush borders. However, when it enters the portal blood it is no longer bound to intrinsic factor but to specific transport proteins called transcobalamins. At some point in the absorption process, the vitamin must separate from intrinsic factor. Most of the recent evidence supports the concept that intrinsic factor is not absorbed (171, 186-188). Further support for the belief that the vitamin is detached from intrinsic factor comes from the data showing that very little cobalamin is found in the lymphatics, which are known to carry large molecular complexes (189).

The unknown factor or factors responsible for the release of the vitamin have been termed "releasing factor." This release probably is the last phase of cobalamin absorption, and unequivocal evidence for its presence has not yet been presented. The fact that the vitamin in blood is bound to a molecule that has neither the biological or immunological characteristics of intrinsic factor and the fact that intrinsic factor is not absorbed provide strong evidence that some process is occurring that separates cobalamin from intrinsic factor.

Role of the Pancreas in Cobalamin Absorption

In the past few years, there has been considerable activity on the important role that the pancreas plays in the absorption of cobalamin in man. The fact that the pancreas might be of importance in the regulation of cobalamin absorption was first noted by McIntyre et al. (104). Veeger et al. (190) and LeBauer et al. (191) first reported that the malabsorption of cobalamin caused by pancreatic disease could be corrected by sodium bicarbonate or pancreatin or both. It was originally believed that this impaired absorption was due to the lowering of the pH of the intestinal contents because of the lack of bicarbonate secretion. However, it was also observed that the pancreatic extract alone, without sodium bicarbonate, could also correct the cobalamin malabsorption.

The recent work of Toskes, Deren, and their co-workers has been instrumental in clarifying the relationship between the pancreas and intestinal absorption of cobalamin. The pH hypothesis of Veeger et al. (190) was studied (192), and it was found that the pH of the ileal contents in patients with pancreatic insufficiency and malabsorption of cobalamin did not differ from the pH of patients with pancreatic insufficiency without cobalamin malabsorption. Known causes of cobalamin malabsorption, such as intrinsic factor deficiency, intrinsic factor antibodies, ileal disease, or bacterial overgrowth of the bowel were also ruled out. Intrinsic factor was present in the gastric juice of the patients studied by Toskes et al. (192), and hog intrinsic factor did not improve absorption. Serum-blocking antibodies could not be detected in any of the patients, and tetracycline did not improve cobalamin absorption. The administration of a single dose of pancreatic extract concurrently with labeled cyanocobalamin to patients with pancreatic insufficiency enhanced the absorption of the vitamin. The failure of the extract to correct the cobalamin malabsorption in patients with pernicious anemia (193) indicated that this response was not due to intrinsic factor contamination of the pancreatic extract.

Studies with rats subjected to 80–90% pancreatectomy also indicate the importance of the pancreas in gastrointestinal absorption of cobalamin (194). The partially pancreatectomized rat appeared healthy and had a growth rate similar to that of control rats, but absorbed significantly less orally administered labeled vitamin compared to control and sham-operated animals. Furthermore, the defect in the absorption was corrected by the administration of exogenous pancreatic extract.

The cobalamin-promoting constituent in pancreatic extract is soluble at $50,000 \times g$, is heat labile, and has a molecular weight of approximately 20,000–25,000 (195). These are physicochemical properties characteristic of several pancreatic proteolytic enzymes. Crystalline trypsin proved to be as effective as the pancreatic extracts. Whether the other proteolytic enzymes contained in the active subfractions also possess the capacity to promote cobalamin absorption has not been investigated.

There appears to be no defect in the binding of intrinsic factor to cyanocobalamin or abnormality in the attachment of the intrinsic factor–cobalamin complex to the ileal receptor that would explain the cobalamin malabsorption observed in patients with pancreatic disease. Very recent studies by Toskes et al. (196) demonstrate that preparations of pancreatic proteases modify crude sources of intrinsic factor to promote normal cobalamin absorption in patients with pancreatic exocrine insufficiency. These proteases appear to contain a low molecular weight contaminant that could facilitate cobalamin absorption in a yet undefined manner.

Several investigators have suggested, however, that pancreatic proteases might inactivate an endogenous inhibitor of cobalamin absorption (147, 148, 196-201). Based on his studies in rats, von der Lippe (200) has proposed that pancreatic extract stimulated the absorption of cobalamin in chronic pancreatic insufficiency by inactivation of nonintrinsic factor-cobalamin-binding substance in the intestinal lumen. One may therefore speculate that the reduced output of exocrine pancreatic secretion in the duodenum in chronic pancreatic insufficiency could lead to the presence of an excess of nonintrinsic factor-cobalamin-binding substance in the intestine. These cobalamin binders could compete with intrinsic factor for the vitamin from the intestine. Kapadia et al. (202) found that, after administering labeled cobalamin orally to control subjects, 11-24% of the radioactivity in the intestinal lumen was bound to nonintrinsic factor-cobalamin binders, but it is not known whether or not the amount of nonintrinsic factor-cobalamin binders in the intestinal lumen is increased in patients with chronic pancreatic insufficiency and malabsorption of the vitamin.

The recent studies of Allen et al. (147, 148) lend support to the proposal of von der Lippe (200). They suggest that the primary defect in cobalamin absorption in pancreatic insufficiency is an inability to partially degrade this nonintrinsic factor-cobalamin protein (probably an R protein) because of a deficiency of pancreatic proteases. Since cobalamin is bound preferentially to these R proteins in the acid milieu of the stomach, rather than to intrinsic factor (also see under "Binding of Cobalamins to Intrinsic Factor"), the cobalamin remains bound to R protein in the slightly alkaline environment of the intestine until pancreatic proteases partially degrade the R proteins and enable cobalamin to become bound exclusively to intrinsic factor. These studies by Allen et al. (147, 148) also suggest that the partial correction of cobalamin malabsorption observed with bicarbonate is due to neutralization of gastric acid, since, at slightly alkaline pH, intrinsic factor can partially compete with R protein for the initial binding and retention of cobalamin.

Allen has tested his hypothesis by determining the ability of a nonradioactive cobalamin analog, cobinamide, that is bound with high affinity to R proteins, but not to intrinsic factor, to correct the malabsorption in patients with pancreatic insufficiency (148). Cobinamide was as effective as trypsin in inhibiting the ability of R proteins to compete with intrinsic factor for cobalamin binding. Cobinamide was equally as effective as trypsin in correcting the malabsorption of cobalamin in patients with pancreatic insufficiency.

Nonintrinsic Factor-Mediated Absorption of Cobalamin

A passive mechanism (not mediated by intrinsic factor) is operative when the amount of administered vitamin is large, usually in excess of the amount

Table 2.   The absorption of a single oral dose of cyanocobalamin in normal human subjects[a]

Oral dose (μg)	Amount absorbed	
	(μg)	(%)
0.1	0.08	80
0.25	0.19	76
0.5	0.35	70
1.0	0.56	56
2.0	0.92	46
5.0	1.4	28
10.0	1.6	16
20.0	1.2	6
50.0	1.5	3

[a]Data from various authors and summarized by Chanarin (70).

available from a normal diet. Absorption probably occurs by diffusion. Only about 1% of an oral dose of 100–5000 μg is absorbed in pernicious anemia patients (203). In addition, the site of cobalamin absorption with these large pharmacological doses is nonspecific (204); some absorption of the vitamin occurs through the nasal mucosa, rectal mucosa, and skin (204–206). The amount of cobalamin that can be absorbed from a single oral dose in normal and pernicious anemia subjects is shown in Tables 2 and 3, respectively. It appears from these data that the average maximum absorption is about 1.5 μg in normal subjects regardless of the size of dose. If doses in excess of 100 μg are given orally to pernicious anemia patients, significant amounts of cobalamin are absorbed. Serum cobalamin levels in the pernicious anemia patients receiving these high doses are in the normal range (208). Since intrinsic factor is absent or deficient in pernicious anemia, large doses must be absorbed by a mechanism independent of intrinsic factor.

Table 3.   The absorption of a single oral dose of cyanocobalamin in pernicious anemia subjects[a]

Oral dose (μg)	Amount absorbed	
	(μg)	(%)
1	0.057	5.7
3	0.108	3.6
10	0.260	2.6
100	1.1	1.1
200	2.0	1.0
400	4.0	1.0
800	8.8	1.1
5000	50.0	1.0

[a]Data from Berlin et al. (207).

The patterns of plasma radioactivity after the administration of small and large oral doses of labeled cyanocobalamin have been studied (124, 125, 128, 141). The level of radioactivity in the blood starts to increase 3–6 h after oral administration of physiological doses and reaches a peak at 8–12 h after ingestion; patients receiving large doses show an early rise in radioactivity 1–2 h after ingestion, with peak values 4–6 h after the dose. In addition, some of the cobalamin appears in the lymph in contrast to observations with small physiological doses (189, 209).

In contrast to the intrinsic factor–mediated absorption, the nonintrinsic factor–mediated absorption of cobalamin does not appear to require calcium ions (59, 145, 210) and is independent of pH (145). Beyond these data, the mechanism of the nonintrinsic factor–mediated absorption is not well defined. It is not certain whether receptors for the large amounts of cobalamin exist in the intestine. Nevertheless, large oral doses of cyanocobalamin have been used for the treatment of pernicious anemia, and full hematopoietic response is obtained in many patients receiving doses in excess of 300 μg/day (208, 211–217).

Intestinal Absorption of Cobalamin Analogs

Except for hydroxocobalamin and possibly adenosylcobalamin, most of the other corrinoids tested appear poorly absorbed compared to cyanocobalamin (62). Sometimes erroneous results can be obtained by using the urinary excretion test to measure absorption; for example, hydroxocobalamin is more strongly bound and retained in tissues than cyanocobalamin (12, 62, 218). Direct measurement of absorption by fecal, hepatic, or whole body counting techniques is necessary in this type of study. Similar findings were obtained when adenosylcobalamin absorption was compared to that observed with cyanocobalamin. Measurement of absorption by the urinary excretion test gave low values with this coenzyme form of vitamin B_{12} because of greater tissue retention (62, 219), but assessment of coenzyme absorption by hepatic uptake or fecal excretion technique showed that it did not differ from cyanocobalamin absorption.

Cyanocobalamin in physiological doses (2 μg) is absorbed by man significantly better than chlorocobalamin, sulfatocobalamin, nitrocobalamin, and thiocyanatocobalamin (220, 221). Absorption was determined by the urinary excretion test, as well as by fecal excretion and hepatic uptake methods. With regard to substitution on the benzimidazole group, only the methoxybenzimidazole derivative (Factor IIIm) is absorbed as well as cyanocobalamin; benzimidazole-5,6-dichlorobenzimidazole analogs were poorly absorbed (127, 222). In addition, 5,6-dimethylbenzimidazole moiety itself does not compete with cyanocobalamin. Pseudovitamin B_{12} does not compete with the vitamin for the physiological absorption of cyanocobalamin (223, 224). This is not surprising, since pseudovitamin B_{12} does not bind to intrinsic factor, nor does it have any hematopoietic activity when given parenterally.

TRANSPORT

In humans, cobalamins are usually not found in the free state. When cobalamins are absorbed from the intestine, they appear to be attached to specific proteins. There are at least two classes of cobalamin-binding proteins in plasma, which were initially distinguished by their electrophoretic mobility (225–227). The binding proteins were found in the α-globulin and β-globulin fractions.

Two binders were initially studied most extensively by Hall and Finkler by using DEAE-cellulose and CM-cellulose chromatography, and were named transcobalamin I and transcobalamin II, respectively (228–231). These terms, originally introduced for the cobalamin-binding components of plasma separated by ion-exchange chromatography and electrophoresis, have also been used for the serum components separated by gel filtration mainly according to difference in molecular size (232–234). Gullberg (235–238) has proposed a different nomenclature for the two major cobalamin-binding protein components in human blood plasma — transcobalamin "large" (TC-L) and transcobalamin "small" (TC-S), referring to molecular size as separated by ion-exchange chromatography. This nomenclature is not widely used. The recent studies on the isolation and physical characterization of the transcobalamins indicate that the molecular weight of transcobalamin I is about 60,000 and that of transcobalamin II is about 38,000, not as widely different in molecular weight as originally thought (45, 46). Gel filtration studies can give falsely high values of molecular weights with proteins containing a high percentage of carbohydrate (239).

Evidence for a third binder (transcobalamin III) in normal human serum has been presented by several investigators (240–246). This protein seems to resemble transcobalamin II in its behavior on DEAE-cellulose and its electrophoretic mobility, and transcobalamin I in antigenic characteristics, behavior on Sephadex G-150, and its inability to stimulate uptake of cobalamin by reticulocytes (245, 246). Transcobalamin I can be separated from transcobalamin III on DEAE-cellulose (241–245) and with isoelectric focusing (247, 248).

Transcobalamin I and III are part of a class of proteins that are antigenically cross-reactive, differ from each other mainly in carbohydrate composition, are present in many body tissues and fluids, and have also been designated as R binders. The term "R binder" was originally used by Gräsbeck (249) to denote a cobalamin-binding protein in human gastric juice that was devoid of intrinsic factor activity and had a rapid mobility on electrophoresis. The R-type cobalamin-binding proteins from other sources do not show rapid mobility. Transcobalamin II is chemically and immunologically distinct from transcobalamin I and III and other R binders. The function of R proteins has not been unequivocally established, whereas transcobalamin II is known to facilitate the uptake of cobalamin by a large number of tissues

(6, 249). The name "transcobalamin" indicates a transport function that transcobalamin II possesses but that Stenman claims the cobalamin-binding proteins of the two R-types do not have. Stenman has therefore proposed the name "cobalophilin," an analogy with siderophilin (250), for the R-type proteins. The function of all the transcobalamins is discussed under "Function of Transcobalamins."

Synthesis and Source of Transcobalamins

In the rat and mouse, transcobalamin II is probably synthesized in the liver (251–256). This belief is based on liver perfusion studies and on the fact that the synthesis of transcobalamin II is decreased after carbon tetrachloride poisoning. In contrast, the concentration and rate of synthesis of transcobalamin II in dogs are not influenced by removal of the liver, implying that the liver is not the only organ responsible for synthesis of this protein (257). Thus, it has been assumed that some extrahepatic synthesis of transcobalamin II occurs and also that it could possibly have a leucocyte origin.

It has been suggested that granulocytes synthesize transcobalamin I and other R-type proteins (258, 259). This evidence is based on the facts that: 1) antibodies to cobalamin-binding protein of granulocytes cross-react with transcobalamin I (260); 2) the content of transcobalamin I is proportional to the total content of granulocytes; and 3) two patients who had a low level of the granulocyte cobalamin-binding protein were deficient in transcobalamin I (261). Recent studies support the concept that the granulocyte is a major source of transcobalamin III (262). This protein is elevated in leukocytosis. If granulocytes were the source of both transcobalamins I and III, some transformation of the protein must occur inside or outside of the cell (263). Alternatively, only certain cells, perhaps the immature ones, may contain transcobalamin I, with the rest containing transcobalamin III.

In tissue culture, synthesis of R-type salivary binders occurs in serous glandular cells from both submandibular and parotid glands (264). Certain human hepatomas contain high concentrations of R proteins, which suggests that these tumors also synthesize these proteins (265).

Purification and Properties of Transcobalamin

The magnitude of the problem with regard to the isolation of transcobalamins is apparent when it is realized that human plasma contains approximately 60 μg of transcobalamin I and 25 μg of transcobalamin II per liter. The isolation of each of these proteins in homogenous form implies, therefore, that transcobalamin be purified almost one million-fold and transcobalamin II more than two million-fold (249). Transcobalamin I of normal plasma can carry about 0.7–0.8 ng of cobalamin per ml, and most of the binding capacity of transcobalamin is normally saturated with endogenous cobalamin. Transcobalamin II can carry an average of 0.1 ng of cobalamin per ml when fully saturated, but is only 10% saturated.

Transcobalamin II has been extensively purified (approximately one million-fold) as its cobalamin complex from human plasma Cohn Fraction III by ion-exchange cellulose and gel filtration (266). A limited amount of chemical data was obtained because of the small amount of final product. This preparation was reported to contain at least 13% carbohydrate but no sialic acid and to have a molecular weight of about 30,000.

Transcobalamin II has been isolated in homogenous form from Cohn Fraction III derived from pooled human plasma by a combination of conventional purification techniques and affinity chromatography (46). The overall purification relative to human plasma was about two million-fold. This apparently pure transcobalamin II binds 28.6 μg of cyanocobalamin per mg of protein and contains one cobalamin binding site per 38,000 g of protein, as determined by amino acid analysis. The molecular weight originally determined by Allen and Majerus (46) was 53,900 and by gel filtration on Sephadex G-150 was 60,000. These higher molecular weights were due to partial aggregation of the protein (6). When cobalamin binds to transcobalamin II there is a shift in the peak of cobalamin absorption from 361 nm to 364 nm. No carbohydrate residues were detected, suggesting that transcobalamin II is not a glycoprotein.

Hall's group (267) has also purified transcobalamin II from Cohn Fraction III by using a modification of the procedure of Allen and Majerus (46). This simplified method incorporated isoelectric precipitation of the transcobalamin II into the purification scheme, which permitted the elimination of two column chromatographic steps originally reported by the above workers. The final product bound 26.7 μg of cyanocobalamin per mg of protein, which is in close agreement with the preparation of Allen and Majerus (46). The absorbancy ratio (A280:A361) of these two preparations was also similar. No amino acid composition was presented by Savage et al. (267).

The method of affinity chromatography described by Allen and Majerus (44) was also used to isolate the cobalamin-binding proteins from granulocytes obtained from patients with chronic granulocytic leukemia (45). In fact, affinity chromatography was the sole purification technique employed in isolating human granulocyte vitamin B_{12}-binding protein in homogenous form in 90% yield. (The relationship and/or identity between transcobalamin I and the granulocyte cobalamin-binding protein is discussed under "Relationship of Transcobalamin I to Other Tissue Cobalamin Binders.")

The human granulocyte vitamin B_{12}-binding protein binds 34.9 μg of cyanocobalamin per mg of protein and has a single cobalamin binding site. Since removal of the vitamin from the protein results in some denaturation of the protein, it was difficult to determine the binding constant between the vitamin and the granulocyte-binding protein. The molecular weight of this protein as determined by sedimentation equilibrium ultracentrifugation was 56,000; by amino acid and carbohydrate analysis, 58,200; by gel filtration and sodium dodecyl sulfate polyacrylamide gel electrophoresis, 121,000–

Table 4.   Carbohydrate content of several R proteins[a]

Protein	Carbohydrate (mol/mol f vitamin B_{12})					
	Sialic acid	Fucose	Galac- tose	Mannose	Galacto- samine	Gluco- samine
Saliva	7	35	47	20	4	37
Milk	6	22	36	20	3	36
Normal granulocyte	11	24	26	20	2	46
Transcobalamin I	18	9	41	24	2	46
Transcobalamin III	11	20	51	22	2	54

[a]Adapted from data of Allen (6).

138,000. Proteins that contain large amounts of carbohydrate often give falsely elevated values for molecular weight when determined by gel filtration (239).

A number of other human R-type cobalamin-binding proteins have been isolated more recently. These are transcobalamins I and III (245), the cobalamin-binding protein from normal granulocytes, (245), milk (268), saliva (268), amniotic fluid (269), and several cobalamin proteins associated with hepatocellular carcinoma (265). Transcobalamin I and transcobalamin III were purified some six million- and three million-fold, respectively, from normal plasma (245). The cobalamin-binding proteins present in human milk and saliva have been isolated in high yield by the use of affinity chromatography on Sepharose as the sole purification technique (268).

All of these R-type proteins have a molecular weight of about 60,000, have identical absorption spectra, are immunologically identical, and have similar amino acid composition, but differ in carbohydrate content. The differences in carbohydrate content of some of these proteins are shown in Table 4. In addition, the amino acid sequences at the NH_2-terminal end have been determined with human saliva and milk vitamin B_{12}–binding proteins and have been shown to be identical. The sequence of the first 13 amino acids at the NH_2-terminal end is Glu-Ile-Ser-Glu-Val-Ser-Glu-Asn-Tyr-Ile-Arg-Leu.

Nexø also used affinity chromatography to purify transcobalamin I (270). Unlike the conventional biospecific affinity chromatography, the ligand in this method is not covalently bound to the matrix, and it is the binding between the ligand and the matrix that is split on desorption. The desorption was induced simply by a shift in temperature.

Independently Nexø et al. (271) purified a cobalamin-binding protein in higher yields from a patient with a hepatoma by using the affinity chromatography techniques described above. The protein had all the physical properties of transcobalamin I. The amino acid sequences of this protein and human transcobalamin were similar to that observed by Allen (see above) (272). The results obtained in this work also support the concept that the protein moiety of all human R binders is the same.

When cyanocobalamin binds to R proteins, the absorbance at 361 nm increases about 30%. In saliva, milk, amniotic fluid, and hepatoma-related R proteins, the spectral maxima shift is from 361 nm to 363 nm, but in transcobalamin I, transcobalamin III, and the normal and chronic myelogenous leukemia granulocyte R protein, only a small shift of 361–361.5 nm is observed.

Relationship of Transcobalamin I to Other Tissue Cobalamin Binders

Antitranscobalamin II serum was found to react only with transcobalamin II, regardless of the source. It did not react with any of the other binders. Antitranscobalamin I and antisaliva cobalamin–binding protein both reacted identically with all the R binders. No cross-reaction between the three groups could be demonstrated.

The variations in sialic acid content of these R proteins are believed to be the cause of the heterogeneity seen in these R proteins when subjected to electrofocusing (263, 264, 273, 274). During the purification of transcobalamin I and cobalamin-binding protein in leucocytes, a reduction on their electrophoretic mobilities occurs, and the same change is produced by sialidase treatment (263).

The difference between the molecular weight estimate of 138,000 obtained for the granulocyte cobalamin–binding protein by gel filtration and the value of approximately 56,000 obtained by sedimentation equilibrium centrifugation and chemical composition is also related to the carbohydrate content of these proteins (6). Proteins that contain a large amount of carbohydrate often give falsely elevated values for molecular weight when determined by gel filtration (239), suggesting that the different molecular weights reported for the individual R-type cobalamin-binding proteins may be the results of differences in carbohydrate content rather than in amino acid composition or sequence.

Before the detection and study of cobalamin transport proteins in plasma, there were many attempts to show that intrinsic factor or a related substance functioned in the circulation as well as in the intestine. Subsequently, it was shown that the component of hog intrinsic factor active in these systems was an R binder and not intrinsic factor. Use was made of this fact in the fractionation of hog intrinsic factor. Nonintrinsic factor was removed from intrinsic factor preparations by heating the latter with an antiserum prepared against hog leucocyte binder, an R-type binder (275).

There is genetic evidence that the R proteins are closely related. These proteins are apparently coded by one gene, and it has been reported that two brothers lacked R proteins (261). Variability among the R proteins could be due to differences in gene expression in different cells. The protein could possibly receive its sialic acid at a late stage of synthesis, perhaps just before it leaves the cell (249). It is evident that the R binders have enough properties in common to form a third group that is quite distinct both functionally and immunologically from transcobalamin II and intrinsic factor.

There is some confusion in the literature with regard to the distinction between transcobalamin I and transcobalamin III. Transcobalamin I and transcobalamin III can be separated from each other by chromatography on DEAE-cellulose (241–245) and by isoelectric focusing (247, 248). Much of the confusion is due to the failure to adequately separate transcobalamin II from transcobalamin III. It is difficult to separate transcobalamin I from transcobalamin III without prior separation of transcobalamin II from transcobalamin III, since these latter two proteins are eluted from DEAE-cellulose in overlapping positions.

It has been proposed that transcobalamin III, although it may occur in plasma, is in a sense an artifact in that it is released from granulocytes in vitro after blood has been collected. This can be inhibited to some extent by collecting the blood in EDTA in the presence of fluoride (245, 276). Purified preparations of transcobalamin III and the normal granulocyte cobalamin–binding protein are indistinguishable from each other in terms of carbohydrate composition, electrophoresis, elution from DEAE-cellulose, absorption spectra, and immunoreactivity. This confirms the proposition that transcobalamin III is derived from granulocytes (244, 262, 276, 277).

It appears that transcobalamin III circulates in vivo in very low amounts, but this does not mean it is only released from granulocytes in vitro. Transcobalamin III has an extremely short plasma survival, and thus one would not expect to find appreciable levels of this protein if it were released from granulocytes in vivo in significant amounts (246). Transcobalamin I has a plasma survival that is 3–4 orders of magnitude greater than that of transcobalamin III (246). Further distinction between transcobalamin I and transcobalamin III comes from their carbohydrate content. Transcobalamin I contains more sialic acid (18 versus 11 residues) and less fucose (9 versus 20 residues) than the transcobalamin III (see Table 3). Transcobalamin I differs from the normal granulocyte cobalamin-binding protein in carbohydrate composition and plasma clearance rate, suggesting that transcobalamin I may not be derived from granulocytes (245).

Binding of Cobalamins to Transcobalamin

The difficulties encountered in measuring and interpreting the affinity of cobalamins to intrinsic factor (see under "Binding of Cobalamins to Intrinsic Factor") also hold for the transcobalamins. Somewhat more methylcobalamin than cyanocobalamin is bound to transcobalamin I and transcobalamin II when excess amounts of these cobalamins are added in vitro to these proteins (278). The ratio of the binding capacity for methylcobalamin to cyanocobalamin was 1.32–1.36 for transcobalamin I and 1.34 for transcobalamin II. The lactone and lactam derivatives can bind to the transcobalamins as efficiently as cyanocobalamin (60). Other than these studies little has been done on the binding of various cobalamins to these different serum cobalamin–binding proteins until the recent work of Kolhouse and Allen (279).

These investigators found that human transcobalamin II is considerably less selective than intrinsic factor and has an affinity only for those analogs missing the b- or b,d,e-amino groups on the corrin ring and those in which the nucleotide moiety cannot coordinate with the cobalt moiety. Human granulocyte-binding protein is the least selective of the cobalamin-binding proteins and appears to bind to a variety of analogs with relatively high affinity.

Most of the cobalamin analogs that were bound to transcobalamin II with high affinity were taken up by a variety of tissues in a manner that was indistinguishable from that of transcobalamin II bound to cyanocobalamin. A variety of analogs bound by the granulocyte-binding protein with high affinity were cleared from plasma by hepatocytes. That intrinsic factor has greater selectivity than transcobalamins for various cobalamins is not unexpected, since the selectivity of intrinsic factor toward cobalamin analogs prevents the absorption of possible "toxic" analogs. The rapid clearance of certain analogs bound to the granulocyte protein, however, shows that there are additional mechanisms that function to prevent the tissue dissemination of cobalamin analogs that do gain access to the body. The enhanced ability of granulocytes to bind cobalamin analogs enables them to be transported exclusively to hepatocytes rather than to other tissues that may be more susceptible to their toxic effects.

It has been suggested that cobalamin analogs be used as antimetabolites in vivo, since transcobalamin II is capable of binding a large number of analogs and transporting them to a variety of tissues (280). In vitro, cyanocobalamin can be dissociated from transcobalamin I and transcobalamin II by raising the pH to 12.9, but transcobalamin II proved to be quite labile; 80% of its cobalamin binding power was destroyed (84). The association constant between pH 4 and pH 11 for transcobalamin II and cyanocobalamin is approximately $10^{11} M^{-1}$. This value is the same as that obtained for R proteins and cyanocobalamin at neutral pH (61).

Sequence of Initial Events during Plasma Transport

Relative to the intrinsic factor–mediated gastrointestinal transport of cobalamins, the state of knowledge regarding the molecular events during plasma transport is poor. Most of the data deal with kinetics rather than molecular and/or physical changes. After the absorption of physiological amounts of cobalamin, the vitamin enters the blood at a slow rate. The vitamin first appears in the blood within 3–4 h after ingestion and reaches a peak level at about 8–12 h (124, 125, 280).

The cobalamin entering the blood after oral ingestion as the vitamin or in food appears to be bound to transcobalamin II (229). More than 8 h after the administration, an increasing proportion of the labeled vitamin becomes bound to transcobalamin I. The amount of vitamin bound to transcobalamin I increases as the amount of the vitamin in transcobalamin II decreases. However, the uptake of cobalamin by transcobalamin II is probably still going on at 24 h (231). Since a normal person usually ingests food several times a day, a small but constant amount of transcobalamin II–cobalamin complex is circulating. The amount of vitamin absorbed to transcobalamin II probably never exceeds 20 pg/ml of plasma (231).

The transfer of the absorbed vitamin from one plasma protein to another has been compared to the fate of copper after oral ingestion. The absorbed copper is bound initially to albumin and is then transported to the liver. In the liver, copper is gradually incorporated into another protein, ceruloplasmin, and the copper appears bound to plasma ceruloplasmin (281).

Alternate explanations, however, have been offered to explain the fact that endogenous cobalamin is bound primarily to an α-globulin, transcobalamin I, but cobalamins fed or injected attach first to a β-globulin (transcobalamin II) (282). Ingested or injected cobalamin could attach to both cobalamin proteins, and that which is attached to transcobalamin II is delivered to tissues rapidly, whereas that attached to transcobalamin I is retained in serum. Very recently, it was shown that all three serum cobalamin binders (transcobalamins I, II, and III) took up cobalamin absorbed from the intestine at about the same rate. Thus, there appears to be an increasing amount of evidence that the transport of cobalamin from the intestine to the blood is not the exclusive function of a single blood protein (283, 284).

Plasma Turnover of Transcobalamins

Cobalamin attached to human transcobalamin II when injected into humans is rapidly cleared, with a $t_{1/2}$ value of approximately 5 min (285). During the following time, a $t_{1/2}$ from 1 to 12 h has been estimated (229, 283). This knowledge was obtained with the aid of cobalt-labeled cyanocobalamin and it has therefore been impossible to determine the fate of the transcobalamin.

Very recently, Allen and his colleagues, using pure transcobalamins, have been able to prepare radioactive iodine–labeled transcobalamins and to study their fate simultaneously with that of the labeled vitamin bound to them (286). The human transcobalamin II, when injected into rabbits, is cleared from the plasma with a half-life of 60–90 min, and the transcobalamin moiety was degraded during this process. A significant amount of the cyanocobalamin originally attached to the transcobalamin recirculated. These more elegant experiments confirm the work of earlier investigators (229, 285) with less pure preparations that transcobalamin II is cleared more rapidly than transcobalamin I (see below). The fact that transcobalamin II is cleared so rapidly tends to support the importance of these proteins in the tissue uptake of cobalamins (see under "Function of Transcobalamins" and "Transport of Cobalamins to Tissue").

The rapid turnover of transcobalamin II, together with rapid recirculation of cobalamins, could be part of a mechanism that is responsible for rapid changes of the cobalamin content of cells. A mechanism of this kind has been suggested as being an important regulatory role of intracellular metabolism of cobalamins (6).

Transcobalamin II plays a dynamic role during the transport of the administered cobalamin. The intravenous administration of cyanocobalamin to normal humans or patients with liver disease causes substantial reductions in total transcobalamin II amounts shortly after injection (287). Larger doses of cyanocobalamin reduce total transcobalamin II to a greater extent than small doses. The injection of cyanocobalamin did not decrease the plasma level of transcobalamin I, which is mostly saturated with endogenous cobalamin and which turns over much more slowly than transcobalamin II (229, 285). Almost identical results are obtained if the cyanocobalamin is injected intramuscularly (288). Therefore, the sequence of events after injection of cyanocobalamin to humans is saturation of transcobalamin II, transfer of saturated transcobalamin II to tissue receptors, and degradation of transcobalamin II, followed by resynthesis of transcobalamin II (recovery of tissue levels).

Human transcobalamin III is also cleared rapidly from rabbit plasma exclusively by the liver after an intravenous injection (246). A small portion of the transcobalamin is excreted intact into the bile during the period from 10 to 80 min after uptake. The remainder of the transcobalamin III is degraded in the liver, and the cobalamin reenters the plasma bound to transcobalamin II. The presence or absence of bound cobalamin has little, if any, effect on the plasma survival of transcobalamin III. Human transcobalamin I and human granulocyte cobalamin–binding protein, in contrast, have a prolonged plasma survival in rabbits and in humans, and it is not certain whether there are specific tissue sites for the uptake of this protein-cobalamin complex (246).

The presence or absence of bound cobalamin also has little, if any, effect on the plasma survival of transcobalamin I. No differences were observed between a control group of patients and a group of patients with pernicious anemia. Cobalamin is liberated from transcobalamin I only when this protein was degraded. Treatment of transcobalamin I with neuraminidase to remove sialic acid results in a rapid clearance of this protein, identical to the rapid clearance of transcobalamin III. The hepatic uptake of transcobalamin and desialyzed transcobalamin I is inhibited by prior injection of large amounts of desialyzed fetuin (246). Therefore, the hepatic uptake is mediated by a general mechanism, described by Ashwell and Morell, that is capable of clearing a variety of glycoproteins from plasma and catabolizing them within lysosomes (289, 290). Ashwell and Morell and their associates (288, 290) have described and elucidated a mechanism by which a large number of asialoglycoproteins, including the asialo forms of orosomucoid, fetuin, ceruloplasmin, haptoglobin, and other glycoproteins, are cleared from plasma and catabolized by the liver. Terminal galactose residues appear to be required for glycoprotein binding to common receptors that are present on hepatocyte plasma membranes, since binding is abolished by modification or removal of galactose residues from the glycoprotein or by the attachment of sialic acid to galactose on the glycoprotein. The plasma survival data appear relevant to what occurs in humans since significant species differences have not been observed in the process described by Ashwell and Morell (289).

Different individual human R-type proteins vary markedly in their plasma survivals in humans. Granulocyte R-type protein is cleared very rapidly, like transcobalamin III and desialyzed transcobalamin I (246). This rapid clearance of granulocyte protein could serve to prevent this protein from accumulating in plasma, where it could reach a very high concentration if it had a prolonged plasma survival similar to that of transcobalamin I. Increased levels of plasma R-type protein are observed frequently in chronic myelogenous leukemia (249, 250, 291, 292) and occasionally in hepatocellular carcinoma (265) and other solid tumors (293).

When physiological quantities of methylcobalamin and cyanocobalamin are injected intravenously in man, both methylcobalamin and cyanocobalamin are cleared at approximately the same rate and distributed in the same way between transcobalamin I and transcobalamin II (278). It would not have been surprising if methylcobalamin, which is the more physiological form of the plasma cobalamins, had been cleared in a different way. The overall behavior of methylcobalamin appears to be identical with that of cyanocobalamin, and previously attained results with regard to transport of radioactive cyanocobalamin appear to be relevant.

Function of Transcobalamins

The function of transcobalamin I is not unequivocally known. It has been suggested that this protein serves the role of a circulating cobalamin reservoir, in equilibrium with tissue stores of cobalamin. A specific transport function has recently been postulated for the granulocyte R protein and transcobalamin III. These proteins, as mentioned previously (see under "Plasma Turnover of Transcobalamins"), deliver cobalamins rapidly only to the liver (246).

Granulocyte cobalamin–binding protein may have antibacterial activity. This protein may play a role in the handling of intra- and extracellular bacteria by leaching cobalamins (237, 294, 295) — i.e., binding cobalamin and preventing its use by bacteria that require the vitamin for growth. The high content of R proteins in leukocytes is consistent with this concept (258). The distribution of R proteins is similar to the protein lactoferrin, again suggesting an antibacterial function for this group of proteins (296–298). Like lactoferrin and lysozyme, the R proteins reach the highest concentration in secretory fluids (299). The granulocyte-binding protein could provide a mechanism by which cobalamin analogs present in areas of cell necrosis are transported rapidly to the liver instead of to other tissues in the body. The relative lack of specificity of R-type proteins for cobalamin analogs enables them to scavenge analogs of bacterial origin that are harmful (6).

Most of the endogenous cobalamin bound to this α-1-globulin has been identified as methylcobalamin (300–302). This finding has led to the speculation that transcobalamin I as well as other R proteins are apoenzymes for methylcobalamin (249). This cobalamin is known to act as a coenzyme in several enzymic reactions.

A deficiency of transcobalamin I causes no apparent abnormality in cobalamin metabolism. Persistent deficiency of serum transcobalamin I was demonstrated in two brothers manifesting primarily low serum cobalamin levels (261). Despite injections of cyanocobalamin, one subject maintained low serum cobalamin levels. The α-globulin binder normally present was virtually absent from saliva and peripheral leukocyte extracts of both subjects, further suggesting the close relationship between R proteins and transcobalamin I.

Possibly transcobalamin I–bound cobalamin is taken up slowly by some tissues not yet studied. There may be a release of cobalamin initially bound to transcobalamin I followed by rebinding to transcobalamin II and then uptake by the cells. Some evidence that transcobalamin I carries cobalamin out of cells comes from the study of the uptake of cobalamin by HeLa cells (303). The labeled vitamin bound to transcobalamin II was incorporated into the HeLa cells. The labeled cobalamin that comes out of the cells was shown to be bound to a protein resembling transcobalamin I. Recent evidence has been published suggesting that human bone marrow cells can take up cobalamin from all three transcobalamins (304). The uptake depends on the presence of calcium ions, cellular respiration, and free sulfhydryl groups.

In contrast to transcobalamin I, transcobalamin II is necessary for normal cellular maturation of the hematopoietic system. Hereditary transcobalamin II deficiency is a rare inborn error of protein metabolism that is inherited as an autosomal recessive condition (305–307). The function of transcobalamin II is to carry cobalamin to recipient tissues. This is supported by its facilitation of uptake by HeLa cells, reticulocytes, erythrocytes, and so on (6, 10, 231) (see under "Transport of Cobalamins to Tissue"). In the absence of transcobalamin II and with normal cobalamin blood levels, megaloblastic anemia and other clinical symptoms are manifest in early life (305–307). Children respond dramatically to high doses (1000 μg weekly) of intramuscular cyanocobalamin with complete clinical and hematological remission.

It is of interest that these children also had decreased contents of transcobalamin I. In addition, the intestinal absorption of cyanocobalamin with or without intrinsic factor was reduced, which lends support to the concept that transcobalamin II is the major protein concerned with newly absorbed cobalamin. The responses of the children to pharmacological doses of cyanocobalamin suggest that the vitamin enters the tissues by passive diffusion, by a mechanism similar to that involved in intestinal transport with high doses of cobalamin in pernicious anemia.

Transport of Cobalamins to Tissue

Although the action of intrinsic factor in promoting the uptake of cobalamins in intestinal tissue is well established, evidence that transcobalamins in human plasma promote the uptake of cobalamins by other tissues is less well known, and investigations on this aspect have only begun in the last 10–15 years. The earliest significant studies in this area were performed by Callender and Lajtha (308), who reported that cyanocobalamin was unable to cause maturation of megaloblasts in vitro, only acting in this manner in the presence of gastric juice or serum.

The importance of cobalamin-binding protein in cobalamin uptake was noted by the early studies showing that intrinsic factor promoted the uptake of cobalamin by rat liver slices (309, 310). In 1961, Cooper and Paranchych found that human serum facilitated the uptake of cobalamins by mouse Ehrlich ascites tumor cells and HeLa cells; intrinsic factor did not show such an effect (311). These investigators subsequently suggested that the cobalamin-binding fraction of ascites fluid was probably a mucoprotein (312). Uptake of cobalamin by the tumor cells was biphasic, consisting of a rapid primary uptake followed by a secondary reaction. It was believed that primary uptake represented a physicochemical reaction between extracellularly bound cobalamin receptors on the cell membrane, and the secondary reaction involved the active transport of cyanocobalamin from these receptors into the cell. This second phase depended on pH, temperature, and energy. This uptake process appeared to be similar to pinocytosis, and a pinocytotic mechanism was suggested for cobalamin uptake by mammalian cells (also see below) (313).

Finkler and Hall (303), in 1967, reported that cobalamin uptake by HeLa cells in tissue culture is increased by transcobalamin II and that liver uptake of cobalamin from plasma occurs more readily when the vitamin is bound to the β-globulin protein (transcobalamin II) than to the α-globulin protein (transcobalamin I). Antitranscobalamin II sera inhibited the uptake of transcobalamin II by HeLa cells. Antitranscobalamin I sera were ineffective in inhibiting the uptake. The transcobalamin II–mediated uptake was inhibited by substances that affect protein synthesis (such as puromycin), oxidative phosphorylation (such as 2,4-dinitrophenol), cell respiration (such as sodium cyanide), or by substances that react with sulfhydryl groups and disulfide groups such as iodoacetamide and dithiothreitol.

Serum enhances the cobalamin uptake of suspensions of erythrocytes containing an increased proportion of reticulocytes (314). Subsequently Retief et al. (315) observed that transcobalamin II had a greater effect in promoting the uptake than did transcobalamin I. Calcium or magnesium ions were required for this reaction, which appears to be a surface absorption phenomenon. It appears that the investigators did not try to distinguish two distinct phases in the uptake, as was done with tumor cells.

Transport of cobalamins into L1210 murine leukemic cells, L51784 murine leukemic cells, human bone marrow cells, isolated rat liver mitochondria, and cultured human fibroblasts is also mediated by transcobalamin II and is reported to be a biphasic process (312, 316–325). This process appears to consist of an initial step in which the transcobalamin II–cobalamin complex binds to the cell surface and a second step in which the cobalamin enters the cell.

From most of the studies described above, evidence has accumulated that the transport process is biphasic. The primary step, which occurs during transport of cobalamins mediated by transcobalamin II, is binding of the complex to the external membrane of the cell. This step is insensitive to temperature, depends on calcium ions, and is inhibited by EDTA. Indeed, specific receptors have been identified and probably mediate this transcobalamin binding (326, 327). The second step appears to involve transport of the vitamin into the cell.

Evidence for the translocation of the cobalamin into the cell is based on subcellular fractionation studies after injection of cobalamin in rats (328–331). Newmark (328, 329) and his co-workers injected rats with labeled cyanocobalamin and measured the radioactivity and cobalamin content of the subcellular fractionation from the kidney. Most of the radioactivity and cobalamin in the kidney was found in the mitochondrial-lysosomal fraction. Microbiological assay of endogenous cobalamins in those two fractions showed adenosylcobalamin predominantly in the mitochondria-rich fraction and hydroxocobalamin in the lysosome-rich one.

Pletsch and Coffey (330, 331) used rat liver to study the subcellular distribution of labeled cobalamin after intracardiac injection. The highest amount of radioactivity was found in the plasma membrane vesicles and microsomes. The radioactivity was associated with a protein that had the characteristics of transcobalamin II. After a couple of hours the microsome-plasma membrane fraction continued to have the largest percentage of cobalamin, but the lysosomal fraction also contained significant amounts of radioactivity. After several days, about half of the mitochondrial cobalamin and most of the supernatant cobalamin were associated with a protein similar in characteristics to transcobalamin II. Pinocytosis and the formation of a secondary lysosomal vacuole in which the cobalamin is split from the transcobalamin is proposed as the mechanism. After the cobalamin is separated from the transcobalamin, the cobalamin accumulates in the mitochondria (328, 330), the probable site of its further metabolism and function.

The uptake of cyanocobalamin by whole cells of *Escherichia coli* is also a biphasic process, consisting of an initial rapid phase that is independent of the energy metabolism of the cell, followed by a slower, secondary, energy-dependent phase (332–334). This is quite similar to many of the transcobalamin-dependent mammalian uptake systems except for the fact that the bacterial system does not have a requirement for the extracellular protein transcobalamin.

In view of the fact that transcobalamin II–cobalamin complex can be found in the cytosol (325) and that transcobalamin II–cobalamin complex promotes mitochondrial uptake of cobalamins, Ostroy and Gams feel that the transcobalamin II–cobalamin complex is incorporated into the cell by a process distinct from pinocytosis with lysosomal fusion (335).

Based on kinetic studies of the interaction of transcobalamin II and its cellular receptor, these investigators have proposed a model for cobalamin incorporation into L1210 cells. Their data indicate that L1210 cells incorporate transcobalamin II–bound cobalamin by a calcium- and temperature-dependent process. They found that the uptake proceeded in a smooth continuous fashion for at least 10 min, not as a biphasic time course, as reported. After its inclusion into the cell, the transcobalamin II–cobalamin can move out of the cell by a calcium-independent process or can bind to mitochondria, where the cobalamin can be used by the mitochondrial enzyme methylmalonyl coenzyme A mutase. After mitochondrial use, the cobalamin is released from the cell onto a new binder, chromatographically similar to transcobalamin III.

The studies by Rosenberg's laboratory with hydroxocobalamin and rat liver mitochondria indicate that this vitamin enters the mitochondrion by diffusion of the free cobalamins without dependence on ionic fluxes or the mitochondrial proteins (336). An intramitochondrial protein, or group of proteins, then specifically binds the cobalamin, allowing its retention and concentration by the mitochondria. Recent studies from Allen's laboratory (184) and from Rosenberg's laboratory (183) indicate that the major intracellular cobalamin-binding proteins are two cobalamin-dependent apoenzymes — methylmalonyl CoA-mutase and methyltetahydrofolate methyltransferase (183, 184). These enzymes are associated with mitochrondria and cytoplasm, respectively. It is significant that adenosylcobalamin, the mutase cofactor, was observed in the mitochondria, and methylcobalamin, the transferase cofactor, was found only in the cytosolic faction. The relative amounts of these cobalamins in liver are similar to those associated with the enzymes (337). It is also significant that the results of both laboratories are in agreement, since Allen's group used the rabbit and Rosenberg's laboratory used the rat for their studies. The schematic representation of transcobalamin binding, uptake degradation, and synthesis of coenzyme is shown in Figure 3.

Studies in rats have demonstrated that after intravenous administration of cyanocobalamin the vitamin is bound rapidly and about 20–30% is concentrated in placental tissue within minutes after injection (338). After a lag period of several hours, the cobalamin enters the fetal circulation, suggesting a specific high affinity binding rate for the transcobalamin II–cobalamin complex. Indeed, Friedman et al. (327) have shown the existence of a specific

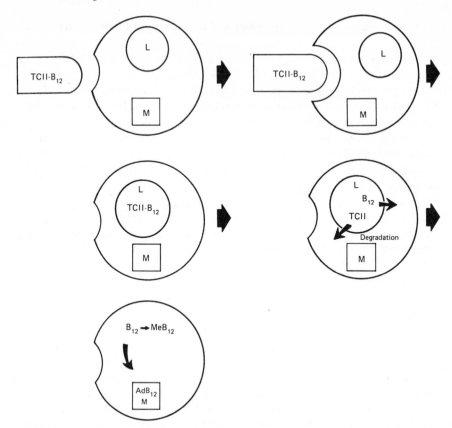

Figure 3.   Incorporation of cobalamins into mammalian cells. The receptor site on the cell has a high affinity for the transcobalamin II–cobalamin complex but not for free transcobalamin. The complex then enters the cell in the lysosomal fraction (L). The transcobalamin II–cobalamin complex is degraded in the lysosome. Some of the cobalamin enters the mitochondrion (M) and is used to synthesize adenosylcobalamin (AdB$_{12}$); some of the cobalamin is also used to synthesize methylcobalamin (MeB$_{12}$) in the cytosol.

high affinity binding site for the transcobalamin II–cobalamin complex in human placental membrane preparations. They succeeded in solubilizing this receptor. The complex binds to a single saturable binding site with an approximate K_a of 7.2 mM^{-1}. The binding requires a divalent cation and is temperature dependent.

More recently, this receptor from human placenta was isolated by Allen's laboratory (339). The receptor appears to have a molecular weight of approximately 50,000, and in contrast to transcobalamin II it is a glycoprotein. However, the amino acid compositions are similar, suggesting that transcobalamin II and the placental receptor may have evolved from a common structural gene, with the former evolving as a nonglycosylated plasma transport protein and the latter as a glycoprotein receptor.

Forms of Cobalamins in Human Plasma

After the isolation of cyanocobalamin it was assumed that serum cobalamin was either cyanocobalamin or a mixture of hydroxocobalamin and cyanocobalamin. Lindstrand and Ståhlberg (340) were the first to show that there were several different cobalamins in human plasma, the major component being methylcobalamin. The various cobalamins, in addition to methylcobalamin, were identified as hydroxocobalamin, 5'-deoxyadenosylcobalamin, and cyanocobalamin (341, 342).

With improved methods of thin layer chromatography and bioautography, followed by photometric scanning or visual assessment, it was also shown by Linnell et al. (337, 343–345) that there may be as many as four different cobalamins in extract of normal plasma. In about 30% of the normal plasma samples, traces of cyanocobalamin, usually less than 5% of the total cobalamins, were found. This was once thought to be associated with the increased cyanide intake caused by smoking, but its presence is not confined to smokers (346).

The use of thin layer chromatography made it possible to apply chromatographic and bioautographic methods for separation of plasma cobalamins to relatively small quantities (5 ml) of blood (343). It therefore was feasible to determine values for individual plasma cobalamins in a large number of healthy people and patients suffering from a variety of disturbances of cobalamin metabolism. In Table 5, the data obtained in normal and pernicious anemia patients are shown (347).

In pernicious anemia subjects methylcobalamin, normally the predominant component, is disproportinately reduced in relation to the other major component so that the ratio of methylcobalamin to hydroxocobalamin falls to less than 1.0. In about 50% of the cases of untreated pernicious anemia, methylcobalamin is undetectable. This abnormal pattern has been seen in several cases of early pernicious anemia in which the total plasma cobalamin was still within normal limits, a finding that may prove to be diagnostically useful (300). Another unusual feature in the pattern of plasma cobalamins in untreated pernicious anemia is the high percentage of cyanocobalamin (up to 40%); therefore, much of the remaining plasma cobalamins in these patients is in an inactive form.

Adenosylcobalamin is the major cobalamin in all cellular tissues (300). Although low on a percentage basis, the concentration of methylcobalamin in liver is about 100 times the concentration in plasma. About 25–35 μg of methylcobalamin is in the liver. One kidney, weighing about 150 g, would contain about six times as much methylcobalamin as there is in the whole volume of plasma (11). Studies in vegans showed a pattern of plasma cobalamins indistinguishable from that of pernicious anemia (300). In folate deficiency, in contrast to cobalamin deficiency, there was no consistent change in the proportions of individual cobalamins.

Table 5. Plasma cobalamins in normal and pernicious anemia patients[a]

Subjects	No. of subjects	Total B_{12} (pg/ml)	Me-B_{12}[b] (pg/ml)	CN-B_{12}[b] (pg/ml)	CO-OH B_{12}[b] (pg/ml)	Ratio of Me:CO-OH B_{12}	CN-B_{12} (% of total)
Normal	28	522±34	364±25	3.2±1.8	155±16	2.9±0.3	0–8
Pernicious anemia	29	64±4.8	9.0±1.9	7.2±1.8	48.8±4.3	0.22±0.05	0–41

[a]Data from Linnell et al. (347).
[b]Me-B_{12} is methylcobalamin; CN-B_{12} is cyanocobalamin; CO–OH B_{12} refers to a mixture of deoxyadenosylcobalamin and hydroxocobalamin.

More recently, the cobalamin distribution of the various transcobalamins has been determined (301, 302). Transcobalamin II contained about equal amounts of methylcobalamin and adenosylcobalamin, whereas methylcobalamin accounted for most of the cobalamin attached to the other transcobalamins. Adenosylcobalamin was the next most abundant cobalamin on transcobalamin I and III. No hydroxocobalamin was observed attached to transcobalamin II. Traces of cyanocobalamin were found to be attached to all the transcobalamins.

REFERENCES

1. Castle, W. B. (1953). N. Engl. J. Med. 249:603.
2. Castle, W. B., and Townsend, W. C. (1929). Am. J. Med. Sci. 178:764.
3. Castle, W. B., Townsend, W. C., and Heath, W. C. (1930). Am. J. Med. Sci. 180:305.
3a. Rickes, E. L., Brink, N. G., Koniuszy, F. R., Wood, T. R., and Folkers, K. (1948). Science 107:396.
3b. Smith, E. L. (1948). Nature 161:638; 162:144.
3c. Pierce, J. V., Page, A. C., Jr., Stokstad, E. L. R., and Jukes, T. H. (1949). J. Am. Chem. Soc. 71:2952.
3d. Ellis, B., Petrow, V., and Snook, G. R. (1949). J. Pharm. Pharmacol. 1:60.
3e. Brink, N. G., Wolf, D. E., Kaczka, E., Rickes, E. L., Koniuszy, F. R., Wood, T. R., and Folkers, K. (1949). J. Am. Chem. Soc. 71:1854.
3f. Brink, N. G., Kuehl, F. A., Jr., and Folkers, K. (1950). Science 112:354.
3g. Jukes, T. H., and Stokstad, E. L. R. (1951). Vitam. Horm. 9:1.
3h. Lichtman, H., Watson, J., Ginsberg, V., Pierce, J. V., Stokstad, E. L. R., and Jukes, T. H. (1949). Proc. Soc. Exp. Biol. Med. 72:643.
4. Barker, H. A., Weissbach, H., and Smyth, R. D. (1958). Proc. Natl. Acad. Sci. USA 44:1093.
5. Weissbach, H., Toohey, J. I., and Barker, H. A. (1959). Proc. Natl. Acad. Sci. USA 45:521.
6. Allen, R. H. (1975). Prog. Hematol. 9:57.
7. Allen, R. H. (1976). Br. J. Haematol. 33:161.
8. Allen, R. H., Burger, R. L., Mehlman, C. S., and Majerus, P. W. (1974). Methods Enzymol. 34B:305.
9. Donaldson, R. H., Jr. (1975). In B. M. Babior (ed.), Cobalamin: Biochemistry and Pathophysiology, p. 335. Wiley Interscience, New York.
10. Ellenbogen, L. (1975). In B. M. Babior (ed.), Cobalamin: Biochemistry and Pathophysiology, p. 215. Wiley Interscience, New York.
11. Glass, G. B. J. (1974). Gastric Intrinsic Factor and Other Vitamin B_{12} Binders: Biochemistry, Physiology and Relation to Vitamin B_{12} Metabolism. Georg Thieme Publishers, Stuttgart.
12. Glass, G. B. J. (1963). Physiol. Rev. 43:529.
13. Mahoney, M. J., and Rosenberg, L. E. (1975). In B. M. Babior (ed.), Cobalamin: Biochemistry and Pathophysiology, p. 369. Wiley Interscience, New York.
14. Toskes, P. P., and Deren, J. J. (1973). Gastroenterology 65:662.
15. Landboe-Christensen, E., and Bohn, C. L. S. (1947). Acta Med. Scand. 127:16.
16. Landboe-Christensen, E., Berk, L., and Castle, W. B. (1952). Am. J. Med. Sci. 224:1.

17. MacDonald, R. M., Ingelfinger, F. J., and Belding, H. W. (1947). N. Engl. J. Med. 237:887.
18. Paulson, M., Conley, C. L., and Gladsden, E. S. (1950). Am. J. Med. Sci. 220:310.
19. Swendseid, M. E., Halsted, J. A., and Libby, R. L. (1953). Proc. Soc. Exp. Biol. Med. 83:226.
20. Glass, G. B. J. (1963). Physiol. Rev. 43:529.
21. Fox, H. J., and Castle, W. B. (1942). Am. J. Med. Sci. 203:18.
22. Landboe-Christensen, E., and Plum, C. M. (1948). Am. J. Med. Sci. 215:17.
23. Meulengracht, E. (1952). Acta Med. Scand. 143:207.
24. Magnus, H. A., and Ungley, C. C. (1938). Lancet 1:420.
25. Meulengracht, E. (1939). Am. J. Med. Sci. 197:201.
26. Motteran, R. (1951). J. Pathol. Bacteriol. 63:389.
27. Wruble, L. D., Cole, G. W., Lessner, H. E., Haidri, S. Z. H., and Kalser, M. H. (1964). Ann. Intern. Med. 60:877.
28. Hurst, H. F. (1923). Lancet 1:111.
29. Paulson, M., and Harvey, J. C. (1954). JAMA 156:1556.
30. Schilling, R. F., Clatanoff, D. V., and Korst, D. R. (1955). J. Lab. Clin. Med. 45:926.
31. MacLean, L. D., and Sundberg, R. D. (1956). N. Engl. J. Med. 254:885.
32. MacDonald, R. M., Ingelfinger, F. J., and Belding, H. W. (1957). N. Engl. J. Med. 237:887.
33. MacLean, L. D. (1957). N. Engl. J. Med. 257:262.
34. Hoedemaeker, P. J., Abels, J., Watchers, J. J., Arends, A., and Nieweg, H. O. (1964). Lab. Invest. 13:1394.
35. Hoedemaeker, P. J., Abels, J., Watchers, J. J., Arends, H., and Nieweg, H. O. (1966). Lab. Invest. 15:1163.
36. Jacob, E., and Glass, G. B. J. (1971). Clin. Exp. Immunol. 8:517.
37. Jacob, E., and Glass, G. B. J. (1971). Proc. Soc. Exp. Biol. Med. 137:243.
38. Taylor, W. H., Mallet, B. J., and Taylor, K. B. (1961). Biochem. J. 80:342.
39. Schwartz, M., and Weber, J. (1971). Scand. J. Gastroenterol. 9(suppl.):57.
40. Bromer, W. W., and Davisson, E. O. (1961). Biochim. Biophys. Res. Commun. 4:61.
41. Gräsbeck, R., Simons, K., and Sinkkonen, I. (1966). Biochim. Biophys. Acta 127:47.
42. Ellenbogen, L., and Highley, D. R. (1967). J. Biol. Chem. 242:1004.
43. Visuri, K., and Gräsbeck, R. (1973). Biochim. Biophys. Acta 310:508.
44. Allen, R. H., and Majerus, P. W. (1972). J. Biol. Chem. 247:7695.
45. Allen, R. H., and Majerus, P. W. (1972). J. Biol. Chem. 247:7702.
46. Allen, R. H., and Majerus, P. W. (1972). J. Biol. Chem. 247:7709.
47. Allen, R. H., and Mehlman, C. S. J. Biol. Chem. 248:3660.
48. Allen, R. H., and Mehlman, C. S. (1973). J. Biol. Chem. 248:3670.
49. Christensen, J. M., Hippe, E., Olesen, H., Rye, M., Haber, E., Lee, L., and Thomsen, J. (1973). Biochem. Biophys. Acta 303:319.
50. Highley, D. R., Davies, M. C., and Ellenbogen, L. J. Biol. Chem. 242:1010.
51. Weiss, J. P., Rothenberg, S. P., and Cotter, R. (1977). FEBS Lett. 78:275.
51a. Francis, G. L., Smith, G. W., Toskes, P. O., and Sanders, E. G. (1977). Gastroenterology 72:1304.
52. Marcoullis, G., Salonen, E.-M., and Gräsbeck, R. (1977). Biochim. Biophys. Acta 495:336.
53. Ternberg, J. L., and Eakin, R. E. J. Am. Chem. Soc. 71:3858.
54. Bunge, M. B., and Schilling, R. F. (1057). Proc. Soc. Exp. Biol. Med. 96:587.
55. Gräsbeck, R. (1958). Acta Chem. Scand. 12:142.

56. Glass, G. B. J., Stephason, L., Rich, M., and Laughton, R. W. (1957). Br. J. Haematol. 3:401.
57. Gräsbeck, R. (1959). Acta Physiol. Scand. 45:88.
58. Gräsbeck, R. (1959). Acta Physiol. Scand. 45:116.
59. Herbert, V. (1959). J. Clin. Invest. 38:102.
60. Hippe, E., Haber, E., and Olesen, H. (1971). Biochim. Biophys. Acta 243:75.
61. Hippe, E., and Olesen, H. (1971). Biochim. Biophys. Acta 243:83.
62. Chosy, J. J., Killander, A., and Schilling, R. F. (1962). In H. C. Heinrich (ed.), Vitamin B_{12} und Intrinsic Factor. 2d Europäisches Symposion, Hamburg, 1961, p. 668. Ferdinand Enke, Stuttgart.
63. Perlman, D., and Toohey, J. I. (1968). Arch. Biochem. Biophys. 124:462.
64. Gallagher, N. D., Foley, K., and Brown, J. (1972). Gastroenterology 63:83.
65. Mathan, V. I., Babior, B. M., and Donaldson, R. M., Jr. (1974). J. Clin. Invest. 54:598.
66. Gottlieb, C. W., Retief, F. P., and Herbert, V. (1967). Biochim. Biophys. Acta 141:560.
67. Gräsbeck, R. (1969). Prog. Hematol. 6:233.
68. Gräsbeck, R. (1967). Scand. J. Clin. Lab. Invest. 95(suppl.):7.
69. Schade, S. G., Abels, J., and Schilling, R. F. (1967). J. Clin. Invest. 46:615.
70. Chanarin, I. (1968). The Megaloblastic Anemias. Blackwell, Oxford.
71. McGuigan, J. E. (1967). J. Lab. Clin. Med. 70:666.
72. Wagstaff, M., Broughton, A., and Jones, F. R. (1973). Biochim. Biophys. Acta 320:406.
73. Hippe, E. (1970). Biochim. Biophys. Acta 208:337.
74. Hippe, E. (1972). Scand. J. Clin. Lab. Invest. 29:59.
75. Okuda, K., and Fujii, T. (1966). Arch. Biochem. Biophys. 115:302.
76. Ellenbogen, L., and Highley, D. R. (1970). Fed. Proc. 29:633.
77. Gräsbeck, R., Kantero, I., and Siurala, M. (1959). Lancet 1:234.
78. Lien, E. L., Ellenbogen, L., Law, P. Y., and Wood, J. M. (1973). Biochem. Biophys. Res. Commun. 55:730.
79. Lien, E. L., Ellenbogen, L., Law, P. Y., and Wood, J. M. (1974). J. Biol. Chem. 249:890.
80. Gregory, M. E., and Holdsworth, E. S. (1957). Biochem. J. 66:456.
81. Highley, D. R., and Ellenbogen, L. (1962). Arch. Biochem. 99:126.
82. McGuigan, J. E., and Peterson, M. L. (1966). Clin. Res. 14:302.
83. Donaldson, R. M., Jr., and Katz, J. H. (1963). J. Clin. Invest. 42:534.
84. Gräsbeck, R., Stenman, U. H., Puutula, L., and Visuri, K. (1968). Biochim. Biophys. Acta 158:292.
85. Ellenbogen, L., Highley, D. R., Barker, H. A., and Smyth, R. D. (1960). Biochem. Biophys. Res. Commun. 3:178.
86. Lengyel, P., Mazumder, R., and Ochoa, S. (1960). Proc. Natl. Acad. Sci. USA 46:1312.
87. Stadtman, T. C. (1962). J. Biol. Chem. 237:2409.
88. Taylor, K. B. (1959). Lancet 2:106.
89. Schwartz, M. (1958). Lancet 2:61.
90. Schwartz, M. (1960). Lancet 2:1263.
91. Jeffries, G. H., Hoskins, D. W., and Sleisenger, M. H. (1962). J. Clin. Invest. 41:1106.
92. Abels, J., Bouma, W., Jansz, A., Woldring, M. G., Bakker, A., and Nieweg, H. O. (1963). J. Lab. Clin. Med. 61:893.
93. Schade, S. G., Abels, J., and Schilling, R. F. (1967). Clin. Exp. Immunol. 2:399.
94. Jeffries, G. H. (1971). In M. Samster (ed.), Immunological Diseases, Vol. II,

p. 1228. Little, Brown & Company, Boston.

95. Samloff, I. M., Kleinman, M. S., Turner, M. D., Sobel, M. V., and Jeffries, G. H. (1968). Gastroenterology 55:575.

96. Wangel, A. G., and Schiller, K. F. R. (1966). Br. Med. J. 1:1274.

97. Rose, M. S., Chanarin, I., Doniach, D., Brostoff, J., and Ardeman, S. (1970). Lancet 2:9.

98. Doniach, D., Roitt, I. M., and Taylor, K. B. (1963). Br. Med. J. 1:1374.

99. Chaiet, L., Rosenblum, C., and Woodbury, D. T. (1950). Science 6:601.

100. Minot, G. R., and Castle, W. B. (1935). Lancet 2:319.

101. Ellenbogen, L. (1963). In A. Albanese (ed.), Newer Methods of Nutritional Biochemistry, Vol. I, pp. 235–287. Academic Press, Inc., New York.

102. Ellenbogen, L., and Highley, D. R. (1963). Vitam. Horm. 21:1.

103. Mollin, D. L. (1959). Br. Med. Bull. 15:8.

104. McIntyre, P. A., Sachs, M. V., Krevans, J. F., and Conley, C. L. (1956). Arch. Intern. Med. 98:541.

105. Doscherholmen, A., and Swaim, W. R. (1973). Gastroenterology 64:913.

106. King, C., Leibach, J., and Toskes, P. (1977). Gastroenterology 72:1080.

107. Schilling, R. F. (1953). J. Lab. Clin. Med. 42:860.

108. Callender, S. T., and Evans, J. R. (1955). Clin. Sci. 14:387.

109. Best, W. R., White, W. F., Robbins, K. C., Landmann, W. A., and Steelman, S. L. Blood 11:338.

110. MacLean, L. D., and Block, H. S. (1954). Proc. Soc. Exp. Biol. Med. 87:171.

111. Ellenbogen, L., Williams, W. L., Rabiner, S. F., and Lichtman, H. C. (1955). Proc. Soc. Exp. Biol. Med. 89:357.

112. Rabiner, S. F., Lichtman, H. C., Messite, J., Watson, R. J., Ginsberg, V., Ellenbogen, L., and Williams, W. L. (1956). Ann. Intern. Med. 44:437.

113. Miller, A., Corbus, H. F., and Sullivan, J. F. (1957). Blood 13:347.

114. Bull, F. E., Campbell, D. C., and Owen, C. A., Jr. (1956). Fed. Proc. 15:509.

115. Rath, C. E., McCurdy, P. F., and Duffy, B. J. (1957). N. Engl. J. Med. 256:111.

116. Dunn, A. L., Walsh, J. R., and Holthaus, J. M. (1958). Arch. Intern. Med. 101:927.

117. Katz, J. H., Dimase, J., and Donaldson, R. M., Jr. J. Lab. Clin. Med. 61:266.

118. McDonald, J. W. D., Barr, R. M., and Barton, W. B. (1975). Ann. Intern. Med. 83:827.

119. Baker, S. J., and Mollin, D. L. (1955). Br. J. Haematol. 1:46.

120. Heinle, R. W., Welch, A. D., Scharf, V., Meacham, G. C., and Prusoff, W. H. (1952). Trans. Assoc. Am. Physicians, 65:214.

121. Pollycove, M., and Apt, L. (1956). N. Engl. J. Med. 255:207.

122. Glass, G. B. J., Boyd, L. J., Gellin, G. A., and Stephanson, L. (1954). Arch. Biochem. Biophys. 51:251.

123. Weisberg, H., and Glass, G. B. J. J. Lab. Clin. Med. 68:163.

124. Booth, C. C., and Mollin, D. L. (1956). Br. J. Haematol. 2:223.

125. Doscherholmen, A., Hagen, P. S., and Liu, M. (1957). Blood 12:336.

126. Doscherholmen, A., and Ripley, D. (1974). Arch. Intern. Med. 134:1019.

127. Heinrich, H. C. (1961). In H. Schwieg and F. Turba (eds.), Kunstkiche Radioactive Isotope in Physiologie, Diagnostik and Therapie, p. 660. Springer, Berlin.

128. Booth, C. C., and Mollin, D. L. (1957). Lancet 2:1007.

129. Cooke, W. T., Cox, E. V., Meynell, M. J., and Gaddie, R. (1959). Lancet 2:123.

130. Clarke, A. C. L., and Booth, C. C. (1960). Arch. Dis. Child. 35:595.

131. Cornell, G. N., Gilder, H., Moody, F., Frey, C., and Beal, J. M. (1961). Bull. N.Y. Acad. Med. 37:675.
132. Allock, E. (1961). Gastroenterology 40:81.
133. Citrin, Y., DeRosa, C., and Halsted, J. A. (1957). J. Lab. Clin. Med. 50:667.
134. Best, W. R., Frenster, J. H., and Zolot, M. M. (1957). J. Lab. Clin. Med. 50:793.
135. Johnson, P. C., and Berger, E. S. (1958). Blood 13:457.
136. Ronnov-Jessen, V., and Hansen, J. (1965). Blood 25:224.
137. Ross, G. I. M., Mollin, D. L., Cox, E. V., and Ungley, C. C. (1954). Blood 9:473.
138. Okuda, K., and Sasayama, K. (1965). Proc. Soc. Exp. Biol. Med. 120:17.
139. Okuda, K., and Takedatsu, H. (1966). Proc. Soc. Exp. Biol. Med. 123:504.
140. Ungley, C. C. (1955). Vitam. Horm. 13:137.
141. Doscherholmen, A., Hagen, P. S., Liu, M., and Olin, L. (1957). J. Clin. Invest. 36:1551.
142. Farquharson, J., and Adams, J. F. (1976). Br. J. Nutr. 36:127.
143. Craft, I. L., Mathews, D. M., and Linnell, J. C. (1971). J. Clin. Pathol. 24:449.
144. Adams, J. F., McEwan, F., and Wilson, A. (1973). Br. J. Nutr. 29:65.
145. Cooper, B. A., and Castle, W. B. (1960). J. Clin. Invest. 39:199.
146. Schade, S. G., and Schilling, R. F. (1967). Am. J. Clin. Nutr. 20:636.
147. Allen, R. H., Seetharam, B., Podell, E., and Alpers, D. H. (1978). J. Clin. Invest. 61:47.
148. Allen, R. H., Seetharam, B., Allen, N. C., Podell, E. R., and Alpers, D. H. (1978). J. Clin. Invest. 61:1628.
149. Abels, J., and Schilling, R. F. (1964). J. Lab. Clin. Med. 64:375.
150. Callender, S. T., Witts, L. J., Allison, P. R., and Gunning, A. (1961). Gut 2:150.
151. Jacob, E., and O'Brien, H. A. W. (1972). J. Clin. Pathol. 25:320.
152. Wilson, T. H., Strauss, E. W., and Hotchkiss, A. (1959). Am. J. Physiol. 197:926.
153. Cooper, B. A. (1964). Medicine 43:689.
154. Herbert, V., and Castle, W. B. (1961). J. Clin. Invest. 40:1978.
155. Sullivan, L. W., Herbert, V., and Castle, W. B. (1963). J. Clin. Invest. 42:1443.
156. England, J. M., and Taylor, K. B. (1966). Clin. Res. 14:135.
157. Carmel, R., Rosenberg, A. H., Law, K. S., Streiff, R. F., and Herbert, V. (1969). Gastroenterology 51:548.
158. Donaldson, R. M., Jr., MacKenzie, I. L., and Tier, J. S. (1967). J. Clin. Invest. 46:1215.
159. Simons, K. (1964). Soc. Sci. Fenn. Comment Biol. 27:5.
160. Hooper, D. C., Alpers, D. H., Burger, R. L., Mehlman, C. S., and Allen, R. H. (1973). J. Clin. Invest. 52:3074.
161. Mackenzie, I. L., and Donaldson, R. M., Jr. (1972). J. Clin. Invest. 51:2465.
162. Katz, M., and Cooper, B. A. (1974). Br. J. Haematol. 26:569.
163. Cotter, R., Rothenberg, S. P., and Weiss, J. P. (1977). Biochem. Biophys. Acta 490:19.
164. Katz, M., Lee, S. K., and Cooper, B. A. (1972). N. Engl. J. Med. 287:425.
165. Katz, M., Mehlman, C. S., and Allen, R. H. (1974). J. Clin. Invest. 53:1274.
166. Herbert, V., Streiff, L., and Sullivan, L. W. (1964). Medicine 43:679.
167. MacKenzie, J. L., Donaldson, R. M., Kopp, W. L., and Trier, J. S. (1968). J. Exp. Med. 128:375.

168. Katz, M., and Cooper, B. A. (1974). J. Clin. Invest. 54:733.
169. Marcoullis, G., and Gräsbeck, R. (1977). Biochim. Biophys. Acta 496:36.
170. Strauss, E. W., Wilson, T. H., and Hotchkiss, A. (1960). Am. J. Physiol. 198:103.
171. Hines, J. D., Rosenberg, A., and Harris, J. W. (1968). Proc. Soc. Exp. Biol. Med. 129:653.
172. Doscherholmen, A., Hagen, P. S., and Olin, L. (1959). J. Lab. Clin. Med. 54:434.
173. Donaldson, R. M., Small, D. M., Robins, S., and Mathan, V. I. (1973). Biochim. Biophys. Acta 311:477.
174. Rosenthal, H. L., Cutler, L., and Sobieszczanska, W. (1970). Am. J. Physiol. 218:358.
175. Peters, T. J., and Hoffbrand, A. V. (1970). Br. J. Haematol. 19:369.
176. Rothenberg, S. P., Weisberg, H., and Ficarra, A. (1972). J. Lab. Clin. Med. 79:587.
177. Latner, A. L., Hodson, A. W., and Smith, P. A. (1962). Lancet 2:230.
178. Peters, T. J., Quinlan, A., and Hoffbrand, A. V. (1971). Br. J. Haematol. 20:123.
179. Peters, T. J., Linnell, J. C., Matthews, D. M., and Hoffbrand, A. V. (1971). Br. J. Haematol. 20:299.
180. Linnell, J. C., Hoffbrand, A. V., Peters, T. J., and Matthews, D. M. (1969). J. Clin. Pathol. 22:742.
181. Gurani, S., Mistry, S. P., and Johnson, B. C. (1960). Biochim. Biophys. Acta 38:187.
182. Stadtman, E. R., Overath, P., Eggerer, H., and Lynen, F. Biochem. Biophys. Res. Commun. 2:1.
183. Mellman, I. S., Youngdahl-Turner, P., Willard, H. F., and Rosenberg, L. E. (1977). Proc. Natl. Acad. Sci. USA 74:916.
184. Kolhouse, J. F., and Allen, R. H., (1977). Proc. Natl. Acad. Sci. USA 74:921.
185. Wilson, T. H. (1963). Physiologist 6:11.
186. Peters, T. J., and Hoffbrand, A. V. (1971). In H. R. V. Arnstein and R. J. Wrighton (eds.), The Cobalamins, p. 61. Churchill-Livingstone, Edinburgh.
187. Yamaguchi, N., Rosenthal, W. S., and Glass, G. B. J. (1970). Am. J. Clin. Nutr. 23:156.
188. Schilling, R. F., and Schloesser, L. L. (1957). In H. C. Heinrich (ed.), Vitamin B_{12} und Intrinsic Factor. 1 Europaisches Symposion, Hamburg, 1956, p. 194. Ferdinand Enke, Stuttgart.
189. Reizenstein, P. G., Cronkite, E. P., Meyer, L. M., Usenik, E., and Driscoll, D. (1960). Proc. Soc. Exp. Biol. Med. 105:233.
190. Veeger, W., Abels, J., Hellemans, N., and Nieweg, H. O. (1962). N. Engl. J. Med. 267:1341.
191. LeBauer, E. K., Smith, K., and Greenberg, N. J. Arch. Intern. Med. 122:423.
192. Toskes, P. P., Hansell, J., Cerda, J., and Deren, J. J. (1971). N. Engl. J. Med. 284:627.
193. Toskes, P. P., Deren, J. J., Fruiterman, J., and Conrad, M. E. (1973). Gastroenterology 65:199.
194. Toskes, P. P., and Deren, J. J. (1972). J. Clin. Invest. 51:216.
195. Toskes, P. P., Deren, J. J., and Conrad, M. E. (1973). J. Clin. Invest. 52:1660.
196. Toskes, P. P., Smith, G. W., Francis, G. M., and Sander, E. G. (1977). Gastroenterology 72:31.
197. Matuchansky, C., Rambaud, J. C., Modigliani, R., and Bernier, J. J. (1974). Gastroenterology 67:406.
198. Okuda, K., Kitazaki, T., and Takamatusu, M. (1971). Digestion 4:35.
199. Gräsbeck, R. (1975). Br. J. Haematol. 30(suppl.):103.

200. von der Lippe, G. V. (1977). Scand. J. Gastroenterol. 12:257.
201. Cotters, R., Rothenberg, S. P., and Weiss, J. Fed. Proc. 36:594.
202. Kapadia, C. R., Bhat, P., Jacob, E., and Baker, S. J. (1975). Gut 16:988.
203. Shinton, W. K., and Singh, A. K. (1967). Br. J. Haematol. 13:75.
204. Monto, R. W., and Rebuck, J. W. (1954). Arch. Intern. Med. 93:219.
205. Monto, R. W., and Rebuck, J. W. (1955). Blood 10:1151.
206. Israels, M. C. G., and Schubert, S. (1954). Lancet 1:341.
207. Berlin, H., Berlin, R., Brante, G., and Sjoberg, S.-G. (1962). *In* H. C. Heinrich (ed.), Vitamin B_{12} und Intrinsic Factor. 2 Europaisches Symposion, Hamburg, 1961, p. 485. Ferdinand Enke, Stuttgart.
208. Chalmers, J. N. M., and Shinton, N. D. (1958). Lancet 2:1069.
209. Taylor, K. B., and French, J. E. (1960). Q. J. Exp. Physiol. 45:72.
210. Cooper, B. A., Paranchych, W., and Lowenstein, L. (1962). J. Clin. Invest. 41:370.
211. Spies, T. D., Lopez, G. G., Milanes, F., Toca, R. L., and Aramburu, T. (1949). South. Med. J. 42:528.
212. Ungley, C. C. (1950). Br. Med. J. 2:905.
213. Conley, C. L., Krevans, J. R., Chow, B. F., Barrows, C., and Lang, C. A. (1951). J. Lab. Clin. Med. 38:84.
214. Unglaub, W. G., and Goldsmith, G. A. South. Med. J. 48:261.
215. Reisner, E. H., Jr., Weiner, L. J., Shittone, M. T., and Henck, E. A. (1955). N. Engl. J. Med. 253:502.
216. Brody, E. A., Estren, S., and Wasserman, L. R. (1959). N. Engl. J. Med. 26:361.
217. McIntyre, P. A., Hahn, R., Masters, J. M., and Krevans, J. R. (1960). Arch. Intern. Med. 106:280.
218. Killander, A., and Schilling, R. F. (1961). J. Lab. Clin. Med. 57:553.
219. Herbert, V., and Sullivan, L. (1964). Ann. N.Y. Acad. Sci. 112:855.
220. Rosenblum, C., Woodbury, D. T., Gilbert, J. P., Okuda, K., and Chow, B. F. (1955). Proc. Soc. Exp. Biol. Med. 89:63.
221. Rosenblum, C. C., Yamamoto, R. S., Wood, R., Woodbury, D. T., Okuda, K., and Chow, B. F. Proc. Soc. Exp. Biol. Med. 91:364.
222. Heinrich, H. C., and Gabbe, E. E. (1964). Ann. N.Y. Acad. Sci. 112:871.
223. Bunge, M. B., Schloesser, L. L., and Schilling, R. F. (1956). J. Lab. Clin. Med. 48:735.
224. Toporek, M. (1960). Am. J. Clin. Nutr. 8:297.
225. Pitney, W. R., Beard, M. F., and Van Loon, E. J. (1954). J. Biol. Chem. 207:143.
226. Miller, A., and Sullivan, J. F. (1958). J. Clin. Invest. 37:556.
227. Heinrich, H. C., Erdmann-Oehlecker, L. S., Sommer, L., and Radel, G. (1956). Clin. Chim. Acta 1:311.
228. Hall, C. A., and Finkler, A. E. (1963). Biochim. Biophys. Acta 78:233.
229. Hall, C. A., and Finkler, A. E. (1965). J. Lab. Clin. Med. 65:459.
230. Hall, C. A., and Finkler, A. E. (1966). Proc. Soc. Exp. Biol. Med. 123:56.
231. Hall, C. A. (1969). Br. J. Haematol. 16:429.
232. Hom, B. L. (1967). Clin. Chim. Acta 18:315.
233. Hom, B. L., and Ahluwalia, B. K. (1968). Scand. J. Haematol. 5:64.
234. Finkler, A. E., Green, P. M., and Hall, C. A. (1970). Biochim. Biophys. Acta 200:151.
235. Gullberg, R. (1970). Clin. Chim. Acta 29:97.
236. Gullberg, R. (1971). Clin. Chim. Acta 33:173.
237. Gullberg, R. (1972). Scand. J. Haematol. 9:639.
238. Gullberg, R. (1972). Scand. J. Haematol. 1:129.
239. Andrews, P. (1969). Biochem. J. 96:595.

240. Hom, B. L., and Olesen, H. (1967). Scand. J. Clin. Lab. Invest. 19:269.
241. Lawrence, C. (1969). Blood 33:899.
242. Gizis, E. J., Dietrich, M. F., Ohoi, G., and Meyer, L. M. (1970). J. Lab. Clin. Med. 75:673.
243. Bloomfield, F. J., and Scott, J. M. (1972). Br. J. Haematol. 22:33.
244. Carmel, R. (1972). Br. J. Haematol. 22:53.
245. Burger, R. L., Mehlman, C. S., and Allen, R. H. (1975). J. Biol. Chem. 250:7700.
246. Burger, R. L., Schneider, R. J., Mehlman, C. S., and Allen, R. H. (1975). J. Biol. Chem. 250:7707.
247. Stenman, U.-H. (1974). Scand. J. Haematol. 13:129.
248. Beagley, J. A., and Hall, C. A. (1975). Blood 45:281.
249. Gräsbeck, R. (1969). Prog. Hematol. 6:233.
250. Stenman, U. H. (1975). Scand. J. Clin. Lab. Invest. 35:147.
251. Tan, C. H., and Hansen, H. J. (1968). Proc. Soc. Exp. Biol. Med. 127:740.
252. England, J. M., Tavill, A. S., and Chanarin, I. (1973). Clin. Sci. Mol. Med. 45:479.
253. Haught, J. E., Strickland, J. E., and Miller, O. N. (1967). Am. J. Clin. Nutr. 20:371.
254. Rapazzo, M. E., and Hall, C. A. (1972). J. Clin. Invest. 51:1915.
255. Savage, C. R., Jr., and Green, P. D. (1975). Fed. Proc. 34:905.
256. Cooksley, W. G. E., England, J. M., Louis, L., Down, M. C., and Tavill, A. S. (1974). Clin. Sci. Mol. Med. 47:531.
257. Sonneborn, D. W., Abouna, G., and Mendez-Picon, G. (1972). Biochem. Biophys. Acta 273:283.
258. Simons, K., and Weber, T. (1966). Biochem. Biophys. Acta 117:201.
259. Corcino, J., Krauss, S., Waxman, S., and Herbert, V. J. Clin. Invest. 49:2250.
260. Hall, C. A., and Finkler, A. E. (1971). Methods Enzymol. 18:108.
261. Carmel, R., and Herbert, V. (1969). Blood 33:1.
262. Carmel, R., and Herbert, V. (1972). Blood 40:542.
263. Stenman, U.-H., Simons, K., and Gräsbeck, R. (1968). Scand. J. Clin. Lab. Invest. 21:202.
264. Hurlimann, J., and Zuber, C. (1969). Clin. Exp. Immunol. 4:141.
265. Burger, R. L., Waxman, S., Gilbert, H. S., Mehlman, C. S., and Allen, R. H. (1975). J. Clin. Invest. 56:1262.
266. Puutula, L., and Gräsbeck, R. (1972). Biochim. Biophys. Acta 263:734.
267. Savage, C. R., Jr., Meehan, A. M., and Hall, C. A. (1976). Prep. Biochem. 6:99.
268. Burger, R. L., and Allen, R. H. (1974). J. Biol. Chem. 249:7220.
269. Stenman, U.-H. (1974). Biochim. Biophys. Acta 342:173.
270. Nexø, E. (1975). Biochim. Biophys. Acta 379:189.
271. Nexø, E., Olesen, H., Christensen, J., Thomsen, J., and Kristiansen, K. (1975). Scand. J. Clin. Lab. Invest. 35:683.
272. Thomsen, J., Bucher, D., Brunfeldt, K., Nexø, E., and Olesen, H. (1976). Eur. J. Biochem. 69:87.
273. Hurlimann, J., and Zuber, C. (1969). Clin. Exp. Immunol. 4:125.
274. Gräsbeck, R., Visuri, K., and Stenman, U.-H. (1972). Biochim. Biophys. Acta 263:721.
275. Gräsbeck, R., and Aro, H. (1971). Biochim. Biophys. Acta 252:217.
276. Scott, J. M., Bloomfield, F. J., Stebbins, R., and Herbert, V. (1974). J. Clin. Invest. 53:228.
277. Gilbert, H. S. (1971). Blood 38:805.

278. Gräsbeck, R., and Puutula, L. (1971). *In* H. V. Arnstein and R. J. Wrighton (eds.), The Cobalamins, p. 143. Churchill-Livingstone, Edinburgh.
279. Kolhouse, J. F., and Allen, R. H. (197). J. Clin. Invest. 60:1381.
280. Heinrich, H. C. (1957). *In* H. C. Heinrich (ed.), Vitamin B_{12} und Intrinsic Factor 1 Europäisches Symposion, Hamburg, 1956, p. 213. Ferdinand Enke, Stuttgart.
281. Bearn, A. G., and Kunkel, H. G. (1954). Proc. Soc. Exp. Biol. Med. 85:64.
282. Herbert, V. (1968). Blood 32:305.
283. Chanarin, I., England, J. M., Rowe, K. L., and Stacey, J. A. (1972). Br. Med. J. 1:441.
284. England, J. M., Clarke, H. G. M., Down, M. C., and Chanarin, I. (1973). Br. J. Haematol. 25:737.
285. Hom, B. L., and Olesen, H. A. (1969). Scand. J. Clin. Lab. Invest. 23:201.
286. Schneider, R. J., Burger, R. L., Mehlman, C. S., and Allen, R. H. (1976). J. Clin. Invest. 57:27.
287. Donaldson, R. M., Jr., Brand, M., and Serfilippi, D. (1977). N. Engl. J. Med. 296:1427.
288. Begley, J. A., Morelli, T. A., and Hall, C. A. N. Engl. J. Med. 297:614.
289. Ashwell, G., and Morell, A. G. (1974). Advan. Enzymol. 41:99.
290. Morell, A. G., Gregoriadis, G., Scheinberg, I. H., Hickman, J., and Ashwell, G. (1971). J. Biol. Chem. 246:1461.
291. Meyer, L. M., Bertcher, R. W., Cronkite, E. P., Suarez, R. M., Miller, I. F., Mulzac, C. W., and Ollvarreta, S. T. (1961). Acta Med. Scand. 169:557.
292. Herbert, V. (1968). Blood 32:305.
293. Carmel, R. (1975). N. Engl. J. Med. 292:282.
294. Gilbert, H. S. (1974). Blood 44:926.
295. Gullberg, R., and Jannerfeldt, E. (1977). Scand. J. Rheumatol. 6:70.
296. Masson, P. L., Heremans, J. F., and Schome, E. (1969). J. Exp. Med. 130:643.
297. Oram, J. D., and Reiter, B. (1968). Biochim. Biophys. Acta 170:351.
298. Bullen, J. J., Rogers, H. J., and Leigh, L. (1972). Br. Med. J. 1:69.
299. Stenman, U.-H. (1975). Scand. J. Haematol. 14:91.
300. Linnell, J. C. (1975). *In* B. M. Babior (ed.), Cobalamin: Biochemistry and Pathophysiology, pp. 287–333. Wiley Interscience, New York.
301. Nexô, E. (1977). Scand. J. Haematol. 18:358.
302. MacDonald, C. M. L. A., Farquharson, J., Bessent, R. G., and Adams, J. F. (1977). Clin. Sci. Mol. Med. 52:215.
303. Finkler, A. E., and Hall, C. A. (1967). Arch. Biochem. Biophys. 120:79.
304. Wickramasinghe, S. N., England, J. M., Saunders, J. E., and Down, M. C. (1975). Acta Haematol. 54:89.
305. Hakami, N., Neiman, P. E., Canellos, G. P., and Lazerson, J. (1971). N. Engl. J. Med. 285:1163.
306. Scott, C. R., Hakami, N., Teng, C. C., and Sagerson, R. N. (1972). J. Pediatr. 81:1106.
307. Hitzig, W. H., Dohmann, U., Pluss, H. J., and Vischer, D. (1974). J. Pediatr. 85:622.
308. Callender, S. T., and Lajtha, L. G. (1951). Blood 6:1234.
309. Miller, O. N., and Hunter, F. M. (1957). Proc. Soc. Exp. Biol. Med. 96:39.
310. Herbert, V. (1950). J. Clin. Invest. 37:646.
311. Cooper, B. A., and Paranchych, W. (1961). Nature 191:393.
312. Paranchych, W., and Cooper, B. A. (1962). Biochim. Biophys. Acta 60:393.
313. Pierce, K., Abe, J., and Cooper, B. A. (1975). Biochim. Biophys. Acta 381:348.

314. Retief, F. P., Gottlieb, C. W., and Herbert, V. (1966). J. Clin. Invest. 415:1907.
315. Retief, F. P., Gottlieb, C. W., and Herbert, V. (1967). Blood 29:837.
316. Ryel, E. M., Meyer, L. M., and Gams, R. A. (1974). Blood 44:427.
317. Meyer, L. M., Gams, R. A., Ryel, E. M., Miller, I. E., and Kumar, S. (1974). Proc. Soc. Exp. Biol. Med. 147:679.
318. Gams, R. A., Ryel, E. M., and Meyer, L. M. (1975). Proc. Soc. Exp. Biol. Med. 149:384.
319. Chello, P. J., and Bertino, J. R. (1973). Cancer Res. 33:1898.
320. DiGirolami, P. M., and Huennekens, F. M. (1975). Arch. Biochem. Biophys. 168:386.
321. Wickramasinghe, S. N., and Carmel, R. (1972). Br. J. Haematol. 23:307.
322. Wickramasinghe, S. N., and Moffatt, B. (1973). Acta Haematol. 49:65.
323. Rosenberg, L. E., Lillhequist, A., and Allen, R. H. (1973). J. Clin. Invest. 52:69A.
324. Youngdahl-Turner, P., Allen, R. H., and Rosenberg, L. E. (1978). J. Clin Invest. 61:133.
325. Gams, R. A., Ryel, E. M., and Ostroy, F. (1976). Blood 47:923.
326. Fiedler-Nagy, C., Rowley, C. R., Coffey, J. W., and Miller, O. N. (1975). Br. J. Haematol. 31:311.
327. Friedman, P. A., Shia, M. A., and Wallace, J. K. (1977). J. Clin. Invest. 59:51.
328. Newmark, P., Newman, G. E., and O'Brien, J. R. P. (1970). Arch. Biochem. Biophys. 141:121.
329. Newmark, P. (197). In H. R. V. Arnstein and R. J. Wrighton (eds.), The Cobalamins, p. 79. Churchill-Livingstone, Edinburgh.
330. Pletsch, Q. A., and Coffey, J. W. (1971). J. Biol. Chem. 246:4619.
331. Pletsch, Q. A., and Coffey, J. W. (1972). Arch. Biochem. Biophys. 151:157.
332. DiGirolomo, P. M., and Bradbeer, C. (1971). J. Bacteriol. 106:745.
333. DiGirolomo, P. M., Kadner, R. J., and Bradbeer, C. (1971). J. Bacteriol. 106:751.
334. White, J. C., DiGirolomo, P. M., Fu, M. L., Preston, Y. A., and Bradbeer, C. (1973). J. Biol. Chem. 248:3978.
335. Ostroy, F., and Gams, R. A. (1977). Blood 50:877.
336. Fenton, W. A., Ambani, L. M., and Rosenberg, L. E. (1976). J. Biol. Chem. 251:6616.
337. Linnell, J. C., Hoffbrand, A. V., Hussein, A. A., Wise, I. J., and Matthews, D. M. (1974). Clin. Sci. Mol. Med. 46:163.
338. Graber, S. E., Scheffel, V., Hodkinson, B., and McIntyre, P. A. (1971). J. Clin. Invest. 50:1000.
339. Seligman, P. A., and Allen, R. H. (1978). J. Biol. Chem. 253:1766.
340. Lindstrand, K., and Stohlberg, K. G. (1963). Acta Med. Scand. 174:665.
341. Lindstrand, K. (1964). Nature 204:188.
342. Ståhlberg, K.-G. (1964). Scand. J. Haematol. 1:220.
343. Linnell, J. C., MacKenzie, H. M., and Matthews, D. M. (1969). J. Clin. Pathol. 22:506.
344. Linnell, J. C., MacKenzie, H. M., Wilson, J., and Matthews, D. M. (1970). J. Clin. Pathol. 22:545.
345. Linnell, J. C., Hussein, H. A. A., and Matthews, D. M. (1970). J. Clin. Pathol. 23:820.
346. Lindstrand, K., Wilson, J., and Matthews, D. M. (1966). Br. Med. J. 2:988.
347. Linnell, J. C., Hoffbrand, A. V., Peters, T. J., and Matthews, D. M. (1971). Clin. Sci. 40:1.

International Review of Biochemistry
Biochemistry of Nutrition IA, Volume 27
Edited by A. Neuberger and T. H. Jukes
Copyright 1979 University Park Press Baltimore

4
Protease Inhibitors and Lectins

I. E. LIENER

College of Biological Sciences, University of Minnesota, St. Paul, Minnesota

Although it is accepted as a general premise in nutrition that the nutritional value of a protein is determined mainly by its amino acid composition, the legumes constitute a valuable source of protein that does not always follow

Table 1.   Effect of heat on the digestibility and protein efficiency ratio of legumes having trypsin inhibitor activity[a]

Legume	Trypsin inhibitor activity ×10⁻⁴ units/g	Digestibility (%) Raw	Heated	Protein efficiency ratio Raw	Heated
Kidney beans (Phaseolus vulgaris)	4.25	56.0	79.5	b	0.8
Hyacinth beans (Dolichos lablab)	4.38	56.5	81.6	b	1.3
Soybeans (Glycine max)	4.15	70.1	85.4	1.3	2.4
Lima beans (Phaseolus lunatus)	4.04	34.0	51.3	b	0.7
Pigeon peas (Cajanus cajan)	2.77	59.1	59.9	0.7	1.6
Cow peas (Vigna sinensis)	1.91	79.0	82.6	1.4	2.2
Lentils (Lens esculenta)	1.78	88.3	92.6	0.4	1.2

[a]Data taken from Jaffé (1) and Kuppuswamy et al. (2).

[b]Loss in weight occurs on these diets.

this rule. It has been recognized for many years that the nutritive value and protein digestibility of legumes are very poor unless subjected to cooking or some other form of heat treatment. The data in Table 1 illustrate the improvement that heat exerts on the digestibility and protein efficiency ratio of some representative legumes. The beneficial effect of heat on the protein value and digestibility of legumes has been generally attributed to the destruction of heat-labile factors that, in one way or another, exhibit deleterious effects when ingested in the diet. In this chapter, two of the most important of these factors, the protease inhibitors and lectins, are discussed in terms of their nutritional significance in the diet of animals and man. The term "protease inhibitors" is used in its broadest sense to include inhibitors of trypsin, chymotrypsin, elastase, etc., bearing in mind that individual inhibitors may differ in their specificity toward one or more proteases (3, 4). The term "lectin" is used interchangeably with such terms as "agglutinins," "hemagglutinins," and "phytohemagglutinins." For the reader who is interested in the physicochemical and biological properties of these factors, excellent reviews on the protease inhibitors (3, 4) and lectins (5–7) are available.

PROTEASE INHIBITORS

Soybeans

Historical Background   The fact that protease inhibitors are so widely distributed among those very plants that constitute an important source of dietary protein throughout the world has stimulated a vast amount of research regarding their possible nutritional significance. Because of the important role that the soybean plays in animal feeding and its potential contribution to human nutrition, the protease inhibitors of this plant have received particular attention. Unfortunately, the literature dealing with this subject is fraught with inconsistencies, claims, and counterclaims, so that a clear-cut picture of the role of the protease inhibitors has yet to emerge. Some of the reasons for this discomforting situation may be attributed to variations in experimental conditions involving such factors as the species of the experimental animal as well as their strain, age, and sex, composition of the diets employed, and the failure to use purified preparations of the protease inhibitors. The situation is perhaps best summed up in the words of one reviewer (8): "In spite of the many experimental approaches (in this field), it appears that the considerable research effort has done more to demonstrate the complexity of the problem than to elucidate the mechanisms involved."

It was not long after soybeans were introduced into the United States, primarily as a source of oil, that Osborne and Mendel (9) made the significant observation that soybeans had to be heated in order to support the growth of rats. With the demonstration of a heat-labile trypsin inhibitor in soybeans (10) and its subsequent crystallization (11), it was generally assumed that the beneficial effect could be attributed to the destruction of this factor, which interfered with the digestion of protein in vivo. Purified soybean fractions high in antitryptic activity were in fact capable of inhibiting the growth of chicks (12), rats (13), and mice (14), an effect that was generally accompanied by low protein digestibility (15, 16). In accordance with the classic concept that the nutritive value of a protein is determined by its amino acid composition, numerous studies were undertaken to determine whether or not supplementation of the raw bean with various amino acids would achieve the same effect as heating. Such experiments showed that the addition of methionine or cystine to unheated soybean meal improves protein utilization to essentially the same extent as proper heating (15, 17, 18). These results were interpreted to indicate that the trypsin inhibitor somehow interfered with the availability or utilization of methionine from the raw bean. It is important to note, however, that additional methionine does not raise the nutritive value of raw soybean to the level of heated soybean similarly supplemented with methionine (19).

Melnick et al. (20) noted that, during the in vitro digestion of raw soybean protein by pancreatin, methionine was released at a slower rate than the other essential amino acids. This led them to postulate that, during the intestinal digestion of raw soybean protein, the release and subsequent absorption of methionine are delayed to the point at which it is no longer available for the mutual supplementation of the other essential amino acids. Although this theory would explain why the trypsin inhibitor interferes with the availability of methionine from raw soybeans, other observations were not in accord with this hypothesis. In vitro studies showed that the trypsin inhibitor does not specifically retard the enzymic release of methionine, but appears to affect all of the amino acids to approximately the same extent (21–23). Goldberg and Guggenheim (24) observed that several amino acids, including lysine, tryptophan, and methionine, were all more slowly absorbed from the gut of rats receiving raw soybeans than were those fed the heated product. Almquist and Merritt (25, 26) have therefore questioned the necessity of postulating a specific interference with the enzymatic release of methionine in order to explain the methionine deficiency provoked by raw soybeans. They believe that the action of this inhibitor involves a general interference with digestion so that a substantial amount of the most limiting amino acid, which in the case of soybean protein happens to be methionine, is excreted unabsorbed or too late to be of value to the animal. In support of this concept, these authors have shown that the addition of the trypsin inhibitor, in the form of raw soybean meal, to rations containing proteins with marginal levels of lysine, arginine, isoleucine, or tryptophan caused chicks to become markedly deficient in these amino acids.

Compelling evidence may be cited that indicates that the growth-retarding effect of the trypsin inhibitor cannot be fully explained by its ability to inhibit protein digestion in intestines. Thus, active antitryptic preparations have been shown to inhibit the growth of experimental animals even when incorporated into diets containing predigested protein or free amino acids (19, 27–29). Such experiments obviously rule out an inhibition of proteolysis as the sole factor responsible for growth inhibition and thus serve to focus attention on some alternate mode of action of the trypsin inhibitor.

Mode of Action   Perhaps the most significant observation that has ultimately led to a better understanding of the mode of action of the soybean trypsin inhibitor was that rats and chicks developed marked hypertrophy of the pancreas (30, 31), an effect that is accompanied by an increased rate of synthesis of pancreatic enzymes (32, 33). Pancreatic hypertrophy can also be produced by feeding animals highly purified preparations of soybean trypsin inhibitors (34–36), although a direct relationship between trypsin inhibitor activity of various soybean fractions and their ability to produce pancreatic hypertrophy cannot always be established (37–39). That the trypsin inhibitors do not account for all of the pancreatic effects observed with raw soybeans is indicated by the experiments of Kakade et al. (40), who found that unheated soybean protein from which the trypsin inhibitors had been removed by affinity chromatography still caused pancreatic hypertrophy and growth inhibition in rats. These authors suggest that the deleterious effects of soy protein observed in the absence of trypsin inhibitors are most likely due to the resistance of the native protein to digestion by proteolytic enzymes in the intestines (see under "Protein Isolates").

Lyman and Lepkovsky (41) were the first to suggest that the growth depression caused by trypsin inhibitor may be a consequence of an endogenous loss of essential amino acids derived from a hyperactive pancreas that is responding in a compensatory fashion in an effort to overcome the depletion of trypsin caused by the inhibitor. Since pancreatic enzymes are particularly rich in the sulfur-containing amino acids (42), pancreatic hypertrophy serves to drain the body tissue of these particular amino acids in order to meet an increased need for the synthesis of these enzymes. This loss in sulfur-containing amino acids accentuates an already critical situation with respect to soybean protein, which is inherently deficient in these amino acids. It is not surprising, therefore, that methionine supplementation effectively counteracts most of the growth depression caused by the trypsin inhibitor despite the persistence of pancreatic hypertrophy (29, 31).

The mechanism whereby the trypsin inhibitor causes pancreatic enlargement is still not fully understood. Lyman and co-workers (43–45) suggest that the level of pancreatic secretion, and hence the size of the pancreas, is normally controlled by a mechanism of feedback inhibition that depends upon the level of trypsin present at any given time in the small intestine. When this level of trypsin falls below a certain threshold value, such as would occur in the presence of trypsin inhibitor or undigested protein (46), the pancreas is induced to produce more enzyme for purposes of repletion. Melmed and Bouchier (47) have also suggested that the secretory activity of the pancreas may be stimulated in a positive fashion by the pancreatic trypsin inhibitor that is released into the intestines. Such a mechanism would serve to reinforce and sustain the stimulatory effect of the negative feedback mechanism involving the trypsin inhibitor and undigested protein.

It is believed that the mediating agent between the level of trypsin in the intestine and the pancreas is humoral in nature (48), and the agent is most likely pancreozymin-cholecystokinin, since repeated injections of these hormones cause an increase in the size of the pancreas and in its secretory activity (49–51).

Unlike its effect on the pancreas of the rat, mouse, and chicks, the trypsin inhibitor fails to cause any pancreatic enlargement in dogs (52), adult guinea pigs (53), calves (54, 55), and pigs (56). Indeed, there appears to be a direct relationship between the size of the pancreas (per unit of body weight) and the sensitivity of their response to raw soybeans or the trypsin inhibitor (see Table 2). Those species of animals in which the pancreas weighs approximately 0.3% of body weight become hypertrophic, whereas those whose weights are below this value are nonresponsive to raw soybeans or the trypsin inhibitor. The guinea pig would appear to be on the borderline in that the adult animal, in contrast to the young animal, is insensitive to the trypsin inhibitor. One would predict from this relationship that the human pancreas would not be sensitive to the stimulatory effects of the soybean trypsin inhibitor, although direct experimental evidence bearing on this point is lacking.

In summary, therefore, it is evident that an inhibition of intestinal proteolysis need not be invoked to explain the growth inhibition produced by the soybean trypsin inhibitor. On the other hand, one cannot ignore the probability that an inhibition of the normal digestive process could play a significant role in determining the overall nutritive properties of the soybean protein. For example, if the quantity of trypsin produced by the pancreas is not

Table 2. Relationship between size of pancreas of various species of animals and the response of the pancreas to raw soybeans or trypsin inhibitor

Species	Size of pancreas (% of body wt)	Pancreatic hypertrophy	References
Mouse	0.06–0.8	+	(33)
Rat	0.5 –0.6	+	(40)
Chick	0.4 –0.6	+	(57)
Guinea pig	0.29	±[a]	(53)
Dog	0.21–0.24	–	(52)
Pig	0.10–0.12	–	(56)
Human	0.09–0.12[b]	(–)[c]	
Calf	0.06–0.08	–	(55)

[a]Observed in young guinea pigs but not in adults.
[b]Taken from Long (58).
[c]Predicted response.

sufficient to neutralize all of the inhibitor present in the intestinal tract, the proteolytic degradation of intact protein will obviously be suppressed. Thus, the increase in fecal nitrogen that is generally observed in animals receiving diets containing the inhibitor (41, 59) may be of dietary as well as of endogenous origin. Experimentally, it may prove difficult to differentiate between these two effects.

Other Plants

To what extent the protease inhibitors may be responsible for the poor digestibility and poor nutritive value of other legumes in their raw state (60–63) is not clear at the present time. In the first place there does not appear to be any clear-cut correlation between the trypsin inhibitor content of various legumes and the beneficial effect of heat treatment (64). Although purified preparations of trypsin inhibitors from the lima bean *(Phaseolus lunatus)* (65, 66), peanuts (67), and *Lathyrus sativus* (68) are capable of inhibiting the growth of rats and even causing pancreatic hypertrophy (67), trypsin inhibitors isolated from the double bean *(Faba vulgaris)* (69, 70), field bean *(Dolichos lablab)* (71), and corn (72) do not inhibit growth. Certain varieties of *Phaseolus vulgaris* that have very low levels of trypsin inhibitor nevertheless have poor growth-promoting properties unless subjected to heat treatment (73). The presence of other growth inhibitors, such as the lectins, which are discussed below, no doubt tends to obscure whatever detrimental effects the trypsin inhibitor per se may have on growth.

Since lima bean fractions high in antitryptic activity inhibit the growth of rats fed acid-hydrolyzed casein (74), it would appear that, as in the case of soybeans, this inhibitor at least does not exert its deleterious effect solely by an inhibition of intestinal proteolysis.

One of the characteristic chemical features of many of the protease inhibitors that are found in legumes other than the soybean is their unusually high content of cystine residues (75). For example, although the protease inhibitors of navy beans and kidney beans comprise only 2.5% of the total protein of these beans, they account for about 30–40% of the total cystine content of the bean protein (76). It is conceivable, therefore, that a dietary loss of cystine from the inhibitor itself could contribute in a significant fashion to the poor quality of these legumes in their native state. Kakade et al. (76) have indeed shown that the cystine of the unheated navy bean protease inhibitor is approximately 50% less available to the chick than the cystine provided by the heat-inactivated inhibitor. In vitro digestibility data suggested that the unavailability of cystine from the unheated inhibitor is most likely the consequence of its resistance to enzymatic attack. Thus, the trypsin inhibitors of some legumes may be a double-edged sword; they not only reduce the digestibility of the protein and cause pancreatic hypertrophy but they may also "lock in" a significant fraction of the total cystine content of the bean protein, which is already marginal.

Effects of Processing

Heat Treatment   It is the relative ease with which the deleterious components of legumes, including the trypsin inhibitor, can be destroyed by heat treatment that has permitted their popular use as an important dietary component. The soybean trypsin inhibitor again has received the most study in this respect. In general, the extent to which the inhibitor is destroyed is a function of the temperature, duration of heating, moisture conditions, particle size, etc. — variables that are closely controlled in the commercial processing of soybeans in order to produce a product having maximum nutritive value. An example of how heat affects the nutritive properties of soybean protein in relation to trypsin inhibitor activity is shown in Figure 1. Not shown in this figure, however, is the fact that excessive heat treatment may damage the nutritive value of the protein, so the absence of inhibitor activity is not always a guarantee that a product will have optimal nutritional quality.

Rackis et al. (78) determined the biological threshold level in rats of trypsin inhibitory activity in soybean meals that had been heat processed to provide varying degrees of destruction of the trypsin inhibitor. Data taken from their paper are shown in Table 3. Maximum body weight and protein efficiency values were obtained with rats fed soy samples in which about 80% of the inhibitor was inactivated. No pancreatic hypertrophy occurred in rats fed soy flour in which 50–60% of the inhibitor activity had been destroyed. These results make it quite evident that complete destruction of trypsin inhibitors is not a prerequisite for obtaining maximum nutritive value of soybean protein. It is not surprising, therefore, that most commercially toasted samples of soybean oil meal, in which 90–92% of the trypsin inhibitor activity has been destroyed, support the growth of rats as well as casein does (79, 80). Although azeotropic extraction of defatted soybean flakes

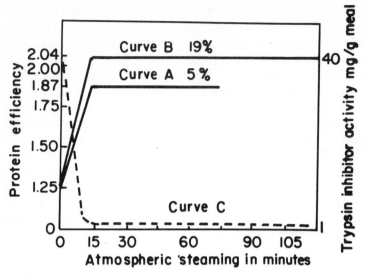

Figure 1.   Effects of autoclaving on protein efficiency and trypsin inhibitor activity of raw soybean meal. Conditions: live steam at atmospheric pressure, 100°C. Curve A, protein efficiency of meals with 5% moisture before autoclaving; curve B, protein efficiency of meals with 19% moisture prior to autoclaving; curve C, decrease in trypsin-inhibitor activity under both conditions. Reproduced from Rackis (77) with permission of the Federation of American Societies for Experimental Biology.

with hexane:alcohol serves to destroy lipoxygenase activity and thus improves the flavor score, this process must be combined with treatment with live steam in order to inactivate more than 90% of the trypsin inhibitor (81). Dielectric heating (82) and microwave radiation (83) have also been used to effect a rapid improvement in nutritional quality of soybeans by destroying over 70% of the trypsin inhibitor activity.

The trypsin inhibitor activity that may be present in soy milk can be effectively eliminated by sterilization of the liquid product or by spray drying

Table 3.   Effect of soy flour containing various levels of trypsin inhibitor (TI) on growth and pancreatic size of rats[a]

TI content		Body weight (g)	Protein efficiency ratio	Pancreas weight (g/100 g of body wt)
mg/100-g Diet	% Destruction			
887	0	79	1.59	0.70
532	40	111	2.37	0.56
282	68	121	2.78	0.50
157	82	134	2.97	0.49
119	87	148	3.08	0.47
71	92	142	3.03	0.45
Casein		145	3.35	0.55

[a]From Rackis et al. (78).

(84, 85). Churella et al. (86) concluded that the low ($<10\%$) residual trypsin inhibitor activity found in some commercially available soy infant formulas had no nutritional significance as judged by growth of rats and by the size of their pancreas. Properly processed soybean milk has a nutritional quality that is essentially equivalent to that of casein whether measured by rat growth studies (87) or by feeding infants (88, 89).

The trypsin inhibitor activity contributed by soybeans used in the preparation of Mexican tortilla is destroyed by treatment with 10% $Ca(OH)_2$ at 80°C for 1 hr (90). The canned frankfurter type of sausage containing 1.5% soy isolate was essentially devoid of any trypsin inhibitor activity after the canning process (91).

Aside from the soybean, comparatively few studies have dealt with the effect of variable heat treatment on the trypsin inhibitor content of other vegetable protein sources. Autoclaving navy beans for 5 min at 121°C destroys about 80% of the trypsin inhibitory activity, and the growth performance of rats fed beans subjected to this heat treatment was considerably improved (92). Longer heating periods, however, were detrimental. The destruction of the inhibitor and improvement in nutritive value were paralleled by an increase in the enzymatic liberation of lysine as measured in vitro (93). Thus, the chemical determination of available lysine is not a very reliable index of the effect of heat on the quality of inadequately heated navy bean protein. About 90% of the trypsin inhibitor activity of the broad bean *(Vicia faba)* is destroyed by autoclaving at 120°C for 20 min, extrusion cooking, or microwave radiation, with a concomitant improvement in the growth performance of chicks (94). Further studies, however, have shown that this improvement in the nutritive value of broad beans is mainly due to the destruction of condensed tannins rather than the trypsin inhibitor (95, 96). The trypsin inhibitor of the cow pea *(Vigna sinensis)* is only partially (10–50%) inactivated by autoclaving, cooking, or toasting (97). Moist heat, 100°C for 15 min, is necessary for the complete inactivation of the trypsin inhibitor of peanuts, although trypsin inhibitor activity could not be directly correlated with the biological value of commercial peanut meals (98).

Fermentation   Fermented soybean preparations such as tempeh and natto are popular food dishes that have been used in the Orient for centuries without any apparent deleterious effects. Van Veen and Schaeffer (99) have reported that the nitrogen of tempeh is readily available, an effect that they assumed to be due to the destruction of the trypsin inhibitor during the preparation of this food. (Soybeans are boiled for at least 30 min prior to fermentation.) This conclusion is corroborated, moreover, by the fact that rats fed diets containing tempeh show no evidence of pancreatic hypertrophy (100). Several reports would suggest that the nutritive value and digestibility of natto are somewhat better than those of the unfermented bean (101–103), but less than those of autoclaved soybeans (104) or casein (105). It is uncertain, however, to what extent the trypsin inhibitor is involved in producing these effects, since no measurements were made of trypsin inhibitor activity in these studies.

Germination   Germination has been reported to effect an improvement in the nutritive value of soybeans (106–108), an effect that cannot be attributed to the trypsin inhibitor since the latter does not appear to change during germination (27, 109). Germination also improves the biological value of black gram *(Phaseolus mungo)* without any significant change in antitryptic activity (110). Conflicting results, however, have been reported for lentil *(Lens esculenta)* and chick pea *(Cicer arietinum)*; an improvement in the nutritive value of these legumes after germination was observed in one instance (110) but not in another (111). Kakade and Evans (112) reported that the germination of navy beans *(P. vulgaris)* did not improve their nutritive value despite the fact that there was a slight transitory decrease in trypsin inhibitor activity during the first 2 days of germination. Palmer et al. (113), on the other hand, found a gradual improvement in the weight gains of rats fed germinated kidney beans *(P. vulgaris)* even though there was a twofold increase in trypsin inhibitor activity. The germination of green gram *(Phaseolus aureus)* and cow pea *(V. sinensis)* did not cause any improvement in the nutritive value, whereas the nutritive value of the chick pea was somewhat enhanced (114, 115). Unfortunately, no measurements of trypsin inhibitor activity were reported in these latter studies. Germination is accompanied by a decrease in the trypsin inhibitor activity of horse gram *(Dolichos biflorus)* (116), moth bean *(Phaseolus aconitifolius)* (116), and field pea *(Pisum sativum)* (117). Although no animal studies have been reported with germinated horse gram and moth bean, curiously enough, the biological value of the field pea decreases during germination (110).

It is obvious from this survey of the literature that there is little correlation between the effect of germination on trypsin inhibitor content of plants and their nutritive value. One can only presume that factors other than the trypsin inhibitors must be responsible for the changes in the nutritive value of the protein induced by germination.

Protein Isolates   A protein isolate represents the major protein fraction of a particular plant source from which much of the other minor components, including the protease inhibitors, have presumably been removed. As such, protein isolates might be expected to exhibit improved nutritional qualities. The major protein fraction of soybeans, glycinin, is in fact capable of supporting good growth in rats (118, 119). Soybean curd or tofu, which is a popular dish in the Orient, is in a sense a protein isolate since it represents the protein that is precipitated with calcium salt from a hot water extract of the whole bean (120). The biological value of tofu is equivalent to that of properly processed soybean meal (121) or casein (105). Since the preparation of tofu involves the cooking or steaming of the beans prior to extraction with water, tofu is believed to be free of the trypsin inhibitor (122), although no specific data on this point are available.

Table 4.   Trypsin inhibitor content of various soybean products and their intermediates[a]

Product	Antitrypsin activity	
	$(TIU^b/g$ dry solids) $\times 10^{-2}$	% of soy flour
Soy flour (unheated)	86.4	100
Soybean isolate	25.5	30
Soybean fiber	12.3	14
Chicken analog	6.9	8
Ham analog	10.2	12
Beef analog	6.5	7

[a]From Liener (124).

[b]TIU, trypsin inhibitor units.

In recent years, a great deal of interest has centered on the use of soybean isolates in the formulation of textured vegetable proteins (123). Soybean protein isolated by extraction and precipitation can be spun into fibers that can be manipulated to give products simulating the texture and flavor of meat products. Data pertaining to the trypsin inhibitor content of various meat analogs are shown in Table 4. It is apparent that the soy isolate used for fabricating these products is quite high in antitryptic activity, containing about 30% of the original activity of unheated soy flour. Subsequent conversion of the soy isolate into fibers and the textured products further reduces the inhibitor content to about 10% of the level of the raw flour. Churella et al. (86) likewise found that some commercial soy isolates contain as much as 30% of the trypsin inhibitor activity of raw soybean meal. This most likely accounts for the fact that heat treatment improves the nutritional quality of a number of commercially available soy isolates (125). In this connection it should be pointed out that, although textured vegetable proteins are almost equivalent in nutritive value to casein or beef (126, 127), the protein isolate from which they were made had poor nutritive value (119). Here again the implication is that soy protein isolates cannot be presumed to be free of growth inhibitory substances such as the trypsin inhibitor.

Only limited information is available on the protease inhibitory activity of protein isolates from plant sources other than soybeans. It has been reported that cooking enhances the nutritive value of the globulin-like protein from the navy bean (128, 129) and the velvet bean (130), an effect that may be related to the known resistance of the globulin fractions from various beans to attack by proteolytic enzymes (129, 131–134), and an enhancement of their digestibility by heat treatment (129, 131). The extent to which residual levels of protease inhibitors may be responsible for these observations is not certain, although in the case of soybeans (40) and navy beans (129) an improvement in digestibility by heat was obtained with protein preparations essentially devoid of trypsin inhibitor activity.

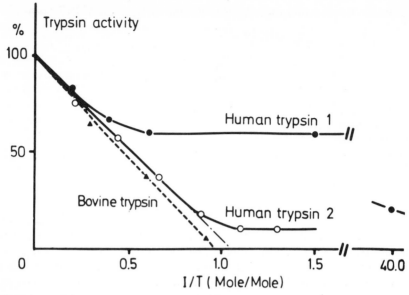

Figure 2.   Inhibition of human trypsins with soybean trypsin inhibitor. Ordinate, remaining trypsin activity is measured on tosyl-DL-arginine methyl ester; abscissa, molar ratio of inhibitor to trypsin. Reproduced from Figarella et al. (137) with permission of Springer-Verlag Publishing Company.

Physiological Significance in Humans

In view of the increasing interest in the use of soybean products for the human diet, it becomes important to assess, if possible, the risk to human health that might be associated with the consumption of soybean preparations in which the protease inhibitors may not have been completely inactivated. Actually, the only report in which human subjects were fed raw soybean flour is that of Lewis and Taylor (135), who found that unheated soybean flour could support positive nitrogen balance, albeit not as efficiently as autoclaved flour. A much more basic question that should be answered is whether the soybean inhibitor is in fact capable of inhibiting human trypsin. Trypsin inhibitor activity in soybeans is invariably measured in vitro on the basis of the extent to which soybean preparations can inhibit bovine or porcine trypsin, since the latter are readily available commercially in pure crystalline form. Human trypsin is known to exist in two forms, a cationic species (trypsin 1) that constitutes the major component of human pancreatic juice (70–80%) and an anionic species (trypsin 2) that accounts for the remainder of the tryptic activity (136–138). The inhibition of these two forms of human trypsin is shown in Figure 2. Although trypsin 2, the minor trypsin component, is inhibited in a 1:1 molar ratio by the soybean inhibitor (as is bovine trypsin), trypsin 1, the major component, is very weakly inhibited. It is perhaps significant to note that ovomucoid, the trypsin inhibitor of egg white, is also a very weak inhibitor of human trypsins (137). This may explain why ovomucoid has virtually no effect on nitrogen balance as measured in human subjects (139).

From these considerations one is tempted to conclude that, despite the considerable body of evidence that implicates the trypsin inhibitors as a factor contributing to the poor nutritive value of raw legumes in animals, their relevance to human nutrition seems dubious. Even if such were not the case, the low levels of trypsin inhibitor activity that might still remain in some commercial soybean products are probably below the threshold level at which they would be expected to exert a deleterious effect (see under "Heat Treatment").

LECTINS

Historical Background

That the seeds of certain plants are highly toxic to man and animals has been known for a long time. During the latter part of the 19th century, when the science of bacteriology was still in its infancy, it was widely believed that the toxicity of such seeds was due to a bacterial toxin. This theory was disproved, however, when, in 1884, Warden and Waddell (140) observed that the toxicity of the jequirity bean, *Abrus precatorius,* resided in fractions that could be precipitated by alcohol from an aqueous extract of the bean. Several years later Dixson (141) obtained a highly toxic concentrate from extracts of the castor bean, *Ricinus communis.* Stillmark (142), however, in 1888 was the first to observe that a protein fraction of the castor bean, which he called ricin, was capable of agglutinating red blood cells, a property that led to the term "phytohemagglutinin," which is still used today in referring to this class of substances. The work of Stillmark attracted the attention of Ehrlich (143), who chose to work with ricin rather than the bacterial toxins that were then so popular among the bacteriologists of that time. The use of these substances led Ehrlich to the discovery of the most fundamental principles of immunology (144, 145).

Landsteiner and Raubitcheck (146), in 1908, showed for the first time that even the seeds of edible species of some common legumes such as navy beans, lentils, and garden peas also contained these so-called phytohemagglutinins. Landsteiner (147) subsequently pointed out that the relative hemagglutinating activities of various seed extracts were quite different when tested with erythrocytes from different animals. It was, in fact, this specificity toward specific types of blood cells that led Boyd and Sharpleigh (148) to coin the word "lectin" (Latin, legere, to choose), a term that is today used interchangeably with phytohemagglutinin.

It has since been found that the lectins are very widely distributed in the plant kingdom, particularly among the legumes, which are known to be very

Table 5.   Some edible plants in which hemagglutinating activity has been detected[a]

Latin name	Common name	Toxicity[b] Peritoneal	Oral	Effect of heat on nutritive value[c]
Arachis hypogaea	Peanut, ground nut	?	?	+
Canavalia ensiformis	Jack bean	+	+	+
Dolichos biflorus	Horse gram	−	+	+
Dolichos lablab	Field bean Hyacinth bean	+	+	+
Glycine max	Soybean	+	+	+
Lathyrus odoratus	Sweet pea	?	?	+
Lens esculenta	Lentil	?	?	+
Phaseolus acutifolius	White tipary bean	+	?	?
Phaseolus aureus	Mung bean	−	?	−
Phaseolus lunatus	Lima bean, double bean	−	+	+
Phaseolus multiflorus	Scarlet runner bean	+	?	?
Phaseolus vulgaris	Kidney bean, navy bean, pinto bean, wax bean	+	+	+
Pisum arvense	Black pea	?	?	?
Pisum sativum	Field pea	−	−	−
Ricinus communis	Castor bean	+	+	+
Vicia faba	Horse bean Broad bean	?	?	+
Vicia sativa	Common vetch	?	?	+

[a]Based on data from refs. 149–153.

[b]Peritoneal toxicity refers to the observation that the intraperitoneal injection of the seed extract or the purified lectin into a test animal produces death. Oral toxicity refers to death or marked inhibition of the growth of animals when purified lectins are incorporated into the diet. + and − denote positive or negative effects respectively; ? denotes that no information is available.

[c]+ indicates that the nutritive value of the plant foodstuff is improved by heat treatment; − indicates that heat does not have any beneficial effect; ? indicates that no information is available.

low in nutritive value unless subjected to some form of heat treatment (Table 5). It is indeed curious that one finds so little information in the literature regarding what would seem to be a possible relationship between the lectins and the poor nutritive value of raw legumes. Perhaps one explanation for this vacuum lies in the fact that the discovery of protease inhibitors in soybeans and other legumes served to direct attention away from the lectins, and nutritionists became preoccupied with studying the role of protease inhibitors, particularly in the soybean. The purpose of this portion of the chapter is to evaluate the role that lectins might play in affecting the nutritional properties of plant proteins.

Soybeans

In 1949 Liener et al. (154) presented evidence that indicated that the trypsin inhibitor did not account for all of the growth inhibition observed with rats on a raw soybean diet. This observation led to the subsequent isolation from raw soybeans of a protein fraction that had hemagglutinating activity and was toxic when injected into rats (155, 156). Since the destruction of this phytohemagglutinin by heat paralleled the improvement in nutritive value of soybean meal (157), the possibility was considered that this protein might be responsible for at least part of the poor nutritive value of raw soybeans. Feeding experiments in which the purified lectin was added to heated soybean meal revealed that this protein was capable of inhibiting growth under conditions of ad libitum feeding (158). However, when the food intake of a control group of animals not receiving the lectin was restricted to that of animals fed diets containing the lectin, no significant growth inhibition was observed. It thus appeared that the growth inhibitory effect of the soybean lectin may have been due to a depressing effect on appetite. A more definitive answer to this problem came from experiments in which a crude soybean extract from which the lectin had been removed by affinity chromatography was fed to rats and compared with a similar preparation from which the lectin had not been removed (159). No significant difference in growth response was observed, from which it was concluded that the soybean lectin has little if any direct effect on the nutritive properties of soybean protein.

Dry Beans *(Phaseolus vulgaris)*

Although the lectins appear to have little significance as far as the soybean is concerned, the situation with respect to some other legumes is quite different. The common bean, *P. vulgaris,* constitutes an important source of dietary protein for large segments of the world's population, and numerous reports may be found in the literature concerning the toxic effects that have sometimes accompanied the ingestion of raw or inadequately cooked beans (160). Although the presence of phytohemagglutinins in *P. vulgaris* had been reported as early as 1908 (146), the toxicity of partially purified preparations of the lectin from this bean was first reported by Jaffé and co-workers (161–163). Honavar et al. (164) fed rats purified preparations of lectins from two varieties of *P. vulgaris,* black bean and kidney bean, and observed that levels as low as 0.5% of the diet caused a definite inhibition of growth; higher levels of these lectins hastened the onset of death (Table 6). These results have more recently been confirmed by Pusztai and Palmer (165) for the kidney bean lectin. These authors also reported that kidney bean protein preparations from which the lectin had been removed by affinity chromatography were nontoxic.

Preliminary soaking prior to autoclaving seemed to be required for the complete elimination of the toxicity of the kidney bean (166), although auto-

Table 6.   Effect of purified hemagglutinin fractions from the black bean and kidney bean on growth of rats[a]

Source of hemagglutinin	Purified hemagglutinin in diet (%)	Gain in weight (g/day)	Mortality[b] (days)
Black bean	0	+2.51	
	0.5	+1.04	
	0.5[c]	+2.37	
	0.75	+0.20	
	1.2	−0.91	15–19
	2.3	−1.61	12–17
	4.6	−1.72	5–7
Kidney bean	0	+2.31	
	0.5	−0.60	13–16
	0.5[c]	+2.29	
	1.0	−0.87	11–13
	1.5	−1.22	4–7

[a]From Honavar et al. (164).

[b]During the period recorded, 100% mortality was observed. No entry indicates no deaths observed.

[c]A solution of hemagglutinin boiled for 30 min and dried coagulum was fed at the level indicated. Hemagglutinating activity was completely destroyed by this treatment.

claving alone for 5 min served to eliminate the toxicity of finely ground navy bean meal (167). However, autoclaving for 30 min was necessary to destroy the hemagglutinating activity of certain African varieties of *P. vulgaris* (168). Of particular significance was the observation that hemagglutinating activity was still detectable after 18 h of dry heat.

One of the complicating factors involved in relating hemagglutinating activity to toxicity is the fact that there are hundreds of different strains and cultivars of *P. vulgaris*. The hemagglutinins present in legumes are known to exhibit different degrees of specificity depending on the species of animal from which the red blood cells have been derived, their blood group in the case of human bloods, and whether or not the cells have been pretreated with proteolytic enzymes or neuraminidase (169). Jaffé and his colleagues (170–172) have made a systematic study of the hemagglutinating activity of a large number of different varieties and cultivars of *P. vulgaris* with respect to their action on the blood from different animals, with and without trypsinization, and the toxicity of these extracts when injected into rats. As shown in Table 7, only those extracts that agglutinated trypsinated cow cells were toxic when injected into rats. Feeding tests confirmed the fact that those varieties that exhibited agglutinating activity toward trypsinated cow cells supported very poor growth when fed to rats (73). Those varieties that were non-agglutinating or agglutinated only rabbit cells were nontoxic when fed. These results serve to emphasize the importance of testing the hemaggluti-

Table 7. Correlation of specific hemagglutinating activity with the intraperitoneal toxicity in rats of extracts of different varieties and cultivars of *Phaseolus vulgaris*[a]

Variety	Rabbit blood	Trypsinated cow blood	Toxicity[b]
Valin de Albenga	+	+	5/4
Merida	+	+	9/9
Negro Nicoya	+	+	5/4
Saxa	+	+	5/5
Peruvita	+	−	5/0
Palleritos	+	−	6/0
Juli	+	−	5/0
Cubagua	+	−	5/0
Porillo	−	+	5/5
Negra No. 584	−	+	5/3
Varnica Saavegra	−	+	10/6
Hallado	−	−	5/0
Madrileno	−	−	5/0
Alabaster	−	−	5/0
Triguito	−	−	6/0

[a]From Jaffé and Brücher (171).
[b]Number of rats receiving injections per number of dead rats.

nating activity of seed extracts against several species of blood cells before one is justified in concluding that a particular bean is toxic or not. The use of trypsinated cow cells would appear to be the most useful system for detecting potentially toxic beans.

Other species of *Phaseolus* that have demonstrated hemagglutinating activity are the lima bean *(P. lunatus),* mung bean *(P. aureus),* white tipary bean *(P. acutifolius),* and the scarlet runner bean *(P. multiflorus)* (see Table 5). The lectins from the lima bean and mung bean have been reported to be nontoxic, however (151, 153). Despite its lack of toxicity, the oral administration of the lima bean lectin severely restricted the growth of rats (153). Similar studies with the mung bean lectin have not been reported. Extracts of the white tipary bean and the scarlet runner bean do display some degree of toxicity when injected into rats (151), but the extent to which they influence the nutritive properties of these beans is not known.

Castor Bean

Ricin, the lectin of the castor bean, *R. communis,* was one of the first lectins to attract the attention of investigators, presumably because of its extreme toxicity; its minimum lethal dose is about 0.001 μg/g (mice), which makes it about 1000 times more toxic than any of the other bean lectins (152). This toxicity persists after oral ingestion, and for this reason detoxification of castor pomace is essential for its safe handling and for its use for animal feeding. Steam heating, as used for the recovery of the solvents employed for the extraction of castor oil, has been found to produce a 1000-fold reduction in toxicity and to render the pomace harmless for sheep, rabbits, and rats when used in the respective diets in a proportion of not more than 10% (173). The steaming of castor bean meal for 1 h at 15 pounds of pressure reduces the toxicity of the meal to 1/2000th of its original value (174). Rats fed 23.9% of the autoclaved meal were in good health after 4 weeks, although growth and food conversion were lower than in the casein controls. Effective detoxification can also be achieved by extraction with hot water (175) or treatment with dilute alkali or formaldehyde (176, 177).

In most of the earlier work dealing with toxicity of ricin it was assumed that toxicity and hemagglutinating activity were associated with the same protein. It is now clear that these are two distinct components — a toxic protein, for which the name ricin has been reserved and which is devoid of hemagglutinating activity, and the so-called castor bean agglutinin, which exhibits agglutinating activity but is nontoxic (178). It may be reasonably assumed that most of the toxic effects observed with castor bean preparations in the past have been due to the toxic component rather than to the agglutinin that may have accompanied it. This, of course, raises the question as to whether the toxicity observed with other lectins may be due to a toxic protein that is not a hemagglutinin but is strongly associated with another protein having hemagglutinating activity. Thus far, however, no evidence for the existence of such a toxin in other legumes (except for *A. precatorius)* has been reported.

Not to be confused with the toxic effects of ricin is the presence of the castor bean allergen and the alkaloid ricinine (174). The latter is generally considered harmless and is growth inhibitory to chicks only when fed in large amounts (179). Individuals handling castor bean pomace that has not been properly processed are known to develop severe symptoms of irritation of eyes, nose, and throat frequently accompanied by asthma, nausea, vomiting, weakness, and pain (180). Although most of these symptoms are most likely due to the castor bean allergen, Cooper et al. (181) attribute at least some of these reactions to ricin.

Jack Bean

Concanavalin A is the name given to the lectin first isolated from the jack bean *(Canavalia ensiformis)* by Sumner in 1919 (182). In recent years this protein has been the object of considerable study because of the many and varied biological effects that it induces in cells because of its interaction with glycoprotein receptor sites on the surface of cell membranes (183). Despite the attention that concanavalin A has received in this regard, very little is known regarding its toxicity. It has been noted that the direct injection of concanavalin A into animals caused the agglutination of red blood cells, followed by hemolysis, and finally death (184–186). Jack bean meal is of poor nutritive value unless heated (64), and consumption of the raw bean has been reported to cause a variety of pathological lesions in rats (187) and cattle

(188). Japanese quail raised under germ-free conditions are able to tolerate the toxic effects of raw jack bean meal or concanavalin A itself much better than conventional birds (189). There appears to be some doubt, however, as to whether the harmful effects that accompany the ingestion of raw jack bean meal are entirely due to concanavalin A. Dennison et al. (190) removed the agglutinating activity of a crude extract of jack bean meal by selective absorption onto Sephadex and observed that the unabsorbed fraction still retained some toxicity, albeit less than the original extract, when injected into rats. This would indicate that a portion of the toxicity of the jack bean meal may reside in a fraction devoid of hemagglutinating activity.

Other Edible Legumes

Although the extracts of peas *(P. sativum)* exhibit hemagglutinating activity, the isolated lectin does not produce any toxic effects when injected into rats (149, 153) or when incorporated into their diet at a level of 1% (150). This may perhaps explain why the nutritive value of peas is not enhanced by heat treatment (152).

The lectin from the field bean *(D. lablab)* is toxic when injected into rats (153) and, when fed at a level of 2.5% in the diet, inhibits the growth of rats and causes zonal necrosis of the liver (191). The lectin presumably accounts for only part of the growth depression and toxicity of the raw field bean, since the effects seen with the purified lectin are less than that noted with raw field bean meal containing an equivalent level of hemagglutinating activity (191). Although the hemagglutinin of the horse gram *(D. biflorus)* is nontoxic when injected, it retarded the growth of rats when administered orally (153).

The broad bean *(V. faba)* is known to contain hemagglutinins, but this activity would appear to have little relationship to the disease in humans known as "favism," which sometimes accompanies the ingestion of this bean by humans (192). Although lectins have been isolated from other edible legumes such as the lentil *(L. esculenta)* and peanuts *(Arachis hypogaea)* (6), their influence on the nutritive value of these legumes is not known.

Nonleguminous Plants

The presence of lectins is not confined to legumes; they are also found in some nonleguminous plants such as the potato, wheat, barley, and rice (5-7, 169). There is very little evidence, however, to indicate that these lectins play any significant role in the nutritive properties of these plants.

Mode of Action

Jaffé and co-workers (161, 163) had proposed many years ago that the toxic effect of lectins when ingested orally may be due to their ability to bind to specific receptor sites on the surface of intestinal epithelial cells, which thus caused a nonspecific interference with the absorption of nutrients across the intestinal wall. This could be reflected in vivo by a decrease in the digestibility of the protein, as evidenced by the fact that the addition of the lectin purified from *P. vulgaris* markedly reduced protein digestibility when added to diets containing casein (193). In vitro experiments with isolated intestinal loops taken from rats fed the purified lectin showed a 50% decrease in the rate of absorption of glucose across the intestinal wall as compared with control animals that had not received the lectin (163). Support for this hypothesis comes from the studies of Etzler and Branstrator (194), who found that a number of different lectins react with the crypts and/or villi of the intestine, but at different regions of the intestine, depending on the specificity of the lectin. Since surface-bound lectins are known to produce profound physiological effects on the cells with which they interact (5–7), one of these effects could be a serious impairment in the ability of these cells to absorb nutrients from the gastrointestinal tract, thus causing inhibition of growth and, in extreme cases, death.

An alternative effect on the intestinal cells is suggested by the studies of Jayne-Williams and Burgess (189, 195), who observed that germ-free Japanese quail were much better able to tolerate the toxic effects of concanavalin A and the navy bean lectin than conventional birds. It was theorized that the binding of lectins to cells lining the intestine may interfere with the normal defense mechanism of these cells whereby normally innocuous intestinal bacteria are prevented from passing from the lumen of the gut into the lymph, blood, and other tissues of the animal body.

Significance in Human Diet

It is difficult, of course, to assess the significance of the lectins in the human diet based on experiments in animals alone. As long as sufficient heat treatment has been applied to ensure destruction of the lectins, there would appear to be little cause for concern. Nevertheless, it should be recognized that conditions may prevail wherein complete destruction of the lectins may not always be achieved. For example, a massive outbreak of poisoning occurred in Berlin in 1948 after the consumption of partially cooked bean flakes (196). Mixtures of ground beans and cereals have been recommended in child-feeding programs in more primitive countries (197). Such mixtures can be prepared locally from easily available foodstuffs and can be formulated in proportions to give an amino acid pattern comparable to that of milk protein. However, cooking such mixtures requires a relatively short heating time to become palatable, so that the lectin may not be completely destroyed (198). Furthermore, primitive cooking is often done in earthen pots on a wood fire, so that with a tough viscous mass like cooked beans heat transfer may be imperfect, and, in the absence of constant and vigorous stirring, the temperature reached in parts of the preparation may well be inadequate for the destruction of the lectins (199). A reduction in the boiling point of water such as would be encountered in certain mountainous regions of the world might also result in incomplete elimination of lectins.

The marked resistance of lectins to inactivation by dry heat (168) deserves special emphasis. Thus, the addition of raw bean flour to wheat flour in bread formulations (200) and in other baked goods (201) should be viewed with caution.

REFERENCES

1. Jaffé, W. G. (1950). Proc. Soc. Exp. Biol. Med. 75:219.
2. Kuppuswamy, S., Srinivasan, M., and Subrahmanyan, V. (1958). Proteins in Foods. Council on Medical Research, New Delhi.
3. Laskowski, M., Jr., and Sealock, R. W. (1971). In P. D. Boyer (ed.), Enzymes, Vol. III, p. 376. Academic Press, Inc., New York.
4. Fritz, H., Tschesche, H., Greene, L. J., and Truscheit, E. (eds.). (1974). Proteinase Inhibitors. Bayer Symposium V. Springer-Verlag, Berlin.
5. Lis, H., and Sharon, N. (1973). Annu. Rev. Biochem. 42:541.
6. Liener, I. E. (1976). Annu. Rev. Plant Physiol. 27:291.
7. Sharon, N. (1977). Sci. Am. 236:108.
8. Anonymous. (1962). Nutr. Rev. 21:19.
9. Osborne, J. B., and Mendel, L. B. (1917). J. Biol. Chem. 32:369.
10. Ham, W. E., and Sandstedt, R. M. (1944). J. Biol. Chem. 154:505.
11. Kunitz, M. (1945). Science 101:668.
12. Ham, W. E., Sandstedt, R. M., and Mussehl, F. E. (1945). J. Biol. Chem. 161:635.
13. Klose, A. A., Hill, B., and Fevold, H. L. (1946). Proc. Soc. Exp. Biol. Med. 62:10.
14. Westfall, R. J., and Hauge, S. M. (1948). J. Nutr. 35:374.
15. Evans, R. J., and McGinnis, J. (1948). J. Nutr. 35:477.
16. Kwong, E., Barnes, R. H., and Fiala, G. (1962). J. Nutr. 77:312.
17. Hayward, J. W., and Hafner, F. H. (1941). Poultry Sci. 20:139.
18. Barnes, R. H., Fiala, G., and Kwong, E. (1962). J. Nutr. 77:278.
19. Liener, I. E., Deuel, H. J., Jr., and Fevold, H. L. (1949). J. Nutr. 39:325.
20. Melnick, D., Oser, B. L., and Weiss, S. (1946). Science 103:326.
21. Riesen, W. H., Clandinin, D. R., Elvehjem, C. A., and Cravens, W. W. (1947). J. Biol. Chem. 167:143.
22. Liener, I. E., and Fevold, H. L. (1949). Arch. Biochem. Biophys. 21:395.
23. Clandinin, D. R., and Robblee, A. R. (1952). J. Nutr. 46:525.
24. Goldberg, A., and Guggenheim, K. (1962). Biochem. J. 83:129.
25. Almquist, H. J., and Merritt, J. B. (1951). Arch. Biochem. Biophys. 31:450.
26. Almquist, H. J., and Merritt, J. B. (1953). Proc. Soc. Exp. Biol. Med. 84:333.
27. Desikachar, H. S. R., and De, S. S. (1947). Science 106:421.
28. Westfall, R. J., Bosshardt, D. K., and Barnes, R. H. (1948). Proc. Soc. Exp. Biol. Med. 68:498.
29. Khayambashi, H., and Lyman, R. L. (1966). J. Nutr. 89:455.
30. Chernick, S. S., Lepkovsky, S. S., and Chaikoff, I. L. (1948). Am. J. Physiol. 155:33.
31. Booth, A. N., Robbins, D. J., Ribelin, W. E., and DeEds, F. (1960). Proc. Soc. Exp. Biol. Med. 104:681.
32. Konijn, A. M., and Guggenheim, K. (1967). Proc. Soc. Exp. Biol. Med. 126:65.
33. Schingoethe, D. J., Gorrill, A. D. L., Thomas, J. W., and Yang, M. G. (1970). Can. J. Physiol. Pharmacol. 48:43.
34. Nesheim, M. C., Garlich, J. D., and Hopkins, D. T. (1962). J. Nutr. 78:89.

35. Gertler, A., Birk, Y., and Bondi, A. (1967). J. Nutr. 91:358.
36. Sambeth, W., Nesheim, M. C., and Serafin, J. A. (1967). J. Nutr. 92:479.
37. Rackis, J. J., Smith, A. K., Nash, A. M., Robbins, D. J., and Booth, A. N. (1963). Cereal Chem. 40:531.
38. Saxena, H. C., Jensen, L. S., and McGinnis, J. (1963). Proc. Soc. Exp. Biol. Med. 112:101.
39. Pubols, M. H., Saxena, H. C., and McGinnis, J. (1964). Proc. Soc. Exp. Biol. Med. 117:713.
40. Kakade, M. L., Hoffa, D. E., and Liener, I. E. (1973). J. Nutr. 103:1772.
41. Lyman, R. L., and Lepkovsky, S. (1957). J. Nutr. 62:269.
42. Neurath, H. (1961). In A. V. S. DeReuck and M. P. Cameron (eds.), The Exocrine Pancreas, p. 76. Little, Brown & Company, Boston.
43. Green, G. M., and Lyman, R. L. (1972). Proc. Soc. Exp. Biol. Med. 140:105.
44. Lyman, R. L., Olds, B., and Green, G. M. (1974). J. Nutr. 104:105.
45. Schneeman, B. O., and Lyman, R. L. (1975). Proc. Soc. Exp. Biol. Med. 148:897.
46. Green, G. M., Olds, B. A., and Lyman, R. L. (1973). Proc. Soc. Exp. Biol. Med. 142:162.
47. Melmed, R. N., and Bouchier, I. A. D. (1969). J. Br. Soc. Gastroenterol. 10:973.
48. Khayambashi, H., and Lyman, R. L. (1969). Am. J. Physiol. 217:646.
49. Rothman, S. S., and Wells, H. (1967). Am. J. Physiol. 213:215.
50. Snook, J. T. (1969). J. Nutr. 97:286.
51. Mainz, D. L., Black, D., and Webster, P. D. (1973). J. Clin. Invest. 52:5300.
52. Patten, J. R., Richards, E. A., and Pope, H., II. (1971). Proc. Soc. Exp. Biol. Med. 137:59.
53. Patten, J. R., Patten, J. A., and Pope, H., II. (1973). Food Cosmet. Toxicol. 11:577.
54. Gorrill, H. D. L., and Thomas, J. W. (1967). J. Nutr. 92:215.
55. Kakade, M. L., Thompson, R. M., Engelstad, W. E., Behrens, G. C., Yoder, R. D., and Crane, F. M. (1976). J. Dairy Sci. 59:1484.
56. Yen, J. T., Jensen, A. H., and Simon, J. (1977). J. Nutr. 107:156.
57. Lepkovsky, S., Bingham, E., and Pencharz, R. (1959). Poultry Sci. 38:1289.
58. Long, C. (1961). Biochemists Handbook, p. 675. Van Nostrand Reinhold Company, New York.
59. Alumot, E., and Nitsan, Z. (1961). J. Nutr. 73:71.
60. Johns, C. O., and Finks, A. J. (1920). Science 52:414.
61. Everson, G., and Heckert, A. (1944). J. Am. Diet. Assoc. 20:81.
62. Richardson, L. R. (1948). J. Nutr. 36:451.
63. Evans, R. J., and Bandemer, S. (1967). Cereal Chem. 44:417.
64. Borchers, R., and Ackerson, C. W. (1950). J. Nutr. 41:339.
65. Klose, A. A., Hill, B., Greaves, J. D., and Fevold, H. L. (1949). Arch. Biochem. 23:215.
66. Tauber, H., Kirshaw, B. B, and Wright, R. D. (1949). J. Biol. Chem. 179:1155.
67. Kwaan, H. C., Kok, P., and Astrup, T. (1968). Experientia 24:1125.
68. Roy, D. N. (1972). J. Agric. Food Chem. 20:778.
69. Apte, U., and Sohonie, K. (1957). J. Sci. Ind. Res. 16C:225.
70. Sohonie, K., Huprikar, S. V., and Joshi, M. R. (1959). J. Sci. Ind. Res. 18C:95.
71. Phadke, K., and Sohonie, K. (1962). J. Sci. Ind. Res. 21C:272.
72. Mitchell, H. L., Parrish, D. B., Corney, M., and Wassom, C. E. (1976). J. Agric. Food Chem. 24:1254.

73. Jaffé, W. G., and Vega Lette, C. L. (1968). J. Nutr. 94:203.
74. Klose, A. A., Greaves, J. D., and Fevold, H. L. (1948). Science 108:88.
75. Birk, Y. (1976). Methods Enzymol. 45:695.
76. Kakade, M. L., Arnold, R. L., Liener, I. E., and Waibel, P. E. (1969). J. Nutr. 99:34.
77. Rackis, J. J. (1965). Fed. Proc. 24:1488.
78. Rackis, J. J., McGhee, J. E., and Booth, A. N. (1975). Cereal Chem. 52:85.
79. Kakade, M. L., and Liener, I. E. (1973). In M. Rechneigl (ed.), Man, Food and Nutrition, p. 231. CRC Press, Cleveland, Ohio.
80. Kakade, M. L., Rackis, J. J., McGhee, E., and Puski, G. (1974). Cereal Chem. 51:376.
81. Rackis, J. J., McGhee, J. E., Honig, D. H., and Booth, A. N. (1975). J. Am. Oil Chem. Soc. 52:249A.
82. Borchers, R., Manage, L. D., Nelson, S. O., and Stetson, L. E. (1972). J. Food Sci. 37:331.
83. Wang, R. W., and Alexander, J. C. (1971). Nutr. Rep. Int. 4:387.
84. Van Buren, J. P., Steinkraus, K. H., Hackler, L. R., El Rawi, I., and Hand, D. B. (1964). J. Agric. Food Chem. 12:524.
85. Hackler, L. R., Van Buren, J. P., Steinkraus, K. H., El Rawi, I., and Hand, D. B. (1965). J. Food Sci. 30:723.
86. Churella, H. R., Yao, B. C., and Thomson, W. A. B. (1976). J. Agric. Food Chem. 24:393.
87. Shurpalekar, S. R., Chandrasekhara, M. R., Swaminathan, M., and Subrahmanyan, V. (1961). Food Sci. 11:52.
88. Kay, J. L., Daeschner, C. W., Jr., and Desmond, M. M. (1960). Am. J. Dis. Child. 100:264.
89. Fomon, S. J. (1962). Proceedings of Conference on Soybean Products for Protein in Human Foods, September 13–15, Peoria, Ill., p. 175. Northern Regional Research Center, U.S.D.A.
90. Cravioto, R., Guzman, J. G., and Massieu, H. G. (1951). Ciencia 11:81.
91. Kotter, L., Palitzsch, A., Belitz, H.-D., and Fischer, K.-H. (1970). Fleischwirtschaft. 8:1063.
92. Kakade, M. L., and Evans, R. J. (1965). Br. J. Nutr. 19:269.
93. Kakade, M. L., and Evans, R. J. (1966). Can. J. Biochem. 44:648.
94. Marquardt, R. R., Campbell, L. D., and Ward, T. (1976). J. Nutr. 106:275.
95. Marquardt, R. R., Ward, A. T., Campbell, L. D., and Cansfield, P. E. (1977). J. Nutr. 107:1313.
96. Ward, A. T., Marquardt, R. R., and Campbell, L. D. (1977). J. Nutr. 107:1325.
97. Elias, L. G., Hernandez, M., and Bressani, R. (1976). Nutr. Rep. Int. 14:385.
98. Woodham, A. A., and Dawson, R. (1968). Br. J. Nutr. 22:589.
99. Van Veen, A. G., and Schaeffer, G. (1950). Documenta Neerl. Indones. Morbis Trop. 2:270.
100. Smith, A. K., Rackis, J. J., Hesseltine, C. W., Smith, M., Robbins, D. J., and Booth, A. N. (1964). Cereal Chem. 41:173.
101. Cheong, T. S., Ke, S. Y., and Yoon, D. S. (1959). Bull. Sci. Res. Inst. (Korea) 4:41.
102. Arimoto, K., Nishihara, A., Tamura, A., and Kobatake, Y. (1962). Kokuritsu Eiyo Kenkyusho Kenkyu Hokoku, p. 40. Cited in Chem. Abst. 66:1688x (1966).
103. Van Veen, A. G., and Steinkraus, K. H. (1970). J. Agric. Food Chem. 18:576.
104. Hayashi, Y., and Ariyama, H. (1960). Tokoku J. Med. Res. 11:171.

105. Standal, B. R. (1963). J. Nutr. 81:279.
106. Everson, G., Steenbock, H., Cederquist, D. C., and Parsons, H. T. (1944). J. Nutr. 27:225.
107. Mattingly, J. P., and Bird, H. R. (1945). Poultry Sci. 24:344.
108. Viswanatha, T., and De, S. S. (1951). Indian J. Physiol. Allied Sci. 5:51.
109. Collins, J. L., and Sanders, G. G. (1976). J. Food Sci. 41:168.
110. Chattapadhgay, H., and Bannerjee, S. (1953). Indian J. Med. Res. 41:185.
111. Devadatta, S. C., Acharya, B. N., and Nadkarni, S. B. (1951). Proc. Indian Acad. Sci. 33B:150.
112. Kakade, M. L., and Evans, R. J. (1966). J. Food Sci. 31:781.
113. Palmer, R., McIntosh, A., and Pusztai, A. (1973). J. Sci. Food Agric. 24:937.
114. Jaya, T. V., Krishnamurthy, K. S., and Venkatamaran, L. V. (1976). Nutr. Rep. Int. 12:175.
115. Venkatamaran, L. V., Jaya, T. V., and Kirshnamurthy, K. S. (1976). Nutr. Rep. Int. 13:197.
116. Subbulakshmi, G., Ganeshkumar, K., and Venkatamaran, L. V. (1976). Nutr. Rep. Int. 13:19.
117. Hobday, S. M., Thurman, D. A., and Barber, D. J. (1973). Phytochemistry 12:1041.
118. Osborne, J. B., and Mendel, L. B. (1912). Z. Physiol. Chem. 80:307.
119. De, S. S., and Ganguly, J. (1947). Nature 159:341.
120. Smith, A. K. (1963). Cereal Sci. Today 8:196.
121. Pian, J. H. C. (1930). Chinese J. Physiol. 4:431.
122. Dean, R. F. A. (1958). In A. M. Altschul (ed.), Processed Plant Protein Foodstuffs, p. 205. Academic Press, Inc., New York.
123. Circle, S. J., and Smith, A. K. (1972). In A. K. Smith and S. J. Circle (eds.), Soybeans: Chemistry and Technology, p. 294. Avi Publishing Company, Westport, Connecticut.
124. Liener, I. E. (1977). In C. E. Bodwell (ed.), Evaluation of Proteins for Humans, p. 284. Avi Publishing Company, Westport, Connecticut.
125. Longnecker, J. B., Martin, W. H., and Sarett, H. P. (1964). J. Agric. Food Chem. 12:411.
126. Bressani, R., Viteri, F., Elias, L. G., DeZaghi, S., Alvarado, J., and O'Dell, A. D. (1967). J. Nutr. 93:349.
127. Kies, C. (1974). Cereal Sci. Today 19:450.
128. Johns, C. O., and Finks, A. J. (1920). J. Biol. Chem. 41:379.
129. Thompson, R. M., and Liener, I. E. (1978). Fed. Proc. 37:264.
130. Finks, A. J., and Johns, C. O. (1921). Am. J. Physiol. 57:61.
131. Waterman, H. C., and Jones, D. B. (1921). J. Biol. Chem. 47:285.
132. Dhonde, S. R., and Sohonie, K. (1960). Ann. Biochem. Exp. Med. 20:261.
133. Pant, G., Rajagopolan, N. C., and Singh, K. S. (1968). Curr. Sci. 37:166.
134. Seidl, D. S., Jaffé, M., and Jaffé, W. G. (1969). J. Agric. Food Chem. 17:1318.
135. Lewis, J. H., and Taylor, F. H. L. (1947). Proc. Soc. Exp. Biol. Med. 64:85.
136. Robinson, L. A., Kim, W. J., White, T. T., and Hadorn, B. (1972). Scand. J. Gastroenterol. 7:43.
137. Figarella, C., Negri, G. A., and Guy, O. (1974). In H. Fritz, H. Tschesche, L. J. Greene, and E. Truscheit (eds.), Proteinase Inhibitors, Bayer Symposium V, p. 213. Springer-Verlag, Berlin.
138. Mallory, P. A., and Travis, J. (1973). Biochemistry 12:2847.
139. Scudamore, H. H., Macy, G. R., Consolazio, C. F., Berryman, G. H., Gordon, L. E., Lightbody, H. D., and Fevold, H. L. (1949). J. Nutr. 39:555.

140. Warden, C. J. H., and Waddell, L. A. (1884). The Non-bacillar Nature of Abrus Poison with Observations on its Chemical and Physiological Properties. Bengal Secretarial Press, Calcutta.
141. Dixson, T. (1886–1887). Aust. Med. Gaz. 6:155.
142. Stillmark, H. (1888). Cited by T. B. Osborne (1909), The Vegetable Proteins, Longmans, Green, and Company, New York, p. 92.
143. Ehrlich, P. (1891). Deutsch. Med. Wochenschr. 17:976.
144. Ehrlich, P. (1891). Deutsch. Med. Wochenschr. 17:1218.
145. Ehrlich, P. (1897). Fortschr. Med. 15:41.
146. Landsteiner, K., and Raubitcheck, H. (1908). Zentralbl. Bakteriol. (Naturwiss.) 45:660.
147. Landsteiner, K. (1945). The Specificity of Serological Reactions, pp. 4–5. Harvard University Press, Cambridge, Mass.
148. Boyd, W. C., and Sharpleigh, E. (1954). Science 119:419.
149. Huprikar, S. V., and Sohonie, K. (1961). J. Sci. Ind. Res. 20(C):82.
150. Liener, I. E. (1962). Am. J. Clin. Nutr. 11:281.
151. DeMuelenaere, H. J. H. (1965). Nature 206:827.
152. Jaffé, W. (1969). In I. E. Liener (ed.), Toxic Constituents of Plant Foodstuffs, p. 69. Academic Press, Inc., New York.
153. Manage, L., Joshi, A., and Sohonie, K. (1972). Toxicon 10:89.
154. Liener, I. E., Deuel, H. J., Jr., and Fevold, H. J. (1949). J. Nutr. 39:325.
155. Liener, I. E. (1951). J. Biol. Chem. 193:183.
156. Liener, I. E., and Pallansch, M. J. (1952). J. Biol. Chem. 197:29.
157. Liener, I. E., and Hill, E. G. (1953). J. Nutr. 49:609.
158. Liener, I. E. (1953). J. Nutr. 49:521.
159. Turner, R. H., and Liener, I. E. (1975). J. Agric. Food Chem. 23:484.
160. Liener, I. E. (1969). Toxic Constituents of Plant Foodstuffs. Academic Press, Inc., New York.
161. Jaffé, W. G., Planchart, A., Paez-Pumas, J. I., Torrealba, R., and Nelly-Franceshi, D. (1955). Arch. Venez. Nutr. 6:195.
162. Jaffé, W. G., and Gaede, K. (1959). Nature 183:1329.
163. Jaffé, W. G. (1960). Arzneim. Forsch. 12:1012.
164. Honovar, P. M., Shih, C.-V., and Liener, I. E. (1962). J. Nutr. 77:109.
165. Pusztai, A., and Palmer, R. (1977). J. Sci. Food Agric. 28:620.
166. Jaffé, W. G. (1949). Experientia 2:81.
167. Kakade, M. L., and Evans, R. J. (1965). Br. J. Nutr. 19:269.
168. DeMuelenaere, H. J. H. (1964). Nature 201:1029.
169. Sharon, N., and Lis, H. (1972). Science 177:949.
170. Brücher, O., Wecksler, M., Levy, A., Palozzo, A., and Jaffé, W. G. (1969). Phytochemistry 8:1739.
171. Jaffé, W. G., and Brücher, O. (1972). Arch. Latinoam. Nutr. 22:267.
172. Jaffé, W. G., Brücher, O., and Palozzo, A. (1972). Z. Immunitaetsforsch. 142:439.
173. Clemens, E. (1963). Landwirtsch. Forsch. 17:202.
174. Jenkins, F. P. (1963). J. Sci. Food Agric. 14:773.
175. Vilkjalmsdottir, J., and Fisher, H. (1971). J. Nutr. 101:1185.
176. Gardner, H. K., Jr., D'Aquin, E. L., Koltun, S. P., McCourtney, E: J., Vix, H. L. E., and Gastrock, E. A. (1960). J. Am. Oil Chem. Soc. 37:142.
177. Fuller, G., Walker, H. G., Jr., Mottola, A. C., Kuzmicky, D. D., Kohler, G. O., and Vohra, P. (1971). J. Am. Oil Chem. Soc. 48:616.
178. Olsnes, I., and Pihl, A. (1978). Trends Biochem. Sci. 3:7.
179. Murase, K. S., Kusakawa, S., Yamaguchi, C., Takahashi, T., Funatsu, M.,

Goto, I., Koya, O., and Ikamoto, S. (1966). J. Agric. Chem. Soc. Jap. 40:61.

180. Perlman, F. (1969). *In* I. E. Liener (ed.), Toxic Constituents of Plant Foodstuffs, p. 319. Academic Press, Inc., New York.

181. Cooper, W. C., Perne, V. B., Scheel, L. D., and Keenan, R. G. (1964). Indian Hyg. Assoc. J. 25:431.

182. Sumner, J. B. (1919). J. Biol. Chem. 37:137.

183. Bittiger, H., and Schnebli, H. P. (1976). Concanavalin A as a Tool. John Wiley & Sons, Inc., New York.

184. Ham, T. H., and Castle, W. B. (1940). Trans. Assoc. Am. Phys. 55:127.

185. Dameshak, W., and Miller, E. B. (1943). Arch. Int. Med. 72:1.

186. Lee, J. S., Prih, C., and Tsai, C. (1944). Proceedings of the Chinese Physiology Society, Chengtu Branch 2:59.

187. Orru, A., and Demel, V. C. (1941). Quad. Nutr. 7:273.

188. Shone, D. K. (1961). Rhodesia Agric. J. 58:18.

189. Jayne-Williams, D. J. (1973). Nature 243:150.

190. Dennison, C., Stead, R. H., and Quicke, G. V. (1971). Agroplantae 3:27.

191. Salgarkar, S., and Sohonie, K. (1965). Indian J. Biochem. 2:197.

192. Mager, J., Razin, A., and Hershko, A. (1969). *In* I. E. Liener (ed.), Toxic Constituents of Plant Foodstuffs, p. 294. Academic Press, Inc., New York.

193. Jaffé, W. G., and Camejo, G. (1961). Acta Cient. Venez. 12:59.

194. Etzler, M., and Branstrator, M. L. (1974). J. Cell Biol. 62:329.

195. Jayne-Williams, D. J., and Burgess, C. D. (1974). J. Appl. Bacteriol. 37:149.

196. Griebel, C. (1950). Z. Lebensm. Unters. Forsch. 90:191.

197. King, K., Fourgere, W., Foucald, J., Dominique, G., and Begkin, I. D. (1966). Arch. Latinoam. Nutr. 16:53.

198. Korte, R. (1972). Ecol. Food Nutr. 1:303.

199. Jaffé, W. G. (1973). *In* W. G. Jaffé (ed.), Nutritional Aspects of Common Beans and Other Legume Seeds as Animal and Human Foods, p. 199. (Caracas, Venezuela: Arch. Latinoamer. Nutr.)

200. Anonymous. (1948). Chem. Industrial Eng. News 26:2516.

201. Marcos, S. K., and Boctor, A. M. (1959). Br. J. Nutr. 13:163.

International Review of Biochemistry
Biochemistry of Nutrition IA, Volume 27
Edited by A. Neuberger and T. H. Jukes
Copyright 1979   University Park Press   Baltimore

5
Naturally Occurring Chemical Carcinogens That May Be Present in Foods

E. C. MILLER and J. A. MILLER

McArdle Laboratory for Cancer Research, Center for Health Sciences, University of Wisconsin, Madison, Wisconsin

The work of the authors and their collaborators in chemical carcinogenesis has been supported by funds from Grants CA-07175, CA-15785, and CA-22484 of the National Cancer Institute, United States Public Health Service.

The occurrence of chemical carcinogens in the human environment has become a subject of wide public concern. Most of this attention has been focused on man-made compounds in the environment, and it is less widely recognized that a variety of chemical compounds with carcinogenic activity are products of living cells. This chapter is devoted largely to the properties of these naturally occurring nonviral and nonradioactive organic chemical carcinogens. Most of these agents are metabolites of microbial and plant cells, but some also occur in animal cells. Although some of these compounds occur in certain common human foods, most of them have been found in either unusual food sources or in contaminated foods. At least 30 naturally occurring chemical carcinogens are now recognized. It is virtually certain that other agents of this type exist among the large number of non-nutritive, lipid-soluble, minor organic components of foods. The great majority of these compounds have yet to be isolated, characterized, and tested for biological activity.

The literature is now too extensive for a review of all the information on the known naturally occurring chemical carcinogens. Accordingly, for each chemical we have tried to select information on its occurrence, the conditions under which tumors are induced, the metabolism of the chemical by animals which appears to be most relevant to its carcinogenic activity, and the electrophilic reactivity of the active forms. In view of the strong direct correlation between the carcinogenic and mutagenic activities of many chemicals and the possible role for mutagenicity in carcinogenesis, references to key mutagenicity data have been included. However, no attempt has been made to provide a comprehensive coverage of the mutagenicity data for these carcinogens.

Where possible, references have been included to previous reviews on the naturally occurring chemical carcinogens. These reviews should be consulted for references to the original literature that could not be included here.

GENERAL ASPECTS OF TUMORS, CARCINOGENS, AND CARCINOGENESIS

The induction and development of cancer in the human and in laboratory animals, whether or not they follow exposures to chemical carcinogens, are complex phenomena that are not yet understood in detail. For these and other reasons the evaluation of the carcinogenic risk of an environmental chemical for humans is a difficult and often impossible task. To put these problems and the naturally occurring chemical carcinogens in better perspective, an outline of current knowledge in chemical carcinogenesis is presented prior to discussion of individual naturally occurring carcinogens. For more detailed information than we could include here, the reader is referred to some comprehensive review articles (1–4).

The Origins and Gross Natures of Tumors

Tumors (a term originally used to mean any swelling of a tissue) or, more accurately, neoplasms (new growths) are abnormal masses of host-derived tissues that grow more or less continuously in a manner uncoordinated with the growth of normal tissues and organs. Although tumors occur in many animal and plant species, they have been studied most extensively in the human and in certain laboratory mammals. Tumors that invade adjacent tissues and spread or metastasize to other parts of the host are termed malignant neoplasms or cancers; these cancers frequently exhibit rapid growth, atypical structures, and many mitotic figures. Benign tumors exhibit fewer of the latter features, are usually encapsulated, and frequently grow only slowly; however, they may kill the host through pressure, gross mass, or other secondary effects (e.g., hemorrhage). Benign tumors may "progress" and become malignant.

Epithelial tumors, derived from ectodermal and endodermal cells, constitute the major share of spontaneous (i.e., without known cause) tumors in the human. The benign epithelial tumors include the wartlike papillomas and the glandlike adenomas, while their malignant counterparts are designated as carcinomas. About 10% of spontaneous tumors in the human are of mesodermal origin. These include fibromas, myomas, lipomas, etc., and their malignant counterparts such as fibrosarcomas, myosarcomas, and liposarcomas. The leukemias are derived from the blood cell–forming tissues. Most of these "spontaneous" tumors occur in the last third of the lifespan of the human or other animals. However, there are some childhood tumors for which the annual incidence is greater in the first 2 or 3 years of the human life than in the next 20–40 years. The incidences of spontaneous tumors depend on a number of factors that include the species, strain, sex, endocrine balance, and nutritional status of the animal.

Carcinogenic Agents

Agents that cause malignant tumors to develop in greater incidences than would occur spontaneously are known as carcinogens or oncogens; the terms carcinogenesis and óncogenesis denote the resulting processes. These terms are both currently used in a broad sense to refer to the induction of tumors of either epithelial or mesodermal origin. No adequately studied agent is known to cause the formation of only benign tumors and, in view of the apparent ability of many benign tumors to progress to malignant neoplasms, it seems likely that few, if any, such agents exist.

There are three principal classes of carcinogenic agents. A relatively large number of DNA- or RNA-containing viruses induce tumors in laboratory animals. Ultraviolet radiation and ionizing continuous and particulate radiations comprise the second class of carcinogenic agents. The third class, the one of particular interest for this chapter, consists of the chemical carcinogens. This class includes a diverse group of nonviral and nonradioactive organic and inorganic structures. Most of these carcinogens are organic molecules with molecular weights below 500. The recognized inorganic chemical carcinogens include a small group of divalent ions (Co^{2+}, Ni^{2+},

Cd^{2+} Be^{2+}, Pb^{2+}, CrO_4^{2-}); relatively few inorganic compounds have been tested for their carcinogenic potential (5, 6).

Certain fibers of asbestos, glass, and alumina (7) and smooth films of a wide variety of organic and inorganic compounds (8) can induce the formation of tumors, usually sarcomas, after prolonged contact with mammalian tissues. Since physical properties (length and diameter of fibers, smoothness and area of films) are much more critical than chemical composition in determining the activities of these carcinogens, it may not be appropriate to regard these agents as chemical carcinogens.

Epidemiologists have concluded that a large fraction of human cancer is determined by environmental factors. Thus, the incidences of many important human cancers vary widely throughout the world, and migrants and their descendants frequently exhibit cancer susceptibilities more similar to those of natives of their new homeland than to those of inhabitants of their native homeland. Solar ultraviolet light is recognized as the main cause of human skin cancer; these cancers occur primarily in light-skinned individuals. On the other hand, the levels of natural background ionizing radiation appear to be too low and probably not variable enough to account for the occurrence and distribution of much, if any, human cancer. Viruses have been identified as causative agents for certain benign tumors (warts) and are suspected of playing a role in other neoplastic diseases such as Burkitt's lymphoma and nasopharyngeal carcinoma. Furthermore, the observed association over a wide species range of specific ribodeoxy viruses with the induction of leukemias suggests that viruses may also be important in the etiology of some human leukemias. There are few instances in which there are data that relate the horizontal transmission of infective virus to the occurrence of human cancers. The role of vertical or germ plasm transmission of carcinogenic viral information in the origin of human cancers is moot.

The above epidemiologic data and the demonstrated occurrence of chemical carcinogenesis in the human (Table 1) strongly support the current belief that certain chemicals to which humans are exposed throughout their lifetimes are major etiologic factors for many human cancers. The chemical carcinogens for the human listed in Table 1 are ones to which individuals have been exposed as a consequence of social habits, industrial situations, or medical treatments. Recognition of these chemicals as human carcinogens has been facilitated by the relatively defined populations that have been exposed, the potencies of the chemicals, and the high levels of exposure. However, with the important exception of cigarette smoke, these agents do not account for more than a small percentage of the total cancer mortality in the human. In addition, a number of other environmental chemicals are under suspicion of being carcinogenic in the human on the basis of their abilities to induce tumors in laboratory animals and, in some cases, from limited epidemiologic evidence for human populations. Epidemiologic

Table 1.   Chemicals generally recognized as carcinogens in the human

Chemical	Site of tumor formation	Reference
Industrial exposures		
2- (or β-)Naphthylamine	Urinary bladder	(9)
Benzidine (4,4′- diaminobiphenyl)	Urinary bladder	(10)
4-Aminobiphenyl and 4-nitrobiphenyl	Urinary bladder	(11)
bis(Chloromethyl)ether	Lungs	(12)
bis(2-Chloroethyl)sulfide	Respiratory tract	(13)
Vinyl chloride	Liver mesenchyme	(14)
Certain soots, tars, and oils	Skin, lungs	(15, 16)
Chromium compounds	Lungs	(17)
Nickel compounds	Lungs, nasal sinuses	(18)
Asbestos	Pleura, peritoneum	(19)
Asbestos plug cigarette smoking	Lungs, pleura, peritoneum	(19)
Medical exposures		
N-N-bis(2-Chloroethyl)-2- naphthylamine (Chlor- napthazine)	Urinary bladder	(20)
Diethylstilbestrol	Vagina	(21)
Societal exposures		
Cigarette smoke	Lungs, urinary tract, pancreas	(22)
Betl nut-tobacco quids	Buccal mucosa	(23)

studies for the detection of human carcinogens in foods may be quite diffi-cult, although as is discussed later, such evidence already implicates at least one naturally occurring carcinogen (aflatoxin B_1) as a probable cause of human liver cancer in certain parts of the world. An important and trouble-some factor in such studies is the long latent period, as long as several decades, in the development of human cancers.

The Metabolic Activation and
Inactivation of Chemical Carcinogens In Vivo

As exemplified by the carcinogens known to be active in the human (Table 1), the synthetic (Figure 1) and naturally occurring chemical carcinogens comprise a very diverse group that have no evident common interclass struc-tural features. However, it is now recognized that most of the carcinogens to which humans or experimental animals are exposed are really precarcino-gens and must be metabolized to ultimate forms that actually induce the tumors (24, 25) (Figure 2). In some cases intermediate proximate carcino-genic metabolites can be identified in the activation pathways. Furthermore, a common structural feature has been recognized for the ultimate forms of

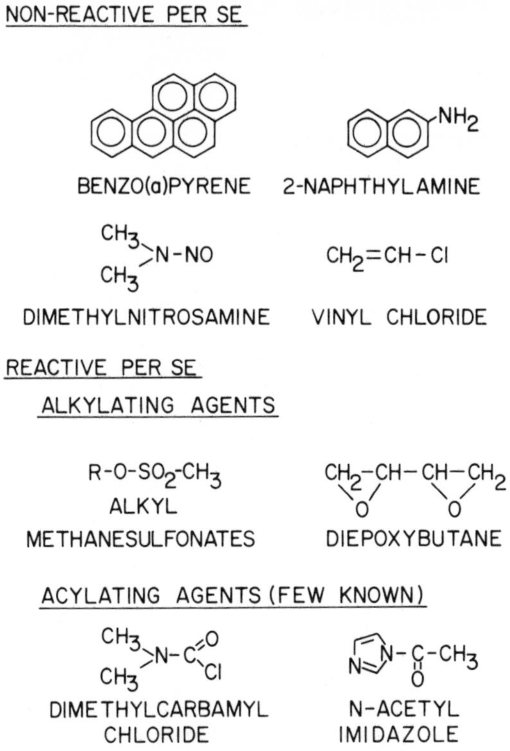
NON-REACTIVE PER SE
NH_2
BENZO(a)PYRENE
2-NAPHTHYLAMINE
CH_3 CH_3 >N-NO
CH_2=CH-Cl
DIMETHYLNITROSAMINE
VINYL CHLORIDE
REACTIVE PER SE
ALKYLATING AGENTS
R-O-SO_2-CH_3
ALKYL
METHANESULFONATES
CH_2-CH-CH-CH_2
O O
DIEPOXYBUTANE
ACYLATING AGENTS (FEW KNOWN)
CH_3 CH_3 >N-C=O Cl
N-C-CH_3 O
DIMETHYLCARBAMYL
CHLORIDE
N-ACETYL
IMIDAZOLE

Figure 1. The structures of representative synthetic chemical carcinogens.

chemical carcinogens — i.e., they all appear to be strong electrophilic (electron-deficient) reactants. The numerically minor groups of carcinogenic alkylating and acylating agents are electrophilic per se and are thus ultimate carcinogens as contacted by animal tissues. In view of their strong electrophilic natures, it is not surprising that the ultimate carcinogens react with nucleic acids and proteins to yield nucleic acid- and protein-bound carcinogen derivatives in target tissues. Genetic and/or epigenetic consequences of these interactions are presumed to initiate the heritable and essentially irreversible changes that are characteristic of neoplastic transformations and of tumors (26).

Chemical carcinogens are also subject to inactivation in vivo. For the ultimate carcinogens, inactivation occurs through reactions with noncritical nucleophiles (e.g., water and glutathione). For precarcinogens or proximate carcinogens, inactivation involves their metabolism to products that are neither strong electrophilic reactants nor precursors of ultimate carcinogens. The relative amounts of a carcinogen that are metabolized by activation and deactivation pathways are important factors in determining its carcinogenic activity in a particular species and tissue.

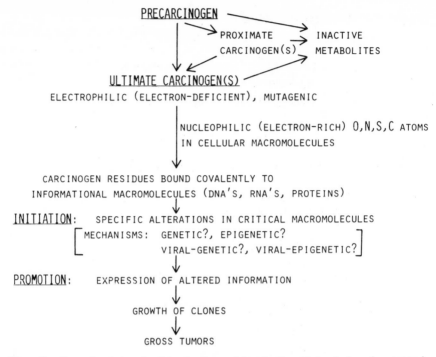

Figure 2.   General pathways for the activation and deactivation of chemical carcinogens and for the development of tumors as a consequence of the reactions of chemical carcinogens.

Mechanisms of Carcinogenesis

The cellular and molecular mechanisms by which spontaneous processes and carcinogenic viruses, chemicals, and radiations lead to the development of tumors are not known, but in a number of situations carcinogenesis has been subdivided into at least two major events (26–30). The first of these is termed initiation; this process appears to occur relatively rapidly and to be essentially irreversible. The second event, promotion, appears, at least in its early stages, to be largely reversible and to take much longer to complete. Initiation must occur before promotion. The most detailed studies of the stages of initiation and promotion have used the mouse skin tumor model, but evidence for similar stages is also available for the development of hepatic, renal, urinary bladder, and other tumors in rodents, as well as for the malignant transformation of fibroblasts in cell cultures. Agents that can initiate tumors usually also possess some tumor-promoting activity, although ethyl carbamate (urethan) and several other compounds appear to be pure initiators for mouse skin. Promoting agents with little or not initiating activity have been identified, e.g., phorbol myristoyl acetate for mouse skin and phenobarbital for rat liver.

   Most of the hypotheses proposed for the molecular mechanisms of carcinogenesis are based on the interactions of these carcinogenic agents with informational cellular constituents (DNAs, RNAs, and proteins), which, directly or indirectly, lead to heritable and at least quasi-irreversible changes in the content or the expression, or both, of genetic information needed for the controlled growth characteristic of normal tissues. While most investigators favor the hypothesis that initiation depends in most, if not all, cases on mutations in DNA, a variety of experiments suggest that mutation may not always be an essential event in the genesis of a tumor (26). The available data suggest that gene activation phenomena are of prime importance in tumor promotion (28, 30), but much more detailed data are needed. Natural selection among the altered cells and their progeny for those cells with proliferative capacities that are relatively unresponsive to host control favors the growth and progression of pretumor or tumor cells into gross tumors.

The Determination of the Carcinogenic Activities of Chemicals

For both ethical and practical reasons the carcinogenic activities of chemicals to which humans may be exposed are determined in laboratory animals. Rats, mice, and hamsters are usually used in these tests because of their relatively short (2–3 years) lifespans and because most of our knowledge of chemical carcinogenesis has been obtained with these species. Protocols for these tests may include administration by oral, topical, injection, or inhalation routes. Since naturally occurring carcinogens are most likely to contact humans via their food, oral administration is usually the most relevant test for determining possible hazard from chemicals made by living cells. The chemicals may be administered at any time in the lifespan from the in utero period to old age; administration early in life frequently appears to be the most efficient for tumor induction by low doses. Administration to preweanling animals or for long periods after weaning (up to the remainder of the lifespan) or combinations of these two are the most common systems for safety evaluation. Multigeneration tests are being proposed for more stringent evaluations. Protocols for such tests, their limitations, and their roles in the evaluation of carcinogenic hazards of chemicals for man have been considered extensively (31, 32).

The incidence of tumors observed as a consequence of the administration of a chemical carcinogen and the latent period (i.e., the time between the first administration of a carcinogen and the time at which a tumor is first detected) depend on a number of factors. The incidence of tumor-bearing animals and the number of tumors per animal generally increase in a sigmoid fashion as the dose of the carcinogen is increased, although doses that are too high may evoke a toxicity that reduces the carcinogenic response. The dose-response curves may or may not be linear over the limited ranges studied. There are no data that unequivocally show the slope or the dose intercept (if any) of dose-response curves for carcinogenic chemicals at the low exposures experienced by most human populations. However, theoretical considerations suggest to some investigators that the dose-response curve at very low doses is linear and that no threshold exists (33).

Marked differences in carcinogenic responses are frequently observed between groups of animals as functions of the species, sex, age at time of administration of the carcinogen, dosage schedule, hormonal status, or nutritional status. Frequently, these factors affect the animals' capacities for the activation and deactivation of the carcinogens. However, some factors (e.g., hormonal and nutritional status) may also influence the abilities of the altered cells to proliferate and to progress to gross tumors. A potentially important example of the latter is the ability of high levels of certain synthetic and naturally occurring retinoids to promote the maintenance of differentiated epithelia and thus inhibit the development of gross tumors derived from epithelial tissues (34, 35).

In some cases carcinogenesis by a chemical is altered by the simultaneous or sequential administration of another chemical that may or may not have carcinogenic activity (29, 36). Additive or synergistic responses for combinations of two or more carcinogens or co-carcinogens are possible. Inhibition of carcinogenesis has been observed in animals administered phenobarbital, certain polycyclic aromatic hydrocarbons, polychlorinated biphenyls, certain antioxidants, and a variety of other compounds at the same time as or shortly before carcinogen administration. Inhibition is not invariable, however, and, in the case of safrole, simultaneous treatment with phenobarbital enhances the hepatocarcinogenic response (37). Alterations in the metabolic activation and deactivation of the carcinogens and the presence of alternate noncritical nucleophilic acceptors for the electrophilic ultimate carcinogens appear to be major factors in these effects on carcinogenesis, but other factors may also play a role. Some of these chemicals, especially phenobarbital and the polychlorinated biphenyls, can increase the incidence of liver tumors when they are administered subsequent to limiting doses of the carcinogen (38, 39). In the latter cases these chemicals are considered to be promoting agents.

It is apparent from the above considerations that the extrapolation of carcinogenic hazards from species to species and under various conditions is very difficult. These extrapolations are even more difficult when they are made to low levels of exposure and when the carcinogens occur in admixture with a wide variety of other chemicals. Yet these are precisely the situations that must be addressed in considering risks of environmental chemicals to the human population.

Short-term Tests for the Detection of Potential Carcinogens

The long experimental periods and the considerable expense of lifetime tests in laboratory animals for the determination of carcinogenic activity have prompted interest in the development of short-term assays with good predictive accuracy (40). Within the past few years mammalian tissue–mediated mutagenicity assays and assays for the malignant transformation of cells in culture have shown much promise as prescreens for this purpose (40–44). Although these end points cannot supplant the induction of tumors in experimental animals for establishing the carcinogenic activity of a chemical, the results of these tests can be used as interim or additional information for estimation of hazard and for deciding which chemicals should be subjected to stringent animal assays.

The basis for the development of mutagenicity assays for the prediction of carcinogenic activity is the finding that most, if not all, ultimate chemical carcinogens are strong electrophilic reactants and that most ultimate chemical mutagens, excluding the numerically small groups of simple nonbinding frameshift mutagens and the base analog mutagens, are also strong electrophilic reactants (45). Furthermore, the recognition that most chemical carcinogens and many chemical mutagens are not active in the forms administered and the elucidation for some chemicals of the metabolic pathways involved in their activation have provided the basis for the supplementation of mutagenicity assays with fortified mammalian tissue preparations. With such fortified systems and with bacterial strains that are particularly sensitive to mutagenesis by chemicals (e.g., strains that are deficient in the repair of damaged DNA and/or are especially permeable to exogenous chemicals), approximately a 90% correlation has been obtained between the carcinogenic and mutagenic activities of chemicals (41–43). It should be noted, however, that this very useful correlation between carcinogenic and mutagenic activities does not provide information on whether or not mutation is an essential step in the initiation of carcinogenesis.

The malignant transformation of cells in culture has been less extensively developed for the prediction of the carcinogenic activities of chemicals in the animal, but the available data are encouraging. A system in which embryos are treated with the test compound in vivo and the cells are cultured in vitro for detection of transformants has the advantage of providing an in vivo metabolic activation system (46). A system in which hamster embryo cells are treated in culture has shown a high correlation between carcinogenic activity and transforming activity for a relatively broad series of carcinogenic and noncarcinogenic chemicals (47). It is possible that the latter type of assay may also be developed with human cells. However, the differences in metabolic capacity between cells of different tissues and between different individuals make it unwise to conclude that an assay for transformation of human cells is necessarily of greater value than a rodent cell system.

Problems in the Extrapolation of Laboratory Data to Yield an Estimation of Possible Hazard for Humans

Evidence that a substance is carcinogenic in one or more test species or that it is mutagenic or induces malignant transformation in cell culture raises the suspicion that the chemical may be carcinogenic in humans. However, care must be observed in the extrapolation of laboratory data for estimation of human risk. Thus, the development of tumors in rodents as a consequence of administration of a chemical at very high levels may not always be validly extrapolated to estimation of the hazard from lower levels of administration. For example, the relative rates of metabolic activation and inactivation may change considerably with the level of the carcinogen as determined by the various kinetic parameters of the enzyme systems involved. Secondary factors may also intervene (26). For instance, high levels of intake of certain chemicals cause the development of stones (e.g., from oxalates, calcium salts, cholesterol) in the urinary bladders of rodents; the presence of stones in turn predisposes the animal to the formation of tumors in the bladder (quite probably as a "promoting" influence). At lower levels that do not predispose to the formation of stones, these chemicals appear to present little risk of the development of urinary bladder tumors. Likewise, although a quantitative relationship appears to exist between carcinogenic and mutagenic activities for some chemicals (48), the mutagenic activities of a wide variety of other carcinogens do not fit the same relationship (44, 49). These exceptions are to be expected from our knowledge of the differences between various cellular and noncellular systems in the metabolic activation of chemicals, the different sensitivities of test bacteria to mutagenicity by different classes of chemicals, and the fact that saturation of the activating and deactivating systems with a test chemical generally does not occur in the whole animal, but is routinely approximated in bacterial and mammalian cell culture systems.

Similarly, negative results in carcinogenicity, mutagenicity, and malignant transformation systems pose uncertainties of extrapolation to the human situation. A major uncertainty in the extrapolation of data from whole animal tests derives from the comparative statistical inadequacy of the sizes of the laboratory groups (rarely over 100 animals per group) that are practical. Such bioassays are therefore incapable of detecting incidences of less than a few percent of the animals, a risk level of great importance to human populations. This problem is usually met by administration of the test chemical at the highest dose that the animals can tolerate and some fractions thereof; thus the exposures of the test animals may greatly exceed the likely human exposure. Mutagenicity and malignant transformation assays in culture are much more sensitive for the detection of these infrequent events because of the large numbers of cells employed in the assays and the possibility of scoring the alterations individually in many cells. As in the case of positive results, the interpretation of negative data from all three types of assays suffers from lack of knowledge of the differences in metabolism of the chemical between cells of various species and of various tissues. Furthermore, it is possible that the development of malignancy in one tissue may depend on the metabolism of the chemical in another tissue of the animal.

In addition to the careful assessment of the laboratory data, evaluation of possible human hazard must include estimation of the possible levels of human exposure. While the shape of the dose-response curve for carcinogenesis by chemicals cannot be determined at very low dose levels, it is clear that the incidence of tumors decreases and the latent period increases as the dose of the carcinogen decreases. Thus, at some low level the risk of malignancy from a given exposure may be relatively unimportant as compared to competing risks and benefits. In the case of naturally occurring chemical carcinogens, one of the possible losses to society that could result from very stringent restraints on the use of certain food supplies would be a loss of nutrients that, under some situations, might be an important health problem.

CARCINOGENESIS BY MICROBIAL PRODUCTS

Fungal Metabolites

Aflatoxin B$_1$ and Related Aflatoxins   Aflatoxin B$_1$ (Figure 3) (50–53), a product of certain strains of *Aspergillus flavus* and of *Penicillium puberulum,* is the most potent hepatocarcinogen known for the rat; it has induced significant incidences of hepatic tumors in this species when fed at 1 ppb with total doses as low as $50\mu g/kg$ of body weight. Aflatoxin B$_1$ is also strongly hepatotoxic and hepatocarcinogenic in most of the species in which it has been studied, although certain species, especially the mouse, are relatively resistant. This toxic metabolite and the less toxic and less carcinogenic related aflatoxins can contaminate a variety of foods, especially grains, peanuts, and cotton (50, 51, 54). This problem is most severe when the crops are grown or stored under warm, humid conditions and less important with good agricultural methods of harvesting, drying, and storage. That contamination of foods by aflatoxins can be a serious human health problem is evident from a recent severe outbreak of aflatoxicosis in western India (55). Furthermore, a strong correlation has been recorded between aflatoxin intake and hepatic tumor incidence for a number of populations in Africa and the Far East (56). While other factors may have contributed to the development of hepatic tumors in the high incidence areas, the human and animal studies strongly implicate aflatoxin B$_1$ as an hepatic carcinogen of practical importance to the human under conditions of relatively high exposures. The significance to human populations of the very low levels of aflatoxin B$_1$ contamination that may occur in certain foods in the United States and other developed countries is not known. The overall incidences of hepatic tumors in these countries are generally low.

The apparent importance of the 2,3-double bond to the toxic and carcinogenic activities of aflatoxin B$_1$ and G$_1$ was first deduced from the much greater toxicities and carcinogenic activities of these compounds as compared to their 2,3-dihydro derivatives (aflatoxins B$_2$ and G$_2$) for the rat and rainbow trout. Subsequently, aflatoxins B$_1$ and G$_1$, which have little toxicity

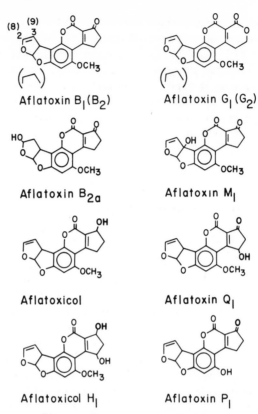

Figure 3.   The structures of the naturally occurring aflatoxins B_1, B_2, G_1, and G_2 and of the major known metabolites of aflatoxin B_1.

or mutagenicity for *Salmonella typhimurium* and *Bacillus subtilis* in the absence of liver preparations, were shown to be strongly toxic and mutagenic when the incubations included NADPH-fortified liver microsomes (41, 57, 58). Aflatoxins B_2 and G_2 are much less active under these conditions.

About 10% of single doses of aflatoxin B_1 injected into male rats is recovered as DNA-, RNA-, and protein-bound adducts in the liver (59, 60), and the incubation of NADPH-supplemented rat, hamster, or human liver microsomes with aflatoxin B_1 and nucleic acids or proteins also results in the formation of nucleic acid– or protein-bound aflatoxin adducts (59, 61) (Figure 4). Hydrolysis with weak acid of the nucleic acid adducts formed either in vitro or in vivo from aflatoxin B_1 yielded 2,3-dihydro-2,3-dihydroxyaflatoxin B_1 (59, 61). From the latter finding it was suggested that the reactive metabolite of aflatoxin B_1 was its 2,3-oxide and that this epoxide reacted at its carbon-2 with either oxygen or nitrogen atoms in the nucleic acids. This deduction was shown to be correct by the isolation and characterization of 2,3-dihydro-2-(guan-7-yl)-3-hydroxyaflatoxin B_1 from acid hydrolysates of aflatoxin B_1-nucleic acid adducts formed in vitro or in vivo

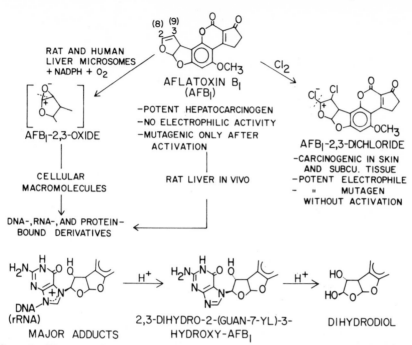

Figure 4.   The metabolic activation of aflatoxin B_1 by liver endoplasmic reticulum and the hydrolysis of the major nucleic acid adducts to 2,3-dihydro-2-(guan-7-yl)-3-hydroxyaflatoxin B_1. The alternate numbering of the 2,3 carbons by the IUPAC system is shown.

by rat or hamster liver (62–65). This adduct accounts for the major share of the DNA- and RNA-bound aflatoxin derivatives formed either in vitro or in vivo. At pH 6.5, at which the dihydrodiol is stable, incubation of aflatoxin B_1 with NADPH-fortified liver microsomes in the absence of added nucleic acids yields 2,3-dihydro-2,3-dihydroxyaflatoxin B_1 as the major product (66). The dihydrodiol is the expected product for the hydrolysis of the 2,3-oxide. Aflatoxin B_1-2,3-oxide is too reactive to permit its isolation from chemical syntheses or metabolic systems, but aflatoxin B_1-2,3-dichloride (Figure 4), synthesized as a model compound for the 2,3-oxide, showed strong carcinogenicity and was mutagenic without metabolic activation (67). The available data suggest that the carcinogenicity of aflatoxin G_1 similarly depends on its 2,3-epoxidation (68).

The toxicity and carcinogenicity of aflatoxin B_2 apparently depend on the desaturation of its 2,3 bond in vivo to yield aflatoxin B_1 and the epoxidation of the latter compound. Appreciable formation of aflatoxin B_2 from aflatoxin B_1 occurs with duck liver homogenates (69), and aflatoxin B_2 has about one-fifth the toxicity of aflatoxin B_1 for day-old ducklings. Injection of aflatoxin B_2 into rats yielded about 1% as much hepatic nucleic acid-aflatoxin adduct as did the injection of aflatoxin B_1; the major adduct isolated from the nucleic acids was the same as that formed from aflatoxin

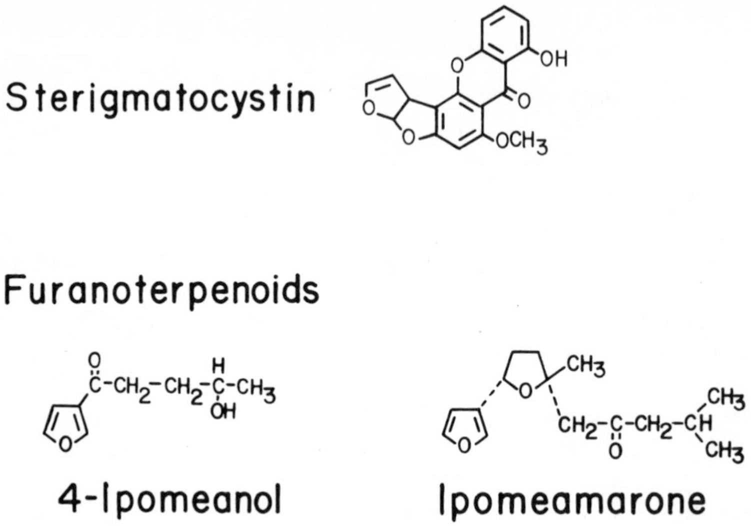

Sterigmatocystin

Furanoterpenoids

4-Ipomeanol

Ipomeamarone

Figure 5.   The structures of sterigmatocysin and of the furanoterpenoids 4-ipomeanol and ipomeamarone.

B_1(60). Aflatoxin B_2 has about 1% of the carcinogenic activity of aflatoxin B_1 in the rat (70).

The metabolism of aflatoxin B_1 at sites on the molecule other than the 2,3 double bond yields derivatives (Figure 3) that are less toxic and less mutagenic (71). Aflatoxicol, formed by reduction of the ketone in the terminal ring to an alcohol, has about one-quarter of the mutagenicity of aflatoxin B_1 for *S. typhimurium* TA98. This metabolite can be oxidized by animal tissues to aflatoxin B_1 and has been suggested as a reservoir of potentially active aflatoxin in the body (72). Aflatoxin M_1, aflatoxicol H_1, and aflatoxin Q_1 were each no more than 3% as mutagenic as aflatoxin B_1 (71). Aflatoxin P_1 and aflatoxin B_{2a} had no detectable mutagenicity. In rats the chronic toxicity of aflatoxin M_1 was similar to that of aflatoxin B_1, but little or no carcinogenic activity was evident in the rat (73). The latter metabolite showed hepatotoxicity and hepatocarcinogenicity similar to that of aflatoxin B_1 in rainbow trout (74).

Sterigmatocystin and Other Furan Derivatives Sterigmatocystin (Figure 5) (75, 76) and several related unsaturated bifuran derivatives are products of several *Aspergillus* and *Penicillium* species. Sterigmatocystin is formed by these molds under conditions favoring the formation of the aflatoxins and can occur at significant levels in foods; its possible role as a human carcinogen has been discussed (76). Sterigmatocystin is acutely hepatotoxic to young ducklings, has approximately one-tenth of the hepatocarcinogenic activity of aflatoxin B_1 when administered orally to rats (77), and induced hepatic damage and hepatic tumors in monkeys (76). Sterigmatocystin is also mutagenic for *S. typhimurium* TA98 and TA100 in the

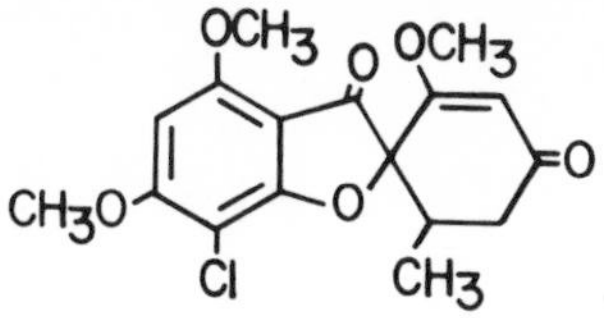

Figure 6.   The structure of griseofulvin.

presence of a NADPH-supplemented liver microsome system (41). The identity of the 2,3 unsaturated furanofuran portion of sterigmatocystin with that of aflatoxin B_1 and the need for metabolic activation by NADPH-fortified hepatic microsomes for its mutagenic activity strongly suggest that sterigmatocystin-2,3-oxide is an ultimate carcinogenic and mutagenic form.

Damaged sweet potatoes *(Ipomoea batatas),* especially those infected with *Fusarium solani,* synthesize a series of toxic unsaturated furanoid metabolites (78) (Figure 5). The marked pulmonary toxicity of the damaged sweet potatoes has been ascribed to a group of four 1,4-dioxygenated-1-(3-furyl)-pentanes (4-ipomeanol, 1-ipomeanol, ipomeanine, and 1,4-ipomeadiol). The hepatoxicity that sometimes occurs appears to be due to the presence of ipomeamarone, a known liver toxin. Occasional nephrotoxicity has been ascribed to 1-ipomeanol and 1,4-ipomeadiol. The toxicity of 4-ipomeanol for the liver and lungs of rats depends on the NADPH-dependent mixed function oxidases of the tissues and is correlated with the extent of binding of the toxin to liver and lung tissues (79–81). In view of these structural and metabolic similarities of the sweet potato toxins to the aflatoxins and sterigmatocystin and because of their occurrence in some marketable sweet potatoes (78), these toxins should be investigated for their possible carcinogenic activities.

Griseofulvin   Griseofulvin (Figure 6) (82, 83) and several of its ring-substituted derivatives are produced by certain *Penicillium* species. The continuous administration of 0.1–1% of griseofulvin in the diet of mice increased the incidence of skin tumors that formed as a result of topical application of the synthetic carcinogen 3-methylcholanthrene (84). Chronic feeding of 0.05–1% of griseofulvin to adult male mice or the subcutaneous injection (total dose, 3 mg) in male preweanling mice yielded liver tumors many months later (85–87). Griseofulvin has been administered in large oral doses for prolonged periods in the therapy of several serious human cutaneous mycoses, but we are unaware of data on its possible occurrence in foods or on adverse effects in humans.

Luteoskyrin and Cyclochlorotine (Yellow Rice Toxins)   Stored rice is quite susceptible to contamination by many fungi, especially *Penicillium* and *Aspergillus* species. The yellow rice that resulted from contamination by *Penicillium islandicum* Sopp caused acute hepatic toxicity and, on chronic administration, hepatic tumors in both rats and mice. The toxicity was found to be largely due to the fungal products luteoskyrin and cyclochloro-

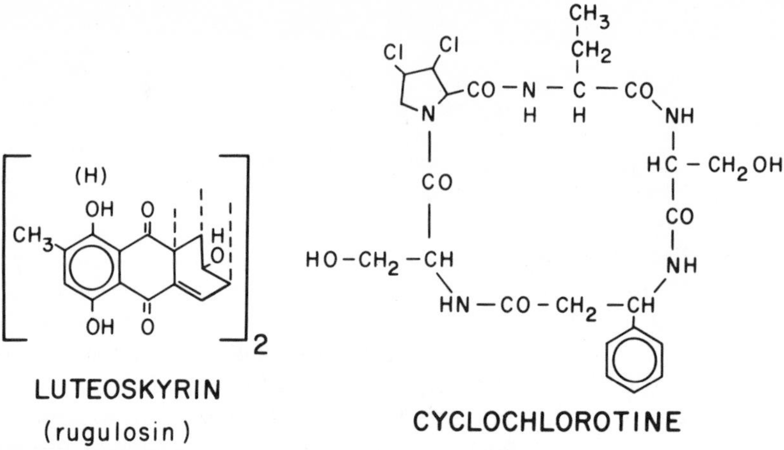

LUTEOSKYRIN
(rugulosin)

CYCLOCHLOROTINE

Figure 7.   The structures of luteoskyrin (rugulosin) and cyclochlorotine.

tine (Figure 7) (88–90). The latter compound was the more toxic and, at levels of 40–60 μg/day for 200 days, caused extensive cirrhosis in mice. Only a few tumors, hepatomas and reticuloendothelial tumors of the liver, were found. Luteoskyrin fed at a dose of 500 μg/day/mouse caused the development of hepatic tumors without cirrhosis within 6 months. Rugulosin, a structurally related mold metabolite, also appears to be hepatocarcinogenic (91).

Hydrazine Derivatives in Mushrooms   Gyromitrin (acetaldehyde *N*-methyl-*N*-formylhydrazone) (Figure 8) and its acid decomposition product, *N*-methyl-*N*-formylhydrazine, have been identified as major poisonous constituents (up to 0.3% and 0.05%, respectively, of the dry weight) of the mushroom *Gyromitra esculenta* (false morel) (92). This mushroom is said to be widely consumed in North American and Europe. Under acidic conditions gyromitrin decomposes via the formation of *N*-methyl-*N*-formylhydrazine to methylhydrazine (93). The half-life of gyromitrin at pH 2 is about 2 h, and methylhydrazine was detected in the stomach after oral administration of gyromitrin to mice. Methylhydrazine induces malignant histiocytomas in hamsters (94) and enhances the induction of lung adenomas in mice (95). Benign and malignant liver and lung tumors developed in mice after long-term administration of 0.008% of *N*-methyl-*N*-formylhydrazine in the drinking water (96). Cooking of the mushrooms in open kettles resulted in decomposition of the gyromitrin and volatilization of the methylhydrazine with a resultant reduction in the toxicity of the mushrooms (92).

The commercially cultivated mushroom *Agaricus bisporus* contains agaritine (β-*N*-(γ-L(+)-glutamyl)-4-hydroxymethylphenylhydrazine) (Figure 8) at levels up to 0.04% (97). Agaritine can be hydrolyzed to 4-hydroxymethylphenylhydrazine by γ-glutamyltransferase in the sporophores of the mushroom or by mild acid (98). Long-term administration of

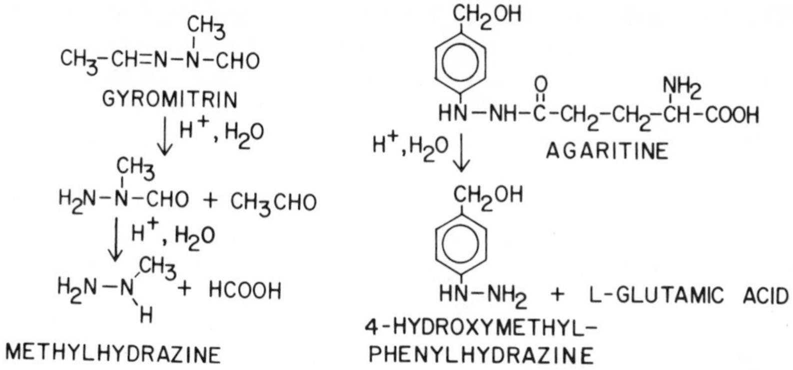

$$CH_3-CH=N-\underset{\underset{CH_3}{|}}{N}-CHO$$

GYROMITRIN

$$\downarrow H^+, H_2O$$

$$H_2N-\underset{\underset{CH_3}{|}}{N}-CHO + CH_3CHO$$

$$\downarrow H^+, H_2O$$

$$H_2N-\underset{\underset{H}{|}}{N}{}^{CH_3} + HCOOH$$

METHYLHYDRAZINE

$$HN-NH-\overset{O}{\overset{||}{C}}-CH_2-CH_2-\underset{\underset{NH_2}{|}}{CH}-COOH$$ AGARITINE

(ring substituent CH_2OH)

$$H^+, H_2O \downarrow$$

$$HN-NH_2 + \text{L-GLUTAMIC ACID}$$

(ring substituent CH_2OH)

4-HYDROXYMETHYL-
PHENYLHYDRAZINE

Figure 8.   The structures of two toxins from mushrooms capable of yielding carcinogenic hydrazines.

0.06% of N'-acetyl-4-(hydroxymethyl)-phenylhydrazine (which is more stable than the nonacetylated compound) in the drinking water of mice resulted in a significant increase in the incidence of lung adenomas and adenocarcinomas and of angiomas and angiosarcomas (97).

Ethyl Carbamate (Urethan)   Ethyl carbamate, $CH_3CH_2-O-CO-NH_2$ (99, 100), has been studied for many years as a synthetic carcinogen that induces tumors in a wide variety of tissues of the rat and mouse; the susceptible tissues include the lung, lymphoid tissue, skin, liver, mammary gland, and Zymbal's gland. In addition to its wide tissue range, this carcinogen has attracted interest because of the simplicity of its chemical structure and because of the much greater (> 100 times) carcinogenic activity of ethyl carbamate as compared to its alkyl homologs. Recent studies in our laboratory (101) have shown that vinyl carbamate, $CH_2=CH-O-CO-NH_2$, is 10–50 times more active than ethyl carbamate for the induction of lung adenomas and for the initiation of skin tumors in the mouse and that, unlike ethyl carbamate, vinyl carbamate is mutagenic for *S. typhimurium* TA100 in the presence of NADPH-fortified microsomes. The ethyl carbon atoms of ethyl carbamate become bound to the liver nucleic acids, but the metabolic intermediate(s) have not been identified (102–104). Ethylation of the phosphate backbone of DNA has been suggested as the major reaction (105, 106), but the lower binding of tritium than carbon-14 from [*ethyl*-1-^{14}C; 1,2-^{3}H]ethyl carbamate is inconsistent with this conclusion (101). Attempts to detect vinyl carbamate as a metabolite in mice have not been successful (101).

The finding of low levels of ethyl carbamate in wines treated with the synthetic sterilant diethyl pyrocarbonate (107), presumably from its reaction with ammonia, led to an investigation of the possible natural occurrence of ethyl carbamate. Detailed studies have shown that naturally fermented foods and beverages such as beers, wines, bread, yogurt, and soy sauce contain detectable but very low levels (usually less than 5μg/kg) of ethyl carbamate (108). A plausible source of the ethyl carbamate is through reaction of ethanol with carbamylphosphate in the yeasts (108). These levels of ethyl carbamate are very low in comparison with the usual levels for the induction of tumors in laboratory animals (frequently a single dose of 0.05–0.5 mg/g of body weight), and their significance to the human population is unknown.

Other Mold Metabolites   Ergot, the dried sclerotia of *Claviceps purpurea,* can contaminate rye and certain other grasses. Administration of ergot as 5% of the diet of rats for 2 years resulted in the development of multiple neurofibromas of the ears that disappeared when the feeding of the ergot was stopped; the tumors reappeared when ergot administration was resumed (109). Ergot contains many alkaloids and physiologically active substances, and there is no information on the metabolite responsible for development of the neurofibromas.

Several mold metabolites have induced sarcomas as a consequence of repeated injections into the subcutaneous tissues of rats. These include various lactones and related compounds, including patulin (110), penicillin G, and penicillic acid (111, 112). Crude extracts of some fungi pathogenic for the human have also induced sarcomas in mice with repeated subcutaneous doses (113).

A number of other mycotoxins have shown mutagenic or DNA-damaging activity (44, 91). These mold toxins include fusarenon X (a product of certain *Fusarium* species), PR toxin (formed by *Penicillium roqueforti*), chaetoglobosin A (from *Chaetomium globosum*), zearalenone and zearalenol-b (from *Fusarium graminearum*), and citrinin (from *Penicillium citrinum*). In a test in which 2 mg of PR toxin was injected subcutaneously into 15 adult male rats twice weekly for 7 weeks, two rats developed sarcomas at the injection site, two developed sarcomas at subcutaneous sites distant from the injection site, and one developed a hepatocellular carcinoma by the termination of the experiment at 19 months. Of 15 control rats that received only the solvent on the same schedule, one developed a malignant lymphoma (E. C. Miller, J. A. Miller, and F. M. Strong, unpublished data). Further studies on these mycotoxins are needed.

Actinomycete Metabolites

The following agents elaborated by various *Streptomyces* species (Figure 9) induce neoplasms in rats or mice when administered parenterally. Tests of these substances by the oral route are needed. Their possible occurrence in foods has not been evaluated.

Actinomycin D (Dactinomycin)   Actinomycin D (114), a cyclic polypeptide lactone-phenoxazone, forms a tight and specific complex with guanine residues in double-stranded DNA and is widely employed as an inhibitor of DNA-directed RNA synthesis. It has induced sarcomas in mice at the sites of repeated subcutaneous injections of small doses. Invasive mesotheliomas developed in rats that received repeated intraperitoneal doses that totaled a few hundred micrograms (115). In the latter experiment tumors

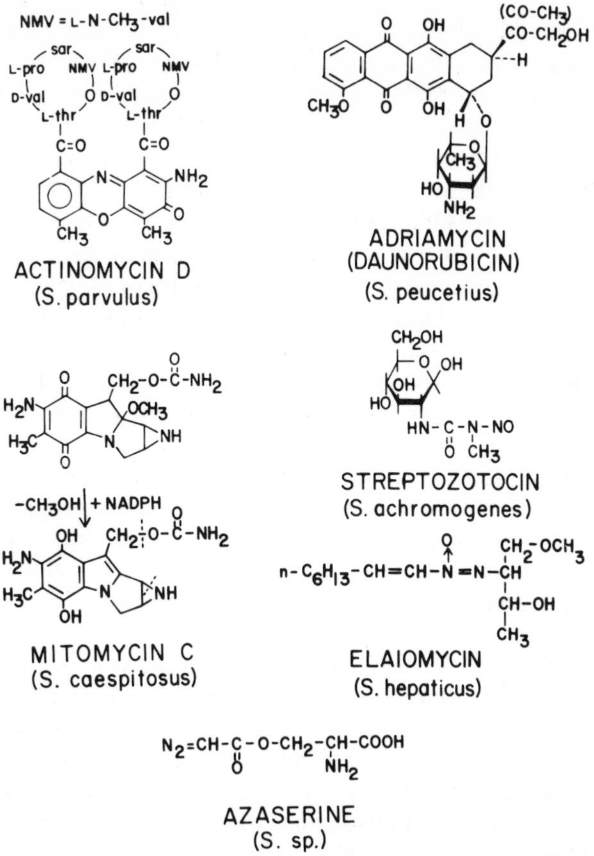

Figure 9.   The structures of some carcinogenic products of actinomycetes.

were not obtained on administration of actinocylgramicidin S, which has the same chromophore as actinomycin D with a different cyclic peptide and does not complex tightly with DNA. Repeated intragastric administration of actinomycin D (48 doses of 1 or 2 mg/kg) to rats did not result in tumors by 1 year (116).

   Adriamycin (Doxorubicin) and Daunorubicin (Daunomycin)   Adriamycin (117) and daunorubicin (118), metabolites of *Streptomyces peucetius,* have induced renal and mammary tumors on intravenous administration to rats (119–121). Adriamycin has also induced malignant transformation of mouse fibroblasts in culture (122). Both compounds are strong frameshift mutagens, and the mutagenicity and oncogenicity of adriamycin in cell culture are decreased on addition of hepatic microsomes (122). These findings, together with the very strong noncovalent binding of adriamycin to DNA, the inability to detect its covalent binding to DNA, and the very weak binding of this metabolite to RNA, suggest that the carcinogenic activity of adriamycin and daunorubicin could result from their noncovalent binding to

DNA. Recent studies showed that adriamycin and daunorubicin facilitate the noncovalent binding of actinomycin D to DNA (123); the possible effect of this interaction on the biological activities of these molecules has not been explored.

Mitomycin C   Repeated subcutaneous injections in mice of microgram quantities of the antibiotic mitomycin C (124) caused the development of sarcomas (125). Of possible importance in its carcinogenic activity is the susceptibility of mitomycin C to reduction by mammalian tissue preparations to a bifunctional alkylating agent that can cross-link DNA (126).

Streptozotocin and Elaiomycin   Streptozotocin (127) and elaiomycin (nitrosamide and azoxy compounds, respectively), like the plant metabolite cycasin (see below), are probably metabolized in vivo to alkylating species. Single intravenous injections in rats of streptozotocin, a metabolite of *Streptomyces achromogenes,* have induced high incidences of tumors of the kidney cortex or, with concurrent administration of nicotinamide, of the pancreas (128–131). Liver damage and benign liver tumors have also developed as a late sequel to streptozotocin administration to rats and Chinese hamsters (132, 133). Low incidences of tumors in a wide variety of tissues of rats were observed 1–2 years after intragastric or parenteral administration of elaiomycin (134).

Azaserine   Rats that received weekly intraperitoneal injections of 5–10 mg/kg of azaserine (*O*-diazoacetyl-*L*-serine) (135) for 6 months developed high incidences of tumors, including adenocarcinomas, of the pancreas and kidney, tissues in which azaserine is concentrated (136). The formation of hyperplastic nodules in the pancreas was potentiated by the administration of raw soya flour, which produces pancreatic hypertrophy (137). Azaserine is also a direct-acting mutagen (136).

Bacterial Metabolites (Ethionine)

Ethionine (138, 139), the *S*-ethyl analog of methionine, was originally synthesized as an antagonist of methionine. It is toxic to several rodent species, in which it causes morphological changes in the liver, pancreas, and other tissues; these changes can be prevented by the administration of methionine. Chronic feeding of 0.25% of ethionine in the diet of rats results in a high incidence of hepatocellular carcinomas (138). Ethionine is incorporated into protein in several tissues through the pathway normally used for the incorporation of methionine. Ethylation of the DNAs and RNAs, especially of tRNAs, occurs in the rat liver (140). Early evidence implicated *S*-adenosylethionine, a metabolite of ethionine, as the ethylating agent; however, more recent data suggest that other intermediates may be important in the in vivo ethylation of nucleic acids (141–143).

The study of ethionine as a synthetic carcinogen antedated the finding that it is a metabolite of several bacteria, including *Escherichia coli,* grown in a salts-glucose medium fortified with sulfate ion or methionine (144). We are

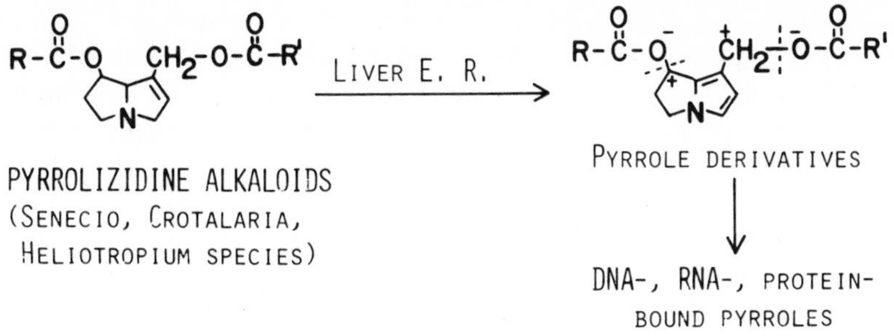

Figure 10.   The metabolic activation of pyrrolizidine alkaloids by the liver endoplasmic reticulum (ER) by dehydrogenation to electrophilic pyrrole derivatives.

not aware of any data on the extent to which the tissues of mammals may be exposed to ethionine formed by intestinal bacteria.

Use of Microbial Cells for Food

Microbial cells (algae, bacteria, and fungi) are being used in increasing amounts as sources of nutrients for both human and animal populations (145). While it is evident that these microorganisms might yield toxic metabolites during their growth, it is presumed that the production of these nutrients would be carried out under rigidly controlled conditions and that any adverse effects would be recognized during the long-term toxicology studies that are required for approval of such foods in the developed countries.

CARCINOGENESIS BY PLANT PRODUCTS

Pyrrolizidine Alkaloids

Pyrrolizidine alkaloids (146–149) occur in many plant species, including the *Senecio, Crotolaria, Heliotropium,* and other genera, in amounts from traces up to as much as 5% of the dry weight. While some pyrrolizidine alkaloids are relatively nontoxic, those members of this group that contain a nuclear double bond alpha to an esterified carbinol (Figure 10) are very potent liver and lung toxins for rodents and certain farm livestock (149). Large doses of these compounds cause acute necrotic and vascular lesions in the liver and lung as well as the development of very large hepatic parenchymal cells (megalocytes). Monocrotaline, retrorsine, lasiocarpine, and heliotrine, all of which are α,β unsaturated esters, are carcinogenic when administered to rats orally or parenterally under conditions that permit long-term survivals (150, 151). The tumors occur most frequently in the liver, but they are also found in a variety of other tissues, including the skin and lungs.

    Plants containing the pyrrolizidine alkaloids may contaminate forages and food grains, and the alkaloids they contain have caused acute and chronic poisoning of livestock in many parts of the world. Acute poisoning of humans from the ingestion of plants or plant extracts that contained the pyrrolizidine alkaloids has also apparently occurred (150). Humans may also be exposed to carcinogenic pyrrolizidine alkaloids through the use of certain herbs or drugs. Thus, the flowers or flower stalks of two varieties of colts-foot, which are used as drugs in the Orient and contain pyrrolizidine alkaloids, induced hemangioendothelial sarcomas in the livers of rats fed dried preparations (152, 153). Although the pyrrolizidine alkaloids have been suggested to have a role in the induction of human liver cancer in some parts of the world, there are no critical data to support this hypothesis (149).

The pyrrolizidine alkaloids are electrophilic at high pH, but their reactivity at neutrality is very low (146). However, the pyrrolizidine alkaloids are dehydrogenated by the mixed function oxidases in liver and lung with the formation of pyrrolic esters (154) (Figure 10). These metabolites have not been isolated, but their presence is inferred from their reactions with 4-dimethylaminobenzaldehyde and from their reaction products with nucleophiles both in vitro and in vivo (154). Their potent electrophilic reactivity makes the pyrrolic esters strong candidates for ultimate carcinogenic derivatives of the pyrrolizidine alkaloids. Synthetic pyrrole esters are short lived in aqueous solutions and are acutely toxic on administration to rats (155). While attempts to induce tumors with the pyrrole esters have been unsuccessful (quite likely because of their instabilities and toxicities), dehydroretronecine (a pyrrole alcohol) induced rhabdomyosarcomas at sites of repeated subcutaneous injections in rats (156).

Safrole and Related Allylic and Propenylic Benzenes

Numerous allylic and propenylic benzene derivatives (149, 157) occur in the essential oils from a wide variety of plants, and some of these plants or plant extracts are used as flavoring agents for human foods, for medicine, or for other purposes. The known naturally occurring allylic arenes include safrole (a major component of oil of sassafras), estragole (present in tarragon and anise), eugenol and acetyl eugenol (found in clove and cinnamon), and myristicin (a component of nutmeg, carrots, parsnips, and bananas) (Figure 11). Known naturally occurring propenylic arenes are cinnamaldehyde (present in cinnamon and cassia), anethole (found in fennel and anise), β-asarone (a major component of oil of calamus), and sinapaldehyde (obtained from wood lignin).

Of these derivatives, safrole (1-allyl-3,4-methylenedioxybenzene) (Figure 12) has received the most study. It was used as a synthetic flavoring agent in the United States prior to the report in 1960 that it caused hepatic damage and a low incidence of liver tumors when fed as 0.5% of the diet to adult rats (158). Safrole is also hepatocarcinogenic in male mice when administered prior to weaning (86, 159, 160). Estragole (1-allyl-4-methoxybenzene) has hepatocarcinogenic activity similar to that of safrole in mice

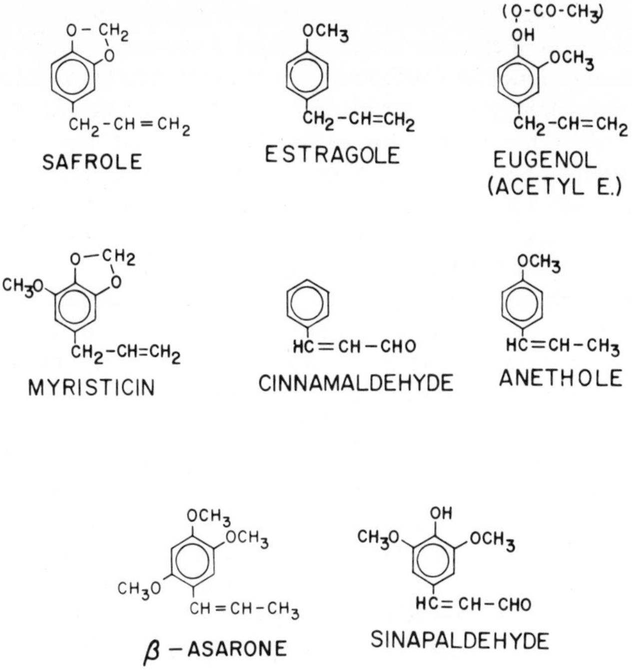

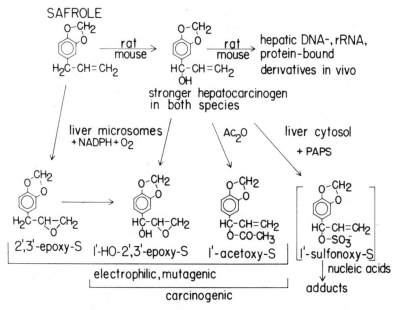

SAFROLE

ESTRAGOLE

EUGENOL (ACETYL E.)

MYRISTICIN

CINNAMALDEHYDE

ANETHOLE

β — ASARONE

SINAPALDEHYDE

Figure 11.   The structures of allylic and propenylic arenes that are products of certain plants.

SAFROLE

rat / mouse → ... rat / mouse → hepatic DNA-, rRNA, protein-bound derivatives in vivo

stronger hepatocarcinogen in both species

liver microsomes + NADPH + O_2

Ac_2O

liver cytosol + PAPS

2',3'-epoxy-S   1'-HO-2',3'-epoxy-S   1'-acetoxy-S   1'-sulfonoxy-S

electrophilic, mutagenic

carcinogenic

nucleic acids adducts

Figure 12.   The metabolic activation of safrole in rat and mouse liver to strong electrophiles.

treated prior to weaning, but its carcinogenicity has not been studied in adult animals (160). Oil of calamus, which contains β-asarone as a major component, induced mesenchymal tumors of the small intestine when fed to rats at a high level for long periods (161). The possible carcinogenicity of certain constituents of wood lignins, such as sinapaldehyde, has been suggested in view of their structural relationships to the above compounds and to 3,4,5-trimethoxycinnamaldehyde; the latter compound was inferred as a cause of nasal squamous cell carcinomas in two rats in a small experiment (162). Nasal tumors have been noted in certain workers exposed to wood dusts (163). A possible association has been noted in another study (164).

Both safrole and estragole are 1′-hydroxylated by rat and mouse liver, and both 1′-hydroxy derivatives are stronger carcinogens than the parent compounds (158–160) (Figure 12). Esterification of the 1′-hydroxy derivatives with acetic anhydride yields in each case an electrophilic ester (158, 160), and 1′-acetoxysafrole is more carcinogenic than safrole or 1′-hydroxysafrole at sites of application (subcutaneous site and forestomach) (159). There is no evidence for the metabolic formation of these acetic acid esters, but rat and mouse livers do synthesize small amounts of the strongly electrophilic ester 1′-sulfonoxysafrole from 1′-hydroxysafrole (165). Metabolic 2′,3′-epoxidation of safrole and estragole and of their 1′-hydroxy derivatives also occurs in rat liver cells or with NADPH-fortified rat or mouse liver microsomes (165–167). Mouse liver microsomes also 1′-hydroxylate the 2′,3′-epoxides of safrole and estragole (167). 1′-Hydroxysafrole-2′,3′-epoxide initiates papilloma formation on the skin of mice; safrole-2′,3′-epoxide, 1′-acetoxysafrole, and the other safrole derivatives studied were not active in this test (37). Of possible relevance to the latter observation is the finding that 1′-hydroxysafrole and 1′-hydroxyestragole are poor substrates for epoxide hydrase as compared to safrole- and estragole-2′,3′-oxide (167). The 1′-acetoxy derivatives of safrole and estragole and the 2′,3′-oxides of safrole and estragole and of their 1′-hydroxy metabolites are each mutagenic for the base substitution mutants S. typhimurium TA100 and/or TA1535 (37, 160, 167, 168).

Whether or not naturally occurring allylic and propenylic benzenes are important in the etiologies of any human cancers is unknown. The data for safrole and estragole indicate that the members of this class are very weak carcinogens as compared to the naturally occurring pyrrolizidine alkaloids and aflatoxins. However, the relatively large number of chemicals of these classes that occur in nature necessitates much further examination of the variety of compounds that exist and of their biological properties.

Cycasin

Cycasin (methylazoxymethanol-β-glucoside) (Figure 13) (169, 170) is one of the more potent plant carcinogens. This compound and at least one related glucoside (macrozamin, in which the sugar is 6-β-D-xylosido-D-glucose) oc-

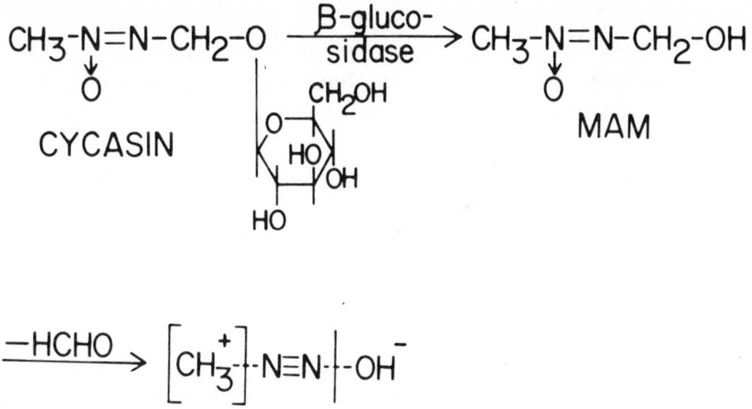

$$CH_3-N=N-CH_2-O \xrightarrow[\text{sidase}]{\beta\text{-gluco-}} CH_3-N=N-CH_2-OH$$

CYCASIN

MAM

$$\xrightarrow{-HCHO} \left[CH_3^+\right]-N\equiv N-\big|-OH^-$$

Figure 13.   The hydrolysis of cycasin to methylazoxymethanol (MAM) by β-glucosidase and the decomposition of methylazoxymethanol to a methylating moiety.

cur in the palmlike cycad trees of the family Cycadaceae. These fern trees have provided food for natives and their livestock in tropical and subtropical regions. The sliced nuts are generally extracted with water prior to use, but acute poisonings have been reported. No evidence has been presented for the carcinogenicity of cycasin in humans.

When administered orally, cycasin is highly carcinogenic for the liver and kidney of rats; it also induces tumors in other species (171). Rat tissues contain low levels of β-glucosidase, and the hydrolysis of cycasin generally depends on the action of intestinal bacteria (172). The product, methylazoxymethanol (MAM), decomposes at neutral pH to an electrophilic intermediate that methylates nucleic acids and proteins both in vitro and in vivo (173). These findings and the carcinogenic activity of methylazoxymethanol (171) have implicated the latter compound as a proximate carcinogenic metabolite of cycasin. The methylating species formed from methylazoxymethanol and cycasin appears to be similar to or identical with that formed in the metabolic activation of the synthetic carcinogen dimethylnitrosamine, and the latter compound has carcinogenic properties similar to those of cycasin (170).

Bracken Fern Toxin(s)

Consumption of bracken fern *(Pteridium aquilinum)* (174) has been known for at least 30 years to cause damage to the bone marrow and intestinal mucosa of cattle. The first evidence for its carcinogenic activity came in 1960 from the finding of polyps of the urinary bladder mucosa in cattle fed high levels of bracken fern for long periods. Since that time ingestion of large amounts of this plant has been noted to induce bladder carcinomas in cattle, urinary bladder carcinomas and intestinal adenocarcinomas in rats, urinary bladder tumors in guinea pigs, pulmonary adenomas in mice, and intestinal adenocarcinomas in Japanese quail (174). The greatest concentration of the toxin(s) occurs in young plants before the fronds have uncurled, and the carcinogenic activity is greatest for the rhizome, less for the stalk, and least in the young fronds. Cooking reduces, but does not eliminate, the toxicity of the fern.

The toxic and carcinogenic component(s) is extractable into methanol (174,175). A product identified as shikimic acid (3,4,5-trihydroxy-1-cyclo-hexene-1-carboxylic acid) was obtained from bracken fern extracts (174). In a limited study the same group of investigators reported the development of precancerous and cancerous lesions of the glandular gastric mucosa and leukemias with shikimic acid; confirmation of this result has not been reported. The latter workers also reported that a fraction not containing shikimic acid had strong carcinogenic activity. More recently, other investigators have reported the induction of intestinal carcinomas in mice with tannin-free aqueous and chloroform-soluble fractions (176). The latter fractions were not mutagenic, but rats given these fractions excreted mutagenic components in the urine.

Carcinogenic compounds are excreted in the milk and urine of cows fed high levels of bracken fern. Rats fed high levels of fresh or powdered milk from bracken fern–fed, but not normal, cows developed carcinomas of the intestine, urinary bladder, and kidney pelvis (177). Implantation of pellets made from cholesterol and extracts of the milk or urine from bracken fern-fed cows caused significant increases in the incidences of carcinomas of the urinary bladder of mice (177, 178).

Bracken fern is used as a human food in several parts of the world, especially in Japan (179). There is no evidence whether or not its ingestion contributes to the induction of human tumors.

Thiourea

Thiourea (180) occurs naturally in laburnum shrubs as well as in certain fungi (*Verticillium albo-atrum* and *Bortrylio cinerea*). Administration of 0.2% of thiourea in the drinking water or diet of rats for periods up to 2 years has resulted in tumors of the thyroid (181), hepatic adenomas (182), and epidermoid carcinomas arising from Zymbal's gland (183). Oral administration of thiourea to mice did not result in a significant tumor incidence, but it did result in the development of follicular cystic changes in the thyroid.

Coumarin

Coumarin (*o*-hydroxycinnamic acid-δ-lactone) (184), which occurs in a number of plants and their essential oils, such as woodruff, Tonka beans, and cassia, has induced bile duct carcinomas in rats fed 3500 or 5000 ppm in the diet for at least 18 months (185).

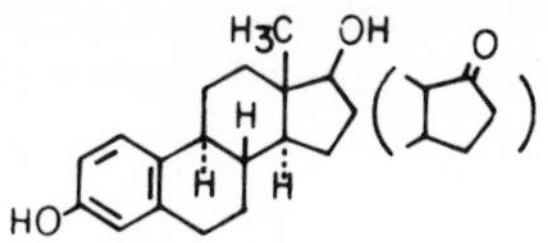

ESTRADIOL (ESTRONE)
(ANIMAL OVARIES, PALM
KERNELS-ESTRONE ONLY)

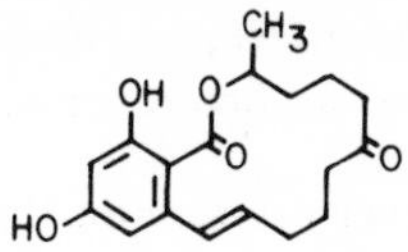

ZEARALENONE
(FUSARIUM MOLDS

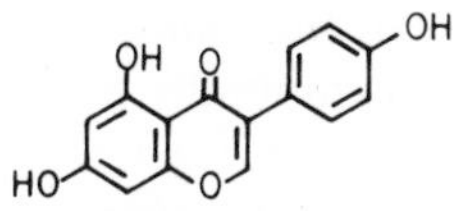

GENISTEIN AND OTHER FLAVONOIDS
(SOY BEANS, OTHER PLANTS)

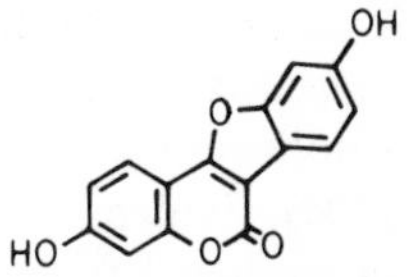

COUMESTROL
(ALFALFA, OTHER
FORAGE CROPS)

Figure 14.   The structures of some naturally occurring estrogenic compounds from plants, animals, and fungi.

Estrogenic Substances

In view of the effects of the repeated administration of large amounts of estrogens in the induction of hyperplasia and neoplasms in the mammary gland and uterus, concern has been expressed for possible carcinogenic hazards from estrogenic substances in plant materials (149, 186) (Figure 14). Although these plant estrogens are generally considerably less active than the animal estrogens, they occur in relatively large amounts and may contribute much more estrogenic activity to foods and feed than the very small amounts of estrogens in animal products. These plant estrogens include estrone in palm kernels, genistein in soy bean, clover, and other plants, coumestrol in alfalfa and other forage crops, and mirestrol in certain legumes. Zearalenone, a product of *Fusarium* molds that can infect grain, also possesses estrogenic activity.

Tannic Acid and Tannins

During World War II, liver damage was observed in humans treated with tannic acid (187) for burns. Subsequent studies showed that repeated subcutaneous injections into rats of a hydrolyzable tannin, gallotannic acid, led to hepatotoxicity and liver tumors (188). Similarly, three condensed nonhydrolyzable tannins produced liver tumors and sarcomas in mice at sites of repeated subcutaneous injections (189). High oral doses of gallotannic acid produced some early hepatic lesions in the livers of rats (188), but tumors have apparently not been induced by orally administered tannins. Beverages such as coffee, tea, and some clarets contain small amounts of tannins. The tannins are heterogeneous substances that are not well characterized (190).

Polycyclic Aromatic Hydrocarbons

Although attempts to detect the endogenous formation of carcinogenic polycyclic aromatic hydrocarbons (191) in animal tissues have been unsuccessful, certain hydrocarbons (e.g., benzo[a]pyrene and benz[a]anthracene) have been found in some plants and plant products at levels of a few parts per billion. Evidence has been presented for the synthesis of small amounts of these hydrocarbons by plants and algae (192, 193), and atmospheric pollution has been implicated as a source of crop contamination by polycyclic hydrocarbons (194). Evidence has also been presented for the synthesis of benzo[a]pyrene in sterilized forest soil inoculated with *Clostridium putride* or *E. coli* (195) and for the synthesis of benzo[a]pyrene and perylene in peptone broths supplemented with naphthalene acetic acid or vitamin K_1 and inoculated with *Bacillus badius* (196).

CARCINOGENESIS BY METABOLITES OF ANIMAL TISSUES

Metabolites of Tryptophan

The increased incidences of tumors of the urinary bladder in rats fed 2-acetylaminofluorene with high levels of tryptophan or indole and the carcinogenic activities of a variety of aromatic amines led to the idea that aromatic amine metabolites of tryptophan might be carcinogenic (197). 3-Hydroxykynurenine, 3-hydroxyanthranilic acid, 2-amino-3-hydroxyacetophenone, and xanthurenic acid-8-methyl ether induced tumors when implanted as pellets in the urinary bladders of mice, but, with the exception of the latter compound, no evidence has been presented for their carcinogenicity in other systems. Dogs fed high levels of tryptophan for long periods developed hyperplasia of the urinary bladder (198), and tryptophan administered after a subcarcinogenic dose of a nitrofuran promoted bladder tumor formation (199). Attempts to relate the development of carcinomas of the human urinary bladder to abnormalities in tryptophan metabolism have not been definitive (197).

Hormones

A number of endogenous protein and steroid hormones are clearly implicated in the development of tumors of the endocrine glands in experimental animals. In view of the very small amounts of hormones in most animal tissues consumed by human populations, hormones from such food sources appear to have little or no significance for the development of human cancer. Accordingly, this subject is not considered here. Reviews on the roles of hormones as etiologic agents in neoplasia (200, 201) provide the interested reader with an entry to this subject.

CARCINOGENIC METALS OR METAL IONS

Certain metal ions (Co^{2+}, Ni^{2+}, Cd^{2+}, Be^{2+}, Pb^{2+}, CrO_4^{2-}) and, possibly, some inorganic arsenic compounds can be viewed as carcinogens that occur naturally in the environment. These inorganic chemicals occur at various levels in foods derived from microorganisms, plants, and animals, but the levels required for the induction of tumors appear to be much greater than the amounts that occur naturally in foods. Furthermore, the induction of tumors by these agents has usually been through administration by parenteral routes, rather than orally. Carcinogenesis by these compounds has been reviewed recently (5, 6, 17, 18, 202–205). This subject is not considered here except to note that the abilities of metal ions to alter the fidelity of DNA synthesis in cells have been suggested as the basis for their carcinogenic and mutagenic activities (206).

CARCINOGENS FORMED DURING PROCESSING OR COOKING OF FOOD

Polycyclic Aromatic Hydrocarbons

In addition to the trace amounts of certain carcinogenic polycyclic aromatic hydrocarbons found in plants and soil as a consequence of endogenous synthesis or environmental contamination (see above), these carcinogens can also be formed at low levels during the cooking of food (191). Broiling of meat directly above burning fuel is apparently the major cooking method that leads to the formation of the hydrocarbons. The contents of benzo[a]-pyrene and of other hydrocarbons were reduced when the meat was cooked at some distance from the flame, at a lower temperature, or with separation of the dripping fat from the flame (207). Similarly, benzo[a]pyrene content of smoked meat was reduced by about 65% if the meat was wrapped in cellulose prior to smoking (208).

The levels of the carcinogenic polycyclic aromatic hydrocarbons in foods are low, and there are no data that implicate dietary intake of the hydrocarbons in the development of human cancer. Nevertheless, in view of the high potencies of many of the hydrocarbons as carcinogens (209), it is only prudent to reduce the formation of these products to the extent that is practical.

Mutagens Formed from Charred Proteins or Amino Acids

Smoke condensates from meat broiled directly over an open fire and the charred flesh have recently been found to contain mutagenic derivatives (49, 210). Further study showed that mutagenic constituents were formed by the pyrolysis ($> 400°C$) of a variety of proteins or of certain amino acids, but not on pyrolysis of carbohydrates, nucleic acids, or vegetable oils (49, 211). The yield of mutagens was greatest on the pyrolysis of tryptophan, and the major mutagenic constituents were characterized as 3-amino-1,4-dimethyl-

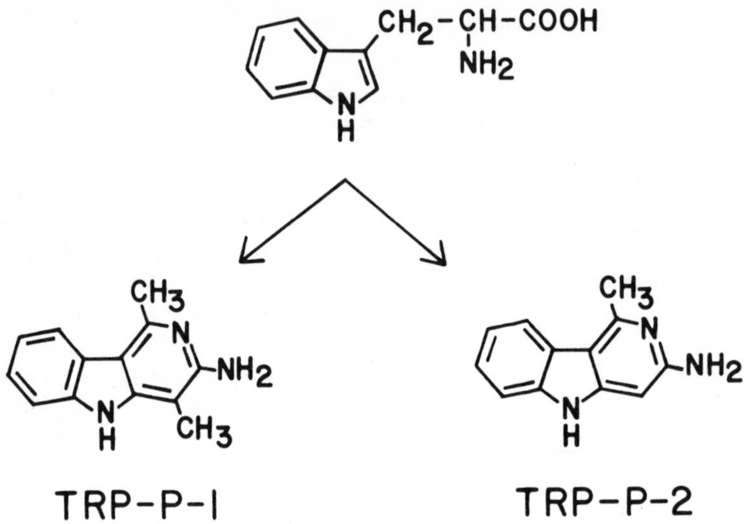

Figure 15.   The structures of Trp-P-1 and Trp-P-2, two mutagenic compounds formed on pyrolysis of tryptophan.

5H-pyrido(4,3-b)-indole   (TRP-P-1)   and   3-amino-1-methyl-5H-pyrido (4,3-b)-indole (TRP-P-2) (212) (Figure 15). Both of these tryptophan pyrolysis products also induced morphological transformation of hamster embryo cells (213). 2-Amino-5-phenylpyridine was isolated as a mutagenic pyrolysis product of phenylalanine (212).

Commoner and his associates (214) have reported on the formation of mutagen(s) on cooking beef at normal frying temperatures without charring.

NITROSAMINES AND NITROSAMIDES AS POTENTIAL CARCINOGENS FORMED IN FOOD OR IN VIVO

Studies on the biological properties of the nitrosamines followed the finding in the 1950s that dimethylnitrosamine caused hepatotoxicity in industrially exposed workers. Experimental studies soon showed that many dialkylnitrosamines, alkylnitrosamides, and alkylnitrosimides are strong carcinogens and/or mutagens under a wide variety of conditions (170, 215). The dialkylnitrosamines require metabolic activation to mutagenic substances, whereas the nitrosamides and nitrosimides are activated by nonenzymic reactions with cellular nucleophiles such as water and glutathione (Figure 16).

Within the past decade concern has been directed to the possible roles of N-nitroso compounds in the etiologies of human cancers in nonindustrial situations (216, 217). An outbreak of serious liver disease in sheep fed fish meal preserved with nitrite stimulated research on the possible occurrence of nitrosamines in foods used for human consumption. The formation of occa-

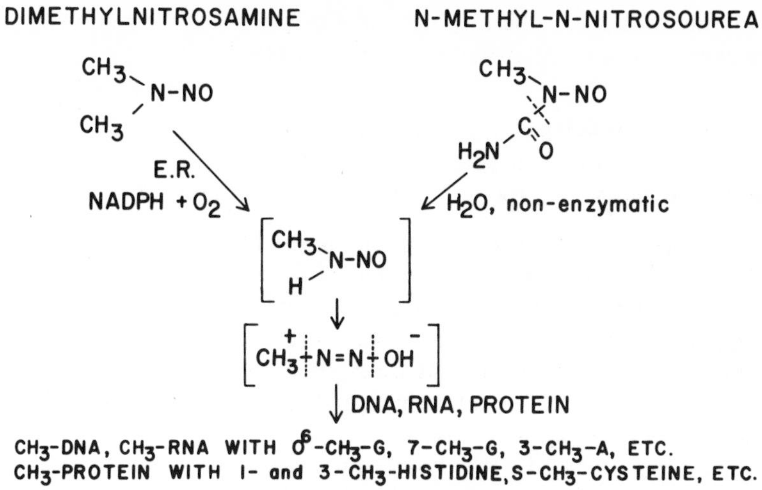

DIMETHYLNITROSAMINE   N-METHYL-N-NITROSOUREA

Figure 16. The activation of dimethylnitrosamine and N-methyl-N-nitrosourea to electrophilic reactants.

sional low levels of dimethylnitrosamine (10 ppb or lower) has been well documented in bacon, hams, and other nitrite-preserved meats (170). N-Nitrosoproline, a compound not shown to be carcinogenic, also occurs in these meats. The latter compound undergoes decarboxylation on heating to yield the carcinogen N-nitrosopyrrolidine, which has been found in cooked, but not raw, bacon (218). Very low levels of nitrosamines have also been reported in a variety of other food products, including cheese, flour, mushrooms, etc. (170).

More concern has been directed to the possible formation in vivo of nitrosamines or nitrosamides from ingested nitrite or nitrate and amines or amides from foods or orally administered drugs. The effects of the concentrations of the reactants and of pH on the nitrosation reactions have been studied in considerable detail, and tumors have been induced in experimental animals given high doses of amine or amide and nitrite simultaneously (219). The levels of nitrite in food are generally very low, but the levels of nitrate may be quite high. Thus, nitrate occurs in water supplies and in almost all vegetable material. Particularly high concentrations of nitrate may occur in leafy vegetables, beets, radishes, carrots, and potatoes (220). The nitrate is readily absorbed from the stomach, circulates in the blood, and is excreted in the saliva. Bacteria in the mouth reduce the nitrate to nitrite, and the nitrite-containing saliva reaches the stomach on being swallowed (220).

There is also concern that N-nitroso compounds may be formed in the human at sites other than the stomach. Recently, mutagenic compounds have been found in some human feces and have been characterized as N-nitroso derivatives (221). Preliminary data show that the levels of these fecal mutagens are reduced under dietary conditions (high fiber, low fat, and low protein) that have been epidemiologically correlated with lower risk to the development of colorectal cancer (222, 223).

OVERALL ASSESSMENT OF NATURALLY OCCURRING CARCINOGENS AND CARCINOGEN PRECURSORS IN THE CAUSATION OF HUMAN CANCER

Much more research is needed to permit an evaluation of the importance of the naturally occurring carcinogens in the development of human cancers. As discussed earlier, the likelihood of the initiation of cancer as a consequence of exposure to a carcinogen depends, as a minimum, on the amount of carcinogen to which the tissues are exposed, the capacities of the tissues to activate and inactivate the carcinogen, and the potencies of the ultimate carcinogenic electrophilic metabolites. The likelihood of the initiation of cancer may also be influenced by the levels of noncritical nucleophilic acceptors in the cells, but these levels probably do not vary markedly from population to population. The development of gross cancers may also be a function of the promoting stimuli to which the initiated cells are exposed and, in some cases, the hormonal environment.

From the foregoing discussion the exposures of most immediate interest to the human population should be those to chemicals known to be potent carcinogens in laboratory animals, especially if the data indicate that human tissues can activate these carcinogens to strong electrophilic reactants (e.g., mutagenicity and related tests) or if they are known to be toxic in humans. Among the mold contaminants the aflatoxins and sterigmatocystin are of particular importance. They are very potent carcinogens in laboratory animals. Aflatoxin contamination of food has caused acute hepatotoxicity in humans, and there are correlations that strongly indicate that the level of aflatoxin exposure is related to the incidence of hepatocellular carcinomas in some human populations (see above). Furthermore, the epidemiologic data provide rough estimates of the levels of aflatoxin exposure that may be associated with the development of hepatic tumors. In spite of our ignorance of the shape of the dose-response curve at very low levels of exposure, these data may be helpful in providing very rough, but reasoned, extrapolations to the possible risks to human populations from the contamination of certain foods where complete elimination is not now technologically or economically practical (224).

Similarly, the toxicities of the pyrrolizidine alkaloids and of the active constituents of bracken fern for farm animals provide evidence that the human intakes of these constituents should be as low as possible. Data on the abilities of human liver preparations to activate these compounds to mutagens might facilitate the estimation of reasonable "permitted" levels, if this appears necessary.

The possible exposures to nitrosamines and nitrosamides, both from natural occurrence and from other sources, have created much interest and concern, since many N-nitroso compounds have high carcinogenic potencies. This situation is even more complicated than those discussed above because of the variety of nitrosated products that might be formed and their range of potencies. Furthermore, the data on the exposures of human populations are limited. There are no generally accepted data that relate exposures to N-nitroso compounds to the development of particular cancers in the human, although both cancer of the stomach and cancer of the colon and rectum are suspected of having such an etiologic relationship because of the possible synthesis of N-nitroso derivatives in the gastrointestinal tract.

On the other hand, safrole and estragole, two naturally occurring arylalkenes, have only weak carcinogenic activities for the rat and mouse. Furthermore, the possible exposures of human populations to arylalkenes from the consumption of essential oils or other plant products appear to be quite low. Thus, the carcinogenic hazard to human populations from naturally occuring arylalkenes seems to be very low, and extreme efforts to reduce exposures of human populations to these compounds do not seem warranted. This evaluation could, however, change rapidly if more carcinogenic members of this class were found in human food sources or if some foods used in large amounts were found to contain much higher levels than are presently recognized.

There is a strong consensus for the desirability of eliminating possible carcinogenic hazards from our food supplies, as witnessed by the concern for the presence of pesticide residues or residues of diethylstilbestrol. Jukes (186) has discussed the unlikelihood of carcinogenic hazards to human populations from the minute residues of diethylstilbestrol that can occur in meat products in comparison to the much larger quantities of estrogens synthesized by the individual. Where there is reason to suspect that some foods contain carcinogens at levels that may increase the human cancer burden, approaches to protection are of great importance. However, attempts to provide absolute protection against cancer for the human population are not scientifically valid or possible. Furthermore, insistence on this level of protection is not consistent with the other risks that all members of the human population take in their daily activities (225, 226).

An important concern in the evaluation of possible carcinogenic hazards is the presumed greater susceptibility to chemical carcinogens of some segments of the population as compared to others. Experimental studies have clearly indicated that in utero or neonatal animals are much more susceptible to certain carcinogens than are older animals of the same species (227, 228). Likewise, individuals with genetic susceptibilities for tumor development (229, 230), those with poor immune capacity (231), and those with impaired capacity for the repair of carcinogen-induced damage (232) may be much more susceptible than others to the adverse effects of low levels of carcinogenic chemicals. Prudent evaluations of hazards for the general population should not put such individuals at great excess risks from cancer. These situations clearly require more study and, as susceptible populations are identified, it may be necessary to provide special standards for their protection. Such extra concern will be important not only with regard to their food supplies, but also to many other aspects of their daily activities.

ADDENDUM

The Ninth International Symposium of the Princess Takamatsu Cancer Research Fund was held January 23–25, 1979, in Tokyo, Japan, to consider "Naturally Occurring Carcinogens — Mutagens and Modulators of Carcinogenesis." The published proceedings of this symposium (233) provide an updating of some of the material presented in this paper. In addition to presenting data on the various naturally occurring carcinogens, the symposium talks presented considerable new data on the pyrolysis products formed from amino acids and on the probable roles of N-nitroso derivatives formed in the gastrointestinal tract in human carcinogenesis. Data were also presented on the relative risks for the development of some human cancers in relation to the consumption of certain foods by Japanese populations.

REFERENCES

1. Becker, F. F. (ed.). (1975). Cancer: A Comprehensive Treatise, Vols. 1, 2, and 3. Plenum Press Publishing Corp., New York.
2. Holland, J. M., and Frei, E. (eds.). (1973). Cancer Medicine. Lea and Febiger, Philadelphia.
3. Hiatt, H. H., Watson, J. D., and Winsten, J. A. (eds.). (1977). Origins of Human Cancer, Books A, B, and C. Cold Spring Harbor Laboratory, Cold Spring Harbor, New York.
4. Searle, C. E. (ed.). (1976). Chemical Carcinogenesis. A.C.S. Monograph No. 173. American Chemical Society, Washington, D. C.
5. Hernberg, S. (1977). In H. H. Hiatt, J. D. Watson, and J. A. Winsten (eds.), Origins of Human Cancer, Book A, p. 147. Cold Spring Harbor Laboratory, Cold Spring Harbor, New York.
6. Sunderman, F. W., Jr. (1971). Food Cosmet. Toxicol. 9:105.
7. Stanton, M. F., and Wrench, C. (1972). J. Natl. Cancer Inst. 48:797.
8. Brand, K. G. (1975). In F. F. Becker (ed.), Cancer: A Comprehensive Treatise, Vol. 1, p. 485. Plenum Press Publishing Corp., New York.
9. IARC Monogr. Eval. Carcinog. Risk Chem. Man. (1974). 4:97.
10. IARC Monogr. Eval. Carcinog. Risk Chem. Man. (1972). 1:80.
11. IARC Monogr. Eval. Carcinog. Risk Chem. Man. (1972). 1:74.
12. IARC Monogr. Eval. Carcinog. Risk Chem. Man. (1974). 4:231.
13. IARC Monogr. Eval. Carcinog. Risk Chem. Man. (1975). 9:181.
14. IARC Monogr. Eval. Carcinog. Risk Chem. Man. (1974). 7:291.
15. IARC Monogr. Eval. Carcinog. Risk Chem. Man. (1973). 3:22.
16. Kipling, M. D. (1976). In C. E. Searle (ed.), Chemical Carcinogens, A.C.S. Monograph No. 173, p. 315. American Chemical Society, Washington, D. C.

17. IARC Monogr. Eval. Carcinog. Risk Chem. Man. (1973). 2:100.
18. IARC Monogr. Eval. Carcinog. Risk Chem. Man. (1973). 2:126.
19. IARC Monogr. Eval. Carcinog. Risk Chem. Man. (1977). 14:106.
20. IARC Monogr. Eval. Carcinog. Risk Chem. Man. (1974). 4:119.
21. IARC Monogr. Eval. Carcinog. Risk Chem. Man. (1974). 6:55.
22. Hammond, E. C. (1966). Natl. Cancer Inst. Monogr. 19:127.
23. Muir, C. S., and Kirk, R. (1960). Br. J. Cancer 14:597.
24. Miller, J. A. (1970). Cancer Res. 30:559.
25. Miller, J. A., and Miller, E. C. (1977). In H. H. Hiatt, J. D. Watson, and J. A. Winsten (eds.), Origins of Human Cancer, Book B, p. 605. Cold Spring Harbor Laboratory, Cold Spring Harbor, New York.
26. Miller, E. C. (1978). Cancer Res. 38:1479.
27. Berenblum, I. (1974). Carcinogenesis as a Biological Problem. Elsevier-North Holland Publishing Company, New York.
28. Boutwell, R. K. (1974). Crit. Rev. Toxicol. 2:419.
29. Van Duuren, B. L. (1976). In C. E. Searle (ed.), Chemical Carcinogens, A.C.S. Monograph No. 173, p. 24. American Chemical Society, Washington, D. C.
30. Slaga, T. J., Sivak, A., and Boutwell, R. K. (eds.). (1978). Mechanisms of Tumor Promotion and Cocarcinogenesis. Raven Press, New York.
31. Weisburger, J. H., and Weisburger, E. K. (1967). In H. Busch (ed.), Methods in Cancer Research, Vol. 1, p. 307. Academic Press, Inc., New York.
32. Weisburger, J. H. (1976). In C. E. Searle (ed.), Chemical Carcinogens, A.C.S. Monograph No. 173, p. 1. American Chemical Society, Washington, D. C.
33. Guess, H., Crump, K., and Peto, R. (1977). Cancer Res. 37:3475.
34. Sporn, M. B., Dunlop, N. M., Newton, D. L., and Smith, J. M. (1976). Fed. Proc. 35:1332.
35. Sporn, M. B. (1977). In H. H. Hiatt, J. D. Watson, and J. A. Winsten (eds.), Origins of Human Cancer, Book B, p. 801. Cold Spring Harbor Laboratory, Cold Spring Harbor, New York.
36. Wattenberg, L. W. (1978). J. Natl. Cancer Inst. 60:11.
37. Wislocki, P. G., Miller, E. C., Miller, J. A., McCoy, E. C., and Rosenkranz, H. S. (1977). Cancer Res. 37:1883.
38. Kimura, N. T., Kanematsu, T., and Baba, T. (1976). Z. Krebsforsch. 87:257.
39. Peraino, C., Fry, R. J. M., Staffeldt, E., and Kisieleski, W. E. (1973). Cancer Res. 33:2701.
40. Stoltz, D. R., Poirier, L. A., Irving, C. C., Stich, H. F., Weisburger, J. H., and Grice, H. C. (1974). Toxicol. Appl. Pharmacol. 29:157.
41. McCann, J., Choi, E., Yamasaki, E., and Ames, B. N. (1975). Proc. Natl. Acad. Sci. USA 72:5135.
42. McCann, J., and Ames, B. N. (1976). Proc. Natl. Acad. Sci. USA 73:950.
43. Purchase, I. F. H., Longstaff, E., Ashby, J., Styles, J. A., Anderson, D., Lefevre, P. A., and Westwood, F. R. (1978). Br. J. Cancer 37:873.
44. Sugimura, T., Nagao, M., Kawachi, T., Honda, M., Yahagi, T., Seino, Y., Sato, S., Matsukura, N., Matsushima, T., Shirai, A., Sawamura, M., and Matsumoto, H. (1977). In H. H. Hiatt, J. D. Watson, and J. A. Winsten (eds.), Origins of Human Cancer, Book C, p. 1561. Cold Spring Harbor Laboratory, Cold Spring Harbor, New York.
45. Miller, E. C., and Miller, J. A. (1971). In A. Hollaender (ed.), Chemical Mutagens — Principles and Methods for Their Detection, Vol. 1, p. 83. Plenum Publishing Corp., New York.
46. DiPaolo, J. A., Nelson, R. L., Donovan, P. J., and Evans, C. H. (1973). Arch. Pathol. 95:380.

47. Pienta, R. J., Poiley, J. A., and Lebherz, W. B., III. (1977). Int. J. Cancer 19:642.
48. Meselson, M., and Russell, K. (1977). *In* H. H. Hiatt, J. D. Watson, and J. A. Winsten (eds.), Origins of Human Cancer, Book C, p. 1473. Cold Spring Harbor Laboratory, Cold Spring Harbor, New York.
49. Sugimura, T., Sato, S., Nagao, M., Yahagi, T., Matsushima, T., Seino, Y., Takeuchi, M., and Kawachi, T. (1976). *In* P. N. Magee, S. Takayama, T. Sugimura, and T. Matsushima (eds.), Fundamentals in Cancer Prevention, p. 191. University of Tokyo Press, Tokyo.
50. Butler, W. H. (1974). *In* I. F. H. Purchase (ed.), Mycotoxins, p. 2. Elsevier-North Holland Publishing Company, New York.
51. Detroy, R. W., Lillehoj, E. B., and Ciegler, A. (1971). *In* A. Ciegler, S. Kadis, and S. J. Ajl (eds.), Microbial Toxins, Vol. VI, p. 3. Academic Press, Inc., New York.
52. IARC Monogr. Eval. Carcinog. Risk Chem. Man. (1976). 10:51.
53. Wogan, G. N. (1976). *In* H. M. Cameron, D. A. Linsell, and G. P. Warwick (eds.), Liver Cell Cancer, p. 121. Elsevier-North Holland Publishing Company, New York.
54. Lillehoj, E. B., Kowlek, W. F., Shannon, G. M., Shotwell, O. L., and Hesseltine, C. W. (1975). Cereal Chem. 52:603.
55. Krishnamachari, K. A. V. R., Bhat, R. V., Nagarajan, V., and Tilak, T. B. G. (1975). Ind. J. Med. Res. 63:1036.
56. Van Rensburg, S. J., Van der Watt, J. J., Purchase, I. F. H., Pereira Coutinho, L., and Markham, R. (1974). S. Afr. Med. J. 48:2508a.
57. Garner, R. C., Miller, E. C., and Miller, J. A. (1972). Cancer Res. 32:2058.
58. Schoenhard, G. L., Lee, D. J., Howell, S. E., Pawlowski, N. E., Libbey, L. M., and Sinnhuber, R. O. (1976). Cancer Res. 36:2040.
59. Swenson, D. H., Miller, E. C., and Miller, J. A. (1974). Biochem. Biophys. Res. Commun. 60:1036.
60. Swenson, D. H., Lin, J.-K., Miller, E. C., and Miller, J. A. (1977). Cancer Res. 37:172.
61. Swenson, D. H., Miller, J. A., and Miller, E. C. (1973). Biochem. Biophys. Res. Commun. 53:1260.
62. Lin, J.-K., Miller, J. A., and Miller, E. C. (1977). Cancer Res. 37:4430.
63. Essigmann, J. M., Croy, R. G., Nadzan, A. M., Busby, W. F., Jr., Reinhold, V. N., Buchi, G., and Wogan, G. N. (1977). Proc. Natl. Acad. Sci. USA 74:1870.
64. Martin, C. N., and Garner, R. C. (1977). Nature 267:863.
65. Croy, R. G., Essigmann, J. M., Reinhold, V. N., and Wogan, G. N. (1978). Proc. Natl. Acad. Sci. USA 75:1745.
66. Lin, J.-K., Kennan, K. A., Miller, E. C., and Miller, J. A. (1978). Cancer Res. 38:2424.
67. Swenson, D. H., Miller, J. A., and Miller, E. C. (1975). Cancer Res. 35:3811.
68. Garner, R. C., Nutman, C. A., Sunman, W., and Martin, C. N. (1978). Proc. Am. Assoc. Cancer Res. 19:171.
69. Roebuck, B. D., Siegel, W. G., and Wogan, G. N. (1978) . Cancer Res. 38:999.
70. Wogan, G. N., Edwards, G. S., and Newberne, P. M. (1971). Cancer Res. 31:1936.
71. Wong, J. J., and Hsieh, D. P. H. (1976). Proc. Natl. Acad. Sci. USA 73:2241.
72. Wong, Z. A., and Hsieh, D. P. H. (1978). Science 200:325.
73. Wogan, G. N., and Paglialunga, S. (1974). Food Cosmet. Toxicol. 12:381.
74. Sinnhuber, R. O., Lee, D. J., Wales, J. H., Landers, M. K., and Keyl, A. C. (1974). J. Natl. Cancer Inst. 53:1285.

75. IARC Monogr. Eval. Carcinog. Risk Chem. Man. (1976). 10:245.
76. van der Watt, J. J. (1974). *In* I. F. H. Purchase (ed.), Mycotoxins, p. 369. Elsevier-North Holland Publishing Company, New York.
77. Purchase, I. F. H., and van der Watt, J. J. (1970). Food Cosmet. Toxicol. 8:289.
78. Boyd, M. R., Burka, L. T., Harris, T. M., and Wilson, B. J. (1974). Biochim. Biophys. Acta 33:184.
79. Boyd, M. R. (1976). Toxicol. Appl. Pharmacol. 33:132.
80. Boyd, M. R. (1977). Proc. Am. Assoc. Cancer Res. 18:246.
81. Boyd, M. R., Burka, L. T., and Wilson, B. J. (1975). Toxicol. Appl. Pharmacol. 32:147.
82. IARC Monogr. Eval. Carcinog. Risk Chem. Man. (1976). 10:153.
83. Wilson, B. J. (1971). *In* A. Ciegler, S. Kadis, and S. J. Ajl (eds.), Microbial Toxins, Vol. 6, p. 460. Academic Press, Inc., New York.
84. Barich, L. L., Schwartz, J., and Barich, D. (1962). Cancer Res. 22:53.
85. Barich, L. L., Schwartz, J., and Barich, D. (1961). Antibiot. Chemother. 11:566.
86. Epstein, S. S., Fujii, K., Andrea, J., and Mantel, N. (1970). Toxicol. Appl. Pharmacol. 16:321.
87. Hurst, E. W., and Paget, G. E. (1963). Br. J. Dermatol. 75:105.
88. Enomoto, M., and Ueno, I. (1974). *In* I. F. H. Purchase (ed.), Mycotoxins, p. 303. Elsevier-North Holland Publishing Company, New York.
89. IARC Monogr. Eval. Carcinog. Risk Chem. Man. (1976). 10:163.
90. IARC Monogr. Eval. Carcinog. Risk Chem. Man. (1976). 10:139.
91. Ueno, Y., and Kubota, K. (1976). Cancer Res. 36:445.
92. Toth, B. (1975). Cancer Res. 35:3693.
93. Nagel, D., Wallcave, L., Toth, B., and Kupper, R. (1977). Cancer Res. 37:3458.
94. Toth, B. (1973). Cancer Res. 33:2744.
95. Toth, B. (1972). Int. J. Cancer 9:109.
96. Toth, B., and Nagel, D. (1978). J. Natl. Cancer Inst. 60:201.
97. Toth, B., Nagel, D., Patil, K., Erickson, J., and Antonson, K. (1978). Cancer Res. 38:177.
98. Levenberg, B. (1961). J. Am. Chem. Soc. 83:503.
99. Mirvish, S. S. (1968). Adv. Cancer Res. 11:1.
100. IARC Monogr. Eval. Carcinog. Risk Chem. Man. (1974). 7:111.
101. Dahl, G. A., Miller, J. A., and Miller, E. C. (1978). Cancer Res. 38:3793.
102. Lawson, T. A., and Pound, A. W. (1973). Chem. Biol. Interact. 6:99.
103. Boyland, E., and Williams, D. (1969). Biochem. J. 111:121.
104. Prodi, G., Rocchi, P., and Grilli, S. (1970). Cancer Res. 30:2887.
105. Pound, A. W., Franke, F., and Lawson, T. A. (1976). Chem. Biol. Interact. 14:149.
106. Lawson, T., and Pound, A. (1978). Proc. Am. Assoc. Cancer Res. 19:184.
107. Ehrenberg, L., Fedorcsák, I., and Solymosy, F. (1976). Prog. Nucleic Acid Res. Mol. Biol. 16:189.
108. Ough, C. S. (1976). J. Agric. Food Chem. 24:323.
109. Nelson, A. A., Fitzhugh, O. G., Morris, H. J., and Calvery, H. O. (1942). Cancer Res. 2:11.
110. IARC Monogr. Eval. Carcinog. Risk Chem. Man. (1976). 10:205.
111. Ciegler, A., Detroy, R. W., and Lillehoj, E. B. (1971). *In* A. Ciegler, S. Kadis, and S. J. Ajl (eds.), Microbial Toxins, Vol. 6, p. 409. Academic Press, Inc., New York.
112. IARC Monogr. Eval. Carcinog. Risk Chem. Man. (1976). 10:211.

113. Blank, F., Chin, O., Just, G., Meranze, D. R., Shimkin, M. B., and Wieder, R. (1968). Cancer Res. 28:2276.
114. IARC Monogr. Eval. Carcinog. Risk Chem. Man. (1976). 10:29.
115. Svoboda, D., Reddy, J., and Harris, C. (1970). Cancer Res. 30:2271.
116. Philips, F. S., and Sternberg, S. S. (1975). Recent Results Cancer Res. 52:29.
117. IARC Monogr. Eval. Carcinog. Risk Chem. Man. (1976). 10:43.
118. IARC Monogr. Eval. Carcinog. Risk Chem. Man. (1976). 10:145.
119. Bertazzoli, C., Chieli, T., and Socia, E. (1971). Experientia 27:1209.
120. Marquardt, H., Philips, F. S., and Sternberg, S. S. (1976). Cancer Res. 36:2065.
121. Sternberg, S. S., Philips, F. S., and Cronin, A. P. (1972). Cancer Res. 32:1029.
122. Marquardt, H., Baker, S., Grab, D., and Marquardt, H. (1977). Proc. Am. Assoc. Cancer Res. 18:13.
123. Krugh, T. R., and Young, M. A. (1977). Nature 269:627.
124. IARC Monogr. Eval. Carcinog. Risk Chem. Man. (1976). 10:171.
125. Ikegami, R., Akamatsu, Y., and Haruta, M. (1967). Acta Pathol. Jap. 17:495.
126. Szybalski, W., and Iyer, V. W. (1967). In D. Gottlieb and P. D. Shaw (eds.), Mechanisms of Action and Biosynthesis of Antibiotics, p. 211. Springer-Verlag Publishing Company, Berlin.
127. IARC Monogr. Eval. Carcinog. Risk Chem. Man. (1974). 4:221.
128. Arison, R. N., and Feudale, E. L. (1967). Nature 214:1254.
129. Mauer, S. M., Lee, C. S., Najarian, J. S., and Brown, D. M. (1974). Cancer Res. 34:158.
130. Rakieten, N., Gordon, B. S., Beaty, A., Cooney, D. A., Davis, R. D., and Schein, P. S. (1971). Proc. Soc. Exp. Biol. Med. 137:280.
131. Horton, L., Fox, C., Corrin, B., and Sönksen, P. H. (1978). Br. J. Cancer 36:692.
132. Berman, L. D., Hayes, J. A., and Sibay, T. M. (1973). J. Natl. Cancer Inst. 51:1287.
133. Feldman, S., Scharp, D., Hirshberg, G., Dodi, G., Ballinger, W., and Lacy, P. (1977). Transplantation 24:152.
134. Schoental, R. (1969). Nature 221:765.
135. IARC Monogr. Eval. Carcinog. Risk Man. (1976). 10:73.
136. Longenecker, D. S., and Curphey, T. J. (1975). Cancer Res. 35:2249.
137. Morgan, R. G., Levinson, H., Hopwood, D. A., Hopwood, D., Saunders, J. H. B., and Wormsley, K. G. (1977). Cancer Lett. 3:87.
138. Farber, E. (1963). Adv. Cancer Res. 7:383.
139. Stekol, J. A. (1963). Adv. Enzymol. 25:369.
140. Swann, P. F., Pegg, A. E., Hawks, A., Farber, E., and Magee, P. N. (1971). Biochem. J. 123:175.
141. Brada, Z., Bulba, S., and Cohen, J. (1975). Cancer Res. 35:2674.
142. Ortwerth, B. J., and Novelli, G. D. (1969). Cancer Res. 29:380.
143. Pegg, A. E. (1972). Biochem. J. 128:59.
144. Fisher, J. F., and Mallette, M. F. (1961). J. Gen. Physiol. 45:1.
145. Litchfield, J. H. (1978). Chemtech. 8:218.
146. Bull, L. B., Culvenor, C. C. J., and Dick, A. T. (1968). The Pyrrolizidine Alkaloids. Elsevier-North Holland Publishing Company, New York.
147. IARC Monogr. Eval. Carcinog. Risk Chem. Man. (1976). 10:265.
148. McLean, E. K. (1970). Pharmacol. Rev. 22:429.
149. Schoental, R. (1976). In C. E. Searle (ed.), Chemical Carcinogens, A.C.S. Monograph No. 173, p. 626. American Chemical Society, Washington, D.C.
150. Schoental, R. (1968). Cancer Res. 28:2237.

151. Rao, M. S., and Reddy, J. K. (1978). Br. J. Cancer 37:289.
152. Hirono, I., Shimizu, M., Fushimi, K., Mori, H., and Kato, K. (1973). Gann 64:527.
153. Hirono, I., Mori, H., and Culvenor, C. C. J. (1976). Gann 67:125.
154. Mattocks, A. R. (1968). Nature 217:723.
155. Mattocks, A. R. (1970). Nature 228:174.
156. Allen, J. R., Hsu, I.-C., and Carstens, L. A. (1975). Cancer Res. 35:997.
157. IARC Monogr. Eval. Carcinog. Risk Chem. Man. (1976). 10:231.
158. Borchert, P., Wislocki, P. G., Miller, J. A., and Miller, E. C. (1973). Cancer Res. 33:575.
159. Borchert, P., Miller, J. A., Miller, E. C., and Shires, T. K. (1973). Cancer Res. 33:590.
160. Drinkwater, N. R., Miller, E. C., Miller, J. A., and Pitot, H. C. (1976). J. Natl. Cancer Inst. 57:1323.
161. Gross, M. A., Jones, W. I., Cook, E. L., and Boone, C. C. (1967). Proc. Am. Assoc. Cancer Res. 8:24.
162. Schoental, R., and Gibbard, S. (1972). Br. J. Cancer 26:504.
163. Acheson, E. D., Cowdell, R. H., Hadfield, E., and Macbeth, R. G. (1968). Br. Med. J. 2:587.
164. Brinton, L. A., Stone, B. J., Blot, W. J., and Fraumeni, J. F., Jr. (1976). Lancet 2:628.
165. Wislocki, P. G., Borchert, P., Miller, J. A., and Miller, E. C. (1976). Cancer Res. 36:1686.
166. Delaforge, M., Janiaud, P., Chessebeuf, M., Padieu, P., and Maume, B. F. *In* A. Frigerio and N. Castaginoli (eds.), Advances in Mass Spectrometry in Biochemistry and Medicine, Vol. 2. Spectrum Publications, New York. In press.
167. Swanson, A. B., Miller, E. C., and Miller, J. A. (1978). Fed. Proc. 37:1383.
168. Dorange, J.-L., Delaforge, M., Janiaud, P., and Padieu, P. (1977). C. R. Soc. Biol. 171:1041.
169. IARC Monogr. Eval. Carcinog. Risk Chem. Man. (1976). 10:121.
170. Magee, P. N., Montesano, R., and Preussman, R. (1976). *In* C. E. Searle (ed.), Chemical Carcinogens, A.C.S. Monograph No. 173, p. 491. American Chemical Society, Washington, D. C.
171. Laquer, G. L., and Spatz, M. (1968). Cancer Res. 28:2262.
172. Matsumoto, H., Nagata, Y., Nishimura, E. T., Bristol, R., and Habner, M. (1972). J. Natl. Cancer Inst. 49:423.
173. Matsumoto, H., and Higa, H. H. (1966). Biochem. J. 98:20C.
174. Evans, I. A. (1976). *In* C. E. Searle (ed.), Chemical Carcinogens, A.C.S. Monograph No. 173, p. 690. American Chemical Society, Washington, D. C.
175. Pamukcu, A. M., Price, J. M., and Bryan, G. T. (1970). Cancer Res. 30:902.
176. Hatcher, J., Pamukcu, A. M., Wang, C. Y., and Bryan, G. T. (1978). Proc. Am. Assoc. Cancer Res. 19:18.
177. Pamukcu, A. M., Erturk, E., Yalciner, S., Milli, U., and Bryan, G. T. (1978). Cancer Res. 38:1556.
178. Pamukcu, A. M., Olson, C., and Price, J. M. (1966). Cancer Res. 26:1745.
179. Pamukcu, A. M., Yalciner, S., Price, J. M., and Bryan, G. T. (1970). Cancer Res. 30:2671.
180. IARC Monogr. Eval. Carcinog. Risk Chem. Man. (1974). 7:95.
181. Purves, H. D., and Griesbach, W. E. (1947). Br. J. Exp. Pathol. 28:46.
182. Fitzhugh, O. G., and Nelson, A. A. (1948). Science 108:626.
183. Rosin, A., and Rachmilewitz, M. (1954). Cancer Res. 14:494.
184. IARC Monogr. Eval. Carcinog. Risk Chem. Man. (1976). 10:113.

185. Hagan, E. C., Hansen, W. H., Fitzhugh, O. G., Jenner, P. M., Jones, W. I., Taylor, J. M., Long, E. L., Nelson, A. A., and Brouwer, J. B. (1967). Food Cosmet. Toxicol. 5:141.
186. Jukes, T. H. (1977). *In* H. H. Hiatt, J. D. Watson, and J. A. Winsten (eds.), Origins of Human Cancer, Book C, p. 1657. Cold Spring Harbor Laboratory, Cold Spring Harbor, New York.
187. IARC Monogr. Eval. Carcinog. Risk Chem. Man. (1976). 10:253.
188. Korpassy, B. (1961). Prog. Exp. Tumor Res. 2:245.
189. Kirby, K. S. (1960). Br. J. Cancer 14:147.
190. Humphries, S. G. (1967). *In* P. Bernfeld (ed.), Biogenesis of Natural Compounds, Ed. 2, p. 801. Pergamon Press, Inc., Oxford.
191. Grasso, P., and O'Hare, C. (1976). *In* C. E. Searle (ed.), Chemical Carcinogens, A.C.S. Monograph No. 173, p. 701. American Chemical Society, Washington, D.C.
192. Borneff, J., Selenka, F., Kunte, H., and Maximos, A. (1968). Environ. Res. 2:22.
193. Gräf, W., and Nowak, W. (1966). Arch. Hyg. Bakteriol. 150:513.
194. Tilgner, D. J. (1970). Food Manuf. 45:47.
195. Mallet, L., and Tissier, M. (1969). C. R. Soc. Biol. 163:64.
196. Niaussat, P., Auger, C., and Mallet, L. (1970). C. R. Acad. Sci. (Paris) 270:1042.
197. Clayson, D. B., and Garner, R. C. (1976). *In* C. E. Searle (ed.), Chemical Carcinogens, A. C. S. Monograph No. 173, p. 366. American Chemical Society, Washington, D. C.
198. Radomski, J. L., Glass, E. M., and Deichmann, W. B. (1971). Cancer Res. 31:1690.
199. Cohen, S. M., Arai, M., and Friedell, G. H. (1978). Proc. Am. Assoc. Cancer Res. 19:4.
200. Clifton, K. H., and Sridharan, B. N. (1975). *In* F. F. Becker (ed.), Cancer: A Comprehensive Treatise, Vol. 3, p. 249. Plenum Publishing Corp., New York.
201. Furth, J. (1975). *In* F. F. Becker (ed.), Cancer: A Comprehensive Treatise, Vol. 1, p. 75. Plenum Publishing Corp., New York.
202. IARC Monogr. Eval. Carcinog. Risk Chem. Man. (1973). 2:48.
203. IARC Monogr. Eval. Carcinog. Risk Chem. Man. (1972). 1:40.
204. IARC Monogr. Eval. Carcinog. Risk Chem. Man. (1972). 1:17.
205. IARC Monogr. Eval. Carcinog. Risk Chem. Man. (1973). 2:74.
206. Loeb, L. A., Sirover, M. A., Weymouth, L. A., Dube, D. K., Seal, G., Agarwal, S. S., and Katz, E. (1977). J. Toxicol. Environ. Health 2:1297.
207. Lijinsky, W., and Ross, A. E. (1967). Food Cosmet. Toxicol. 5:343.
208. Rhee, K. S., and Bratzler, L. J. (1970). J. Food Sci. 35:146.
209. Dipple, A. (1976). *In* C. E. Searle (ed.), Chemical Carcinogens, A.C.S. Monograph No. 173, p. 245. American Chemical Society, Washington, D. C.
210. Nagao, M., Honda, M., Seino, Y., Yahagi, T., and Sugimura, T. (1977). Cancer Lett. 2:221.
211. Matsumoto, T., Yoshida, D., Mizusaki, S., and Okamoto, T. (1978). Mutat. Res. 56:281.
212. Sugimura, T., Kawachi, T., Nagao, M., Yahagi, T., Seino, Y., Okamoto, T., Shudo, K., Kosuge, T., Tsuji, K., Wakabayashi, K., Iitaka, Y., and Itai, A. (1977). Proc. Jpn. Acad. 53:58.
213. Takayama, S., Katoh, Y., Tanaka, M., Nagao, M., Wakabayashi, K., and Sugimura, T. (1977). Proc. Jpn. Acad. 53:126.
214. Commoner, B., Vithayathil, A., Dolara, P., Nair, S., Madyastha, P., and Cuca, G. (1978). Science 201:913.

215. Magee, P. N., and Barnes, J. M. (1967). Adv. Cancer Res. 10:163.
216. Hawksworth, G., Hill, M. J., Gordillo, G., and Cuello, C. (1975). IARC Sci. Publ. 9:229.
217. Correa, P., Haenszel, W., Cuello, D., Tannenbaum, S., and Archer, M. (1975). Lancet 2:58.
218. Lijinsky, W., and Taylor, H. W. (1977). In H. H. Hiatt, J. D. Watson, and J. A. Winsten (eds.), Origins of Human Cancer, Book C. p. 1579. Cold Spring Harbor Laboratory, Cold Spring Harbor, New York.
219. Mirvish, S. S. (1977). J. Toxicol. Environ. Health 2:1267.
220. Tannenbaum, S. R., Archer, M. C., Wishnok, J. S., Correa, P., Cuello, C., and Haenszel, W. (1977). In H. H. Hiatt, J. D. Watson, and J. A. Winsten (eds.), Origins of Human Cancer, Book C, p. 1609. Cold Spring Harbor Laboratory, Cold Spring Harbor, New York.
221. Wang, T., Kakizoe, T., Dion, P., Furrer, R., Varghese, A. J., and Bruce, W. R. (1978). Nature 276:280.
222. Hill, M. J. (1977). In J. D. Watson, H. H. Hiatt, and J. A. Winsten (eds.), Origins of Human Cancer, Book C, p. 1627. Cold Spring Harbor Laboratory, Cold Spring Harbor, New York.
223. Weisburger, J. H., Cohen, L. A., and Wynder, E. L. (1977). In H. H. Hiatt, J. D. Watson, and J. A. Winsten (eds.), Origins of Human Cancer, Book A, p. 567. Cold Spring Harbor Laboratory, Cold Spring Harbor, New York.
224. Jukes, T. H. (1978). Nature 271:449.
225. Lowrance, W. W. (1976). Of Acceptable Risk: Science and the Determination of Safety. William Kaufmann, Inc., Los Altos, California.
226. Pochin, E. E. (1975). Br. Med. Bull. 31:184.
227. Tomatis, L., Mohr, U., and Davis, W. (eds.). (1973). IARC Sci. Publ. 4:180.
228. Toth, B. (1968). Cancer Res. 28:727.
229. Mulvihill, J. J. (1975). In J. F. Fraumeni, Jr. (ed.), Persons at High Risk of Cancer: An Approach to Cancer Etiology and Control, p. 3. Academic Press, Inc., New York.
230. Anderson, D. E. (1975). In J. F. Fraumeni, Jr. (ed.), Persons at High Risk of Cancer: An Approach to Cancer Etiology and Control, p. 39. Academic Press, Inc., New York.
231. Kama, I., and Friedman, H. (1977). Adv. Cancer Res. 25:271.
232. Cleaver, J. E., and Bootsma, D. (1975). Annu. Rev. Genet. 9:19.
233. Miller, E. C., Miller, J. A., Takayama, S., Sugimura, T., and Hirano, I. (eds.) (1979). Naturally Occurring Carcinogens — Mutagens and Modulators of Carcinogenesis. Proceedings of the Ninth Annual International Symposium of the Princess Takamatsu Cancer Research Fund, January 23–25, Tokyo, Japan. Japan Scientific Societies Press, Tokyo, and University Park Press, Baltimore. In press.

International Review of Biochemistry
Biochemistry of Nutrition IA, Volume 27
Edited by A. Neuberger and T. H. Jukes
Copyright 1979   University Park Press   Baltimore

6
Vitamin C: Conservative Human Requirements and Aspects of Overdosage

G. N. SCHRAUZER

University of California, San Diego, Revelle College, La Jolla, California

The publication of the book *Vitamin C and the Common Cold* by Pauling in 1970 (1) led to an enormous increase in the consumption of vitamin C in many of the industrialized countries. The idea that vitamin C prevents or ameliorates infections of the upper respiratory tract is not new and has previously resulted in sporadic episodes of vitamin C overconsumption. One such episode occurred during the Great Flu Epidemic of 1952–1953 (2), but did not draw much attention. In 1970, however, all past records of vitamin C overdosage were surpassed. Vitamin C received such worldwide acclaim as a cold remedy that the demand for it continues to rise and it is now regarded by many as a drug rather than a vitamin. As a consequence of these developments it has become difficult, in the United States, to obtain vitamin C tablets that contain only 100 mg or less. Instead, pounds of ascorbic acid are offered either in bulk or in 500–1000-mg tablets in supermarkets and drugstores because the consumption of large doses has become rather universal. In a monthly journal published by the American Chemical Society in February, 1978 (3), an interview of a physician by the editor was published in which use of the vitamin at "maintenance doses" of 4–15 g/day was advocated for the prevention of colds, high serum cholesterol, cancer, and hayfever, and during a cold the consumption of 100 g/day was recommended. In a somewhat ironic description of a self-experiment, the magazine's editor stated that he fought his cold by intermittently "popping 1000 mg (vitamin-C) pills like bar peanuts," consuming a total of 400 g in 1 week (3). Rational discussion of the pharmacological efficacy of a drug becomes difficult at such dosage levels, and, even though ascorbic acid is relatively nontoxic, the safety of intakes corresponding to 1000 times the recommended daily or dietary allowances must be considered in the light of the unabated growth of this abuse.

CONSERVATIVE USES OF VITAMIN C

Intakes Recommended for Normal, Healthy Individuals

After the isolation of vitamin C (L-ascorbic acid) by Zilva, Bezsonoff, and Agopian in 1925, numerous investigations demonstrated the value of small doses of the compound in the prevention and cure of scurvy. A reasonable consensus was reached that for adults 10 mg or even less of ascorbic acid are sufficient to prevent the outbreak of symptoms of vitamin C deficiency. Daily allowances of ascorbic acid that in most countries now range between 30 and 75 mg per adult were recommended. The Food and Nutrition Board justified its recommended dietary allowance (RDA) of 45 mg as follows: "Evidence has been presented and confirmed that a daily intake of 10 mg of ascorbic acid is sufficient to alleviate and cure the clinical signs of scurvy in human subjects. This amount, however, may not be satisfactory for the maintenance of optimal health over long periods of time" (4).

Experiments have shown that a daily intake of 45 mg of ascorbic acid maintains a body pool of 1500 mg. The United States Food and Drug Administration (5) proposed a recommended daily allowance of vitamin C of 60 mg for an adult, basing its higher estimate on the concept that "the Recommended Dietary Allowances are the levels of intake of essential nutrients considered, in the judgement of the Food and Nutrition Board, on the basis of available scientific knowledge to be adequate to meet the known nutritional needs of practically all healthy persons." To allow for a reasonable safety margin, the Committee of Food and Nutrition, National Research Council (U.S.A.), in 1941 recommended 70–75 mg of ascorbic acid per day for the healthy, moderately active adult. Their philosophy was summarized in a statement that is quoted here since it illustrates the fact that the RDAs are not meant to be scientifically precise values: "The allowances are designed to afford a margin of sufficiency above average physiological requirements to cover variations among essentially all individuals in the general population. They provide a buffer against the increased needs during common stresses and permit full realization of growth and productive potential."

In a survey of the diets of 15,000 Americans from 1950–1968, 55% were found to ingest somewhat less than the RDA of vitamin C, 28% received less than two-thirds, 12% received below one-half (6). With the use of a number of biochemical indices, another study suggested that 39% of a representative number of Americans obtained vitamin C in amounts "below acceptable level," and 19% at a "deficient or poor level." Hemoglobin, hematocrit, vitamin A, carotene, thiamine, and riboflavin values were also judged as below acceptable in 24–50% of the subjects tested, and deficient or poor in 3–24% (6). It is a matter of opinion whether these results reflect the nutrition problems in the population of the United States or the safety margins of the RDAs. Without entering into a detailed discussion of this complex issue, it may be stated that as far as vitamin C is concerned dietary intakes prior to 1970 were on the whole adequate if judged on the basis of clinically observed cases of frank vitamin C deficiency. Scurvy is still observed occasionally — for example, among elderly men living alone and on poorly balanced diets — but is otherwise quite rare.

Intakes Recommended Under Special Conditions

Modifications of the RDAs are justified to meet variations in the requirements as they occur at different ages, in pregnancy, during lactation and high physical activity, etc. For infants, the RDA of 35 mg/day was justified from the vitamin C content of normal human milk. In adolescence, 80–100 mg/day have been recommended; during pregnancy, 100 mg/day; and during lactation, 150 mg/day.

Even under stress or during high physical activity, the vitamin C requirement is not markedly increased. Several studies revealed that maximal physical activity can be maintained for extended periods even at vitamin C intakes far below the RDA (7). Some authors have recommended higher doses of vitamin C for athletes to improve performance. Jakovliev (8), in 1961, suggested 300 mg/day. Howald et al. (9) reported that doses of 1 g caused slight improvements of cardiovascular and metabolic parameters, but warned against the intakes of larger amounts because these might have a negative effect on athletic performance by disturbing the equilibrium between oxygen transport and use. However, even intakes of 1 g were found by Howald et al. (9) to have a negative effect on energy supply to the working muscle. One would accordingly have to conclude that vitamin C in larger than the recommended amounts has no beneficial effects on athletic performance. The higher vitamin demands of athletes are better met by means of a well-balanced diet.

Therapeutic Dosage Prior to 1970

For the treatment of manifest scurvy past recommendations of dosage levels remained in the 250–1,000-mg range per day (10), although lower doses will suffice (11). Infantile scurvy, which was observed among infants that were fed boiled milk for extended periods, was treated with 50-mg doses of ascorbic acid administered 3 times per day per os or with 35-mg intramuscular injections twice per day, together with an improvement of the diet by the use of fresh milk and small additions of vegetable or fruit juices. To stimulate wound repair in surgical patients whose serum ascorbic acid levels are low, 150–200 mg of vitamin C was recommended per day to assure adequate tissue saturation during the postoperative period. Patients exhibiting steatorrhea may suffer from a vitamin C malabsorption syndrome and also respond favorably to vitamin C (10).

ASCORBIC ACID UPTAKE, METABOLISM, AND EXCRETION

Healthy adult men have an average body pool of 1.5 g of ascorbic acid. In healthy human volunteers, scurvy was induced by allowing the body pool to fall to a level of 300 mg or less. Under these conditions the plasma ascorbic acid concentrations become extremely low. However, low plasma levels of ascorbic acid are not necessarily indicative of vitamin C deficiency. Only if the plasma level remains at 0.1 mg/100 ml for extended periods and does not recover do characteristic symptoms of scurvy appear, as was demonstrated in the classical studies by Hodges et al. (11). Sauberlich (12) showed in 1973–1975 that serum vitamin C concentrations reach 0.6 mg/100 ml at a daily ascorbic acid intake of 45 mg. The regular administration of ascorbic acid in amounts corresponding to the recommended dietary allowance (Food Nutrition Board) thus assures adequate tissue saturation as reflected by the reasonably high plasma ascorbate levels. With increasing dosage, plasma ascorbic acid concentrations continue to rise until the concentration of 1.4

mg/100 ml is reached. At and above this concentration renal clearance rises sharply. Typically, plasma ascorbate levels between 0.8 and 1.1 mg/100 ml are observed in normal subjects receiving vitamin C in doses of between 200–500 mg/day (13).

Kübler and Gehler (14) investigated the kinetics of enteral resorption of vitamin C at doses of 1.5, 3, 6, and 12 g. A single dose of 1.5 g caused a temporary rise of the plasma ascorbate levels to 1 mg/100 ml. At dosages of 3, 6, and 12 g maximum plasma concentrations of about 1.5, 1.9, and 2.2 mg/100 ml, respectively, were reached 3 h after administration. In all cases the plasma concentrations were back to nearly the starting concentrations 14 h after the start of the experiment. Ascorbic acid resorption declined with increasing dosage, from 49.5% after administration of 1.5 g to 16% after the 12-g dose. These authors concluded that ascorbic acid resorption remains dose proportional only up to 180 mg per dose. At this dosage, nearly 71% of the total vitamin C is absorbed.

Mašek, Hrubá, and Novák (15) measured the urinary excretion of vitamin C of normal individuals receiving 0.5–1.5 g of ascorbic acid/day for up to 38 days. Each day during the experimental period between 55–90% of the dose was excreted. These authors noted an initial increase of the serum vitamin C concentrations during the first 9 days of their experiment. In the following days, during continued dosing of 1.5 g/day, they observed a decline of the serum ascorbate concentration that persisted in spite of the increased dosage until the experiment was terminated. The conclusion was reached that the decline or fluctuation of the ascorbic acid levels was due to enhanced metabolism and not increased retention, since leucocyte ascorbic acid levels remained unchanged. The same authors also stated that there obviously exists a certain rational upper dosage that for healthy adults was estimated to lie between 80 mg and 100 mg/day.

Ascorbic acid is apparently not metabolized to CO_2 in the human organism, although this was once believed and has been observed in certain primates. In man, catabolism to oxalate occurs instead. Lamden and Chrystowski (16) showed in 1954 that the daily ingestion of about 4–9 g of ascorbic acid significantly increased urinary oxalate. Atkins et al. (17) subsequently found that about 60% of the urinary oxalate arises from ascorbic acid or glycine metabolism; the origin of the remainder is unknown.

UNORTHODOX USE OF VITAMIN C

Therapeutic Applications Against the Common Cold

The idea that vitamin C could have prophylactic or therapeutic effects against infections of the upper respiratory tract probably has its origin in certain folk remedies for the common cold and the belief in the ability of vitamin C to increase resistance against infection. In Central Europe, gargling with unsweetened lemon juice at the onset of a cold was still a common practice about 30–40 years ago. Korbsch (1938) (18) may have been the first to describe some positive results in the control of colds through the oral administration of 1 g of vitamin C per day. He reported that injections of 500 mg of ascorbic acid were even more effective, although one must wonder about the actual efficacy in view of statements such as "It was necessary to repeat injections during the next days, although in the majority of cases the colds disappeared spontaneously without reappearing." His claims were later criticized by Dahlberg et al. (19), who studied the effect of vitamin C on developing colds with 2500 soldiers of the Swedish army in 1942. The diet was the regular one for troops stationed in northern Sweden and care was taken that no bias was introduced. The experimental subjects receiving vitamin C were first saturated with 200 mg of ascorbic acid daily for 24 days before the study was begun and were maintained on 50 mg/day for the duration of the experiment. Dahlberg et al. reported, "No difference could be found as regards to frequency or duration of colds, degrees of fever, etc....Military competitions...disclosed no difference between the two groups" (19). The Swedish authors took the position that an apparent vitamin C deficit as measured by low plasma ascorbate levels does not necessarily indicate symptoms of disease, impaired constitution, or increased disposition to diseases: "The idea of vitamin C as a prophylactic is still very widespread in Sweden...largely thanks to unreliable advertisements from abroad.... The prescribing of extra vitamin C calls in each case for other symptoms which can be assumed to be associated with vitamin C hypovitaminosis, or which usually precede manifest scurvy."

Tebrock et al. (20) in 1956 also disclaimed subjective or objective effects of ascorbic acid on incidence and duration of colds among 1900 persons. Bibile (21) noted no positive effects of ascorbic acid at dosage levels of 500 mg/day in a study involving 250 students. Even 3 g of ascorbic acid per day for 3 days failed to protect against infections with viruses known or suspected to cause colds (22); there also was no noticeable increase of resistance against virus infections in tissue cultures under the influence of ascorbic acid.

Statistical data accumulated in the Cincinnati General Hospital over the years 1935–1963 indicate a maximum of scurvy admissions between the months of March and May (23), not during the winter months in which infections of the upper respiratory tract occur with high frequency. This lack of correlation shows that the incidence of colds is not an index of vitamin C deficiency in a population.

Among other studies that may be quoted in this context is that of Ritzel (24), which involved participants of a ski camp, all schoolchildren. Ritzel did observe beneficial effects of vitamin C, but his conclusions were based on subjective evaluations ("fever and chills" were listed among the symptoms, but no temperature measurements were made) and thus cannot be accepted. Most other investigators were similarly unable to prove the efficacy of vitamin C in controlled studies. Glazebrook and Thompson (25) in 1942 saw no significant decrease in the intensity and course of infections of the upper respiratory tract after the administration of vitamin C. Neither did Cowan, Diehl, and Baker (26), who summarized their findings as follows: "This controlled study yields no indication that either large doses of vitamins A, B_1, B_2, C, D and nicotinic acid have any important effect on the number or severity of infections of the upper respiratory tract when administered to young adults who presumably are already on a reasonably adequate diet."

The renewed interest in the prophylactic effects of ascorbic acid stimulated the conduct of several new studies to assess its efficacy in preventing colds. Among these field trials the best known are that of Lewis et al. (27), involving 311 subjects, that of Coulehan et al. (28) with 868 Navaho schoolchildren, and that of Anderson (29) in Canada with 2349 adults. Most of the investigators discuss the numerous problems with experiments involving such large numbers of patients. They are formidable and introduce numerous sources of possible error that cannot be discussed here. The overall impression from these experiments is that vitamin C probably has no or at best a very slight effect on developing or manifest minor infections of the upper respiratory tract. Anderson believes his studies justify a daily dose of 100–200 mg (29). Coulehan et al. feel that "vitamin C is unlikely to have widespread usefulness as a cold remedy" (28). Lewis et al. (27) concluded from experience gathered with a large population of well-motivated volunteers that "taking two capsules three times a day was too much bother for the possible small benefit received." Some believers in the efficacy of vitamin C have tended in the past to underscore the value of their regimen by stating that they had "no cold worth mentioning in years." Yet, Crandon, Lund, and Hill (30) in 1940 also reported almost complete freedom from respiratory infections during 8 months of a vitamin C–depletion self-experiment during which the plasma vitamin C level reached zero in 120 days, as was pointed out by Goldberg (31). Vrana (32) described the case of a male patient with manifest scurvy characterized by perifollicular hemorrhages and petechiae that responded to vitamin C; he stated: "This patient denied any manifestations of upper respiratory tract illness for at least two years before admission to the hospital with vitamin C deficiency."

Vitamin C may have become a people's remedy against respiratory infections because the topical application of an acidic substance on affected areas in the mouth during a cold affords some sort of physical comfort, a possibility that should be tested. However, the popularity of vitamin C may be in part attributed to psychosocial motivating factors emerging in many countries around 1970. These factors shifted public demand away from drugs toward more "natural" methods of healing. However, by now vitamin C itself is being used as a drug.

Vitamin C in the Treatment of Mental Illness

VanderKamp (33) in 1966 reported results suggesting that schizophrenic patients can metabolize more vitamin C than normal subjects. Later, Herjanic and Moss-Herjanic (34) published similar observations in a loading test designed to observe the appearance of the first trace of ascorbic acid in the urine upon oral administration of therapeutic doses. They found that schizophrenics required considerably larger amounts of vitamin C than normal healthy individuals. One patient reportedly required an oral dose of 110 g; the majority of patients started renal clearance of ascorbic acid after doses of between 5 g and 30 g. This was much more than observed with normal controls, who required only 5 g. These results suggested to them "significant difference in the amount of ascorbic acid needed by psychotic patients as compared to normal controls in order to produce a positive saturation test in the urine" (34).

In a more quantitative study, Milner (35) measured the urinary excretion of schizophrenics receiving 1.0 g of ascorbic acid per day for 19 days. He noted a statistically significant improvement in the depressive, manic, and paranoid states of the patients. He also claimed that his patients were in a "clinical state of subscurvy." During a loading test in which his schizophrenic patients were given 1 g of vitamin C per day, the average urinary excretion reached 79% of the total dose on the 9th day. When his results are compared with published data on excretion by normal subjects during a similar loading test, one finds no significant differences between the two groups after saturation was reached. Thus, the mentally ill patients excreted 72.6% of the daily dose between day 5 and day 19 of loading, whereas the healthy subjects studied by Mašek et al. (15) excreted on the average 73.4% of the daily 1 g dose administered. This comparison seems to disprove the notion of abnormal ascorbic acid metabolism in Milner's patients. On the other hand, it is obviously possible that vitamin C deficiency occurs among hospitalized patients in certain mental institutions.

Ascorbic Acid in Neoplastic Disease

Bauer (36) quotes work of Stepp and Schroeder in 1936 that revealed that cancer patients are frequently vitamin C deficient. However, he considers this deficiency to be caused by poor nutrition and suggests the administration of vitamin C to correct any deficiencies prior to major surgery or intensive radiation therapy. He also recommends vitamin C supplements as an adjuvant in the treatment after chronic infections or for regeneration of the organism. Cameron and Pauling (1974) suggest, in stronger terms, that vitamin C offers promise of "general improvement in the results of cancer management, including prophylaxis in general, supportive treatment when standard methods of therapy are being used, and palliative treatment in advanced terminal cancer" (37). Cameron and Pauling (37, 38) found that a majority of patients with terminal cancer experienced some degree of subjective benefit, which was usually first evident approximately the 5th to 10th day after the administration of 10 g of ascorbic acid per day. A small number of patients exhibited some objective signs of improvement in their condition. These included relief of pain from skeletal metastases, relief of other pressure effects, and reduction of malignant ascites and malignant pleural effusions. However, these improvements occurred in only a small number of patients, and in some patients opposite results were also observed. Although it is probably not to be disputed that, in certain cases, "the administration of ascorbic acid can bring about a fractional, albeit significant, improvement in cancer morbidity and mortality" (38a), the suggestion that ascorbic acid also produced some retardation of expansile metastatic growth was criticized by Alcantara and Speckmann (39, 40), who noted that, of 50 advanced cancer patients treated with vitamin C, 17 (34%) had no response, while in four patients (8%) the administration of ascorbic acid was followed by widespread tumor hemorrhage and necrosis, with disastrous results. It would seem, therefore, that indiscriminate ascorbic acid treatment of cancer patients cannot be recommended. Taking into account the lack of suitable controls in the Cameron-Pauling experiments and the above discussion, one would tend to agree with Alcantara's conclusion that the benefits derived in some of the patients may be part of a spectrum of correcting various nutritional deficiencies in the cancer patient. One might add to this that the large doses of ascorbic acid administered also elicit nonspecific effects such as diuresis, diarrhea, changes in electrolyte balance, and water content of tissues, etc., all of which could contribute to the subjective improvements of the condition of some of the patients.

Presently, several authors are proposing that ascorbic acid also has a prophylactic value in cancer prevention. This belief is based on the observed diminution of the formation of carcinogenic metabolites of 3-hydroxyanthranilic acid and of β-naphthylamine in vitamin C-exposed animals (41-43). Some of this work has since been criticized on statistical grounds and because of results of experiments with another potent urinary carcinogen, N-formamide, which produced carcinoma of the bladder in mice receiving large amounts of ascorbic acid in their drinking water (44). Ascorbic acid also had no effect on the carcinogenic action of nitrosamines or nitrosamides and of 4-biphenylamine (45). The belief in the anticarcinogenic value of ascorbic acid has its origin in the recognition of the strongly reducing properties of the compound, which render it an "antioxidant." Theories of carcinogenesis involving free radical metabolites of procarcinogens have been proposed; hence it is logical to expect that a reducing agent such as ascorbic acid might help to destroy such free radicals and diminish the carcinogenic action of certain compounds. The validity of this concept for cancer prophylaxis remains doubtful, however, if only in view of the absorption-excretion characteristics of vitamin C, which give rise to large fluctuations of the urinary ascorbic acid concentrations unless extremely high intakes are maintained at all times, in addition to the uncertain etiology.

The value of vitamin C as a palliative in radiation therapy has not been established. In fact, Miller and Sokoloff (46) have recommended the opposite, i.e., complete elimination of vitamin C during radiotherapy of tumors. They were able to show that the radiosensitivity of Crocker rat carcinoma could be increased in animals maintained on low ascorbic acid diets. It was suggested that the increased fragility of the vascular system of a tumor in vitamin C deficiency may enhance its radiosensitivity. The same authors reported results of a clinical study involving 26 cases in which four patients with Hodgkin's disease demonstrated full recurrence of tumor growth after radiotherapy under normal dietary conditions. A much better control of the disease was accomplished by placing the patients on an ascorbic acid–free diet prior to or during radiotherapy. Reducing the ascorbic acid blood level to near zero in the preradiation, radiation, and postradiation periods caused the patients to remain asymptomatic for 15–20 months. Because vitamin C is so readily accessible, many cancer patients currently take large doses on their own; at least one patient (47) with diagnosed Hodgkin's disease has followed advice offered by proponents of the megavitamin therapy to ingest 20 g of vitamin C per day. Recently, Karkar et al. (48) demonstrated that the ascorbic acid concentrations in the leukocytes and plasma of cancer patients increased after radiotherapy. They feel that vitamin C–free diets during cancer therapy deserve further study, especially since patients can be maintained on such diets for several months without inducing any symptoms of scurvy.

The indiscriminate administration of large doses of vitamin C to patients with leukemia must be rejected because of observed differences in the distribution of ascorbic acid in blood from patients with different forms of the disease. For example, the concentration of ascorbic acid in leucocytes is higher than normal in chronic lymphatic leukemia, but not in chronic myeloid leukemia (49). Such differences may be important in the management of leukemic patients. Since ascorbic acid accelerates the conversion of folic acid into citrovorum factor and deficiency of the vitamin may inhibit this conversion, Sokoloff recommended a vitamin C–free diet, in combination with small doses of cortisone (50) for the treatment of chronic leukemia. A number of authors [Andrews and Brook (51), Loh and Wilson (52), and Krassner and Dymock (53)] have reported that leukocyte as well as plasma ascorbic acid concentrations are subnormal in cancer patients. Krassner and Dymock treated patients with vitamin C supplements and observed a clear clinical benefit, whereas untreated patients demonstrated increased mortality. However, these authors point out that the use of megadoses of vitamin C should not be confused with the replacement of the vitamin to its physiological level.

Just as important as the demonstration of the beneficial effects of vitamin C in the maintenance of cancer patients are observations that suggest that certain tumor cells require vitamin C for growth. The experiments by Magliozzi (54) are of interest in this context. This author demonstrated that guinea pigs of an inbred strain on a scorbutic diet showed diminished tumor growth as compared with animals receiving 10 or 1000 mg of ascorbic acid per kg of body weight. Roberts and Dalton (55) observed that the growth of liposarcoma in guinea pigs on a vitamin C-free diet was much slower than that of normally fed controls. After 30 days the average tumor weight was 7.4 g in the vitamin C-deficient animals, while in those receiving 40 mg of ascorbic acid it was 26.5 g. The tumors in the high ascorbic acid animals were more malignant and demonstrated a tendency to invade the surrounding muscle and connective tissue capsule. On the other hand, immunological response mechanisms are weakened in vitamin C deficiency (56), suggesting greater susceptibility to carcinogenic stress; obviously the induction of a prescorbutic state is not recommended for cancer prophylaxis, although it may be beneficial in cancer therapy.

The ability of ascorbic acid to inhibit the formation of nitrosamines from nitrite and alkylamines under simulated gastric conditions has led to the proposal of the use of vitamin C in the prophylaxis of stomach cancer (57-59). In these applications, vitamin C would function as a chemical reducing agent and would have to be ingested in massive amounts whenever nitrite-cured foods are eaten or nitrite-contaminated water is consumed. There are obvious practical difficulties for the successful application of this method. It is also not known what, if any, role nitrosamines play in the etiology of human gastric cancer.

Last but not least it should be mentioned that weekly injections of massive doses of ascorbic acid from the period of weaning to the age of 12 months had no significant effect on the incidence and development of spontaneous mammary adenocarcinoma in an inbred strain of female C_3H mice carrying the Bittner virus (60). Under normal conditions of maintenance, these mice develop spontaneous mammary tumors with 80–100% incidence, beginning at the age of about 12 months. Vitamin C was ineffective in preventing or retarding the appearance of tumors, however.

In summary, it would seem that the restoration of vitamin C deficiency in cancer patients may or may not have beneficial effects, depending on the case. The advantage of massive overdosage over more conservative applications is not convincing. It is hoped that eventually vitamin C will again find its place in the nutritional maintenance of the healthy and the ill at dosage levels that can be justified scientifically.

Miscellaneous Therapeutic Applications

Ascorbic acid has been used to promote wound healing in surgical patients; in the treatment of burns, traumatic shocks, jaundice, polio, polyarthritis, asthma, hay fever; to improve capillary resistance; to enhance iron utilization in anemic patients; to treat megaloblastic anemias (together with folic acid) in children; and in heavy metal detoxification (often together with calcium-EDTA or 2,3-dimercaptopropanol). It is not necessary in this chapter to discuss these various applications in any great detail. In some cases their efficacy has been questioned. In others, better methods have become available.

Industrial Applications

Ascorbic acid and its derivatives are used in industry to prevent spoilage of a variety of food products, to maintain the red color of canned meat, and to prevent rancidity of fats or the browning of cut apple slices. It is also used as a stabilizer of such foods as milk and milk products. The reducing properties of ascorbic acid form the chemical basis of these applications, endowing the compound with powerful antioxidant properties. Use of the term "antioxidant" has also become popular in attempts to describe the biological functions of ascorbic acid as well as of a number of other naturally occurring compounds. While appropriate in food technology, the term should be used with caution when dealing with enzymatic processes in vivo.

SAFETY CONSIDERATIONS WITH HIGH ASCORBIC ACID DOSAGE

Toxicity

In the rat, the LD 50 of free ascorbic acid on oral administration has been determined to be about 5 g/kg of body weight (61). In chronic feeding experiments (62) with young rats exposed to feed that contained 25% of ascorbic acid, all animals were dead within 2-3 weeks. Lang has pointed out that the toxicity of ascorbic acid depends on whether the free acid or its salts are administered (62). Since the renal excretion of free ascorbic acid is not possible because of the acidic nature of the compound, disturbances of the electrolyte balance may occur unless the loss of sodium is compensated. Lang accordingly performed feeding studies with sodium ascorbate and found that rats began to show symptoms of toxicity only after administration of about 25 g/kg of body weight. Taking into account various safety factors, the maximum tolerated dose was determined to be about 10 g/kg of body weight (62). Extrapolating these results to man, it may be estimated that the oral ingestion of 100 g of free ascorbic acid by an adult is still "safe" so far as acute toxicity is concerned, but, if such high ascorbic acid intakes are considered at all, at least the sodium salt should be taken.

  In the newer medical literature an interesting fatal case of ascorbic acid–induced hemolysis has been described by Campbell et al. (63). After admission for treatment of acute renal failure and of second-degree burns of the hand, a 68-year-old black man was given 80 g of ascorbic acid intravenously on each of 2 consecutive days. He developed extensive hemolysis and died on the 22nd hospital day. The authors (63) related the fatal outcome of the ascorbic acid treatment of their patient to a cellular deficiency in glucose-6-phosphate dehydrogenase (G-6-PD), causing inadequate response to oxidative stress. Infection and exposure to various types of drugs have been linked with hemolysis in patients with G-6-PD deficiency. The authors caution against the use of large doses of ascorbic acid and report that mild degrees of hemolysis were observed in patients with G-6-PD deficiency even after the administration of only 1500 mg.

Irrespective of G-6-PD deficiency, which was assumed to be the ultimate cause of death, one must wonder whether the outcome would have been the same had sodium ascorbate been injected rather than free ascorbic acid. Stewart et al. (64) in 1941 did not observe adverse effects in animal experiments with high intravenous doses of sodium ascorbate. They demonstrated that the intravenous administration of sodium ascorbate (0.2–2 g/kg of body weight) prolonged the survival time of cats bled of 50% of their original blood volume. The rationale of these studies was to use ascorbate to secure a more adequate supply of oxygen to the tissues under stress. It is known (65) that ascorbate accelerates the oxygen consumption of rat liver homogenates to which lactate has been added as the substrate; ascorbic acid acts as a catalyst of oxygen consumption under these conditions.

Effects of Vitamin C on High Altitude Resistance

Before World War II moderate doses of vitamin C were shown (66, 67) to temporarily increase the "high altitude resistance" in experimental animals and human subjects and it was therefore recommended for pilots, airplane passengers, mountaineers, etc. However, subsequent studies revealed that larger doses of vitamin C severely diminish the high altitude resistance. When rabbits were given 200 mg of sodium ascorbate intravenously 30 min prior to exposure to simulated high altitude conditions, an acceleration of oxygen use was observed as compared with untreated controls (68, 69). Animals pretreated with a threefold amount of sodium ascorbate (4 × 100 mg/day intramuscularly for 4 days prior to the experiment plus 200 mg of ascorbate 30 min before the experiment) developed convulsions typical of hypoxia with unprecedented violence and sooner than the untreated animals. A similar diminution of the high altitude resistance was also demonstrated in experiments with human volunteers.

Pfannenstiel (68) and Doerholt (69) found that ascorbate-treated human subjects failed to perform adequately in writing down numbers in descending order, beginning with 1000, 999, 998, etc., and required oxygen supplements at "altitudes" that were well tolerated by untreated controls. Schrauzer et al. (70) confirmed these findings in 1975. The adverse effects of ascorbic acid in their experiment appeared in subjects receiving 3 g of vitamin C per os for 6 days prior to the tests in a low pressure chamber. The observed diminished resistance of vitamin C–saturated subjects to hypoxic stress demonstrates that massive doses of vitamin C are undesirable and not conducive to good health. Vitamin C overdosage is especially counterindicated under conditions of diminished oxygen supply. (Goldstein (70a) describes a case of a 40-year-old patient with sickle cell thallasemia who had taken high doses of ascorbic acid during a cold and experienced crises of undetermined origin.) It would be of interest to establish the extent to which large doses of vitamin C also interfere with the oxygen economy under normal conditions of life. The apparent beneficial effects of low or moderate doses of vitamin C on high altitude resistance or oxygen use, on the other hand, are probably real but not yet adequately explained.

Effects on the Reproductive System

In attempts to produce an experimental "hypervitaminosis C," Altmann (71) treated young dogs with ascorbic acid (intramuscular, 4.1 g per animal, distributed over a period of 28 days) but observed only weight gains and no toxicity effects. Similar experiments with guinea pigs produced only one sign that was considered relevant: the animals littered only once and produced only four young. This pathological sign was linked with the excessive amounts of vitamin C administered (72, 73). The effect on reproduction may be related to the experiments of Russian workers (74, 75) who induced abortions in pregnant women through large doses of intravenously injected vitamin C. On oral administration, abortions have not been reported to occur. However, Neuweiler (76) and Mouriquand and Edel (77) have shown that massive doses of vitamin C have indeed a damaging effect on the reproductive capacity of guinea pigs — they produce dead fetuses and less possibility of conception.

Effects of Long-term Intakes

Observations that suggested the occurrence of systemic conditioning in response to high ascorbic acid intakes were probably made first by Jakovliev during the siege of Leningrad in World War II (78). The incidence and severity of scurvy in the civilian population during the stress were higher among individuals that had previously received extradietary supplements of vitamin C than in subjects that had never received vitamin C other than with their diet. Jakovliev subsequently showed that guinea pigs that were maintained on a high vitamin C diet for 6 months developed scurvy more rapidly if placed on a vitamin C-free diet than animals that never received excessive amounts of ascorbic acid. He accordingly stated in 1958 (78): "It is necessary on the one hand to set detailed vitamin C requirements depending on the metabolic intensity, on the other hand it is also necessary to strictly maintain these set requirements."

Gordonoff (79) repeated Jakovliev's experiment with guinea pigs but chose to inject 0.5 g of ascorbic acid subcutaneously per day and per animal for 4 weeks prior to placing them on a scurvy diet. The average survival time of the vitamin C-"supersaturated" animals on the scorbutogenic feed was

24.88 days, that of untreated controls, 38.6 days; the difference in the survival times was statistically significant ($P = 0.01$). In all animals dying of scurvy the bones were tested for pathological signs. The vitamin C–pretreated animals exhibited more severe signs than the controls. Gordonoff concluded his paper in 1960 by stating that "We have at any rate proven that patients that previously received vitamin C in large doses are in a worse condition to withstand vitamin C deficiency than those maintained on a normal diet. . . . It appears that there is a vitamin C regulating mechanism. It is therefore not recommended to administer large doses (grams per day), over a long period of time."

Schrauzer and Rhead (80) demonstrated the conditioning effect of vitamin C by examining blood levels and urinary ascorbate excretion in a group of individuals who had been ingesting ascorbic acid regularly in gram amounts per day for extended periods. Their plasma and erythrocyte ascorbic acid concentrations were lower, and their urinary excretion rates higher, than in control subjects during a short-term ascorbic acid loading test. The authors also described the effects of abrupt cessation of ascorbic acid overdosage and concluded that this may lead to unexpected outbreaks of ascorbic acid deficiency symptoms. Qualitative observations from a self-experiment leading to prescorbutic symptoms after cessation of vitamin C overdosage were reported. Elsewhere (81), the same authors published the case history of an individual who took 1 g of ascorbic acid per day regularly for 1 year and who developed symptoms of scurvy 2 years after termination of the regimen. A Swede who had been working on a citrus plantation in Florida and drinking excessive amounts of orange juice for several years became scorbutic while subsisting on a normal diet in Sweden. Schrauzer and Rhead (80) summarize their study as follows: "Long-term ascorbic acid overdosage on the gram- or higher scale is without merit and leads to systemic conditioning, while adequate ascorbic acid saturation is achieved without excessive supplements."

The concept of systemic conditioning to vitamin C was independently expressed by Wachholder (82), but his experimental results were statistically insignificant. Lang (62) later failed to demonstrate the conditioning effect with guinea pigs by using sodium ascorbate instead of ascorbic acid, and also because he allowed several days for a more gradual adaptation of his animals to the scorbutogenic diet. These results thus are not directly comparable to those of Gordonoff (79). Sorensen et al. (83) in 1974 reported results that clearly demonstrated systemic conditioning in young male guinea pigs maintained on an experimental diet containing 86 g of ascorbic acid per kg of feed for 275 days. The experimental animals maintained higher tissue stores of ascorbic acid than the control animals. However, this difference was significant only in the testes. When subjected to a scorbutogenic diet the experimental animals were depleted of ascorbic acid faster than the control animals. Catabolism of ascorbic acid was increased in the experimental group, as was urinary excretion. The authors reported, "The results are in agreement with the hypothesis that the regular ingestion of massive doses of ascorbic acid leads to accelerated ascorbic acid metabolism, i.e. systemic conditioning. The accelerated catabolism was not reversible by subnormal intakes of the vitamin" (83).

Cochrane (84) in 1965 postulated prenatal conditioning of the human fetus to high intakes of ascorbic acid by the mother and suggested that this effect can be produced experimentally with guinea pigs. Norkus and Rosso (85) demonstrated the prenatal conditioning effect with guinea pigs on a high (0.5%) versus a low (0.05%) ascorbic acid diet during the last half of pregnancy. The pups from the mother animals fed a high ascorbic acid diet showed a higher rate of ascorbic acid catabolism as measured by the formation of CO_2 than the controls. When the weaned pups were placed on a scorbutogenic diet, the experimental animals developed scurvy and died sooner. A linear inverse correlation between the excretion of CO_2 and the time-span at which scurvy appeared was also observed.

Postsaturation hypovitaminosis C among previous takers of ascorbic acid will not become manifest at all if high basal vitamin C intakes are maintained after cessation of the regimen. However, conditioned individuals may have permanently higher vitamin C requirements. Consistent with the observations of Sorensen et al. (83) that accelerated catabolism of vitamin C was not reversible in prenatally conditioned guinea pigs (see above), it thus may be expected that former vitamin C takers will no longer receive adequate amounts of vitamin C if maintained on normal diets without vitamin C supplementation. The subject who was described by Rhead and Schrauzer (81) developed scurvy 2 years after the termination of a self-imposed regimen of 1 g of ascorbic acid per day for 1 year and informed the author of this chapter that he had a second episode of scurvy and from this time is taking vitamin C supplements daily. Advocates of high vitamin C dosage may use this as an example of an individual with a genetically higher vitamin C requirement. However, a genuine genetic hypoascorbemia is more likely to become acutely noticeable in early infancy than after years of normal life. Schrauzer (80), who developed symptoms of scurvy after a vitamin C overdosage selfexperiment, again developed classical symptoms of hypovitaminosis C in 1978 (8 years after his overdosage experiment) following a 2-year attempt to subsist on a normal diet without vitamin C supplements. This time there was no swelling or bleeding of gums or loosening of the teeth. The main symptoms observed were muscular pain, impaired functioning of joints with swelling and pain, roughness and sensitivity of skin, and impaired wound healing. The symptoms remained unaffected by adequate intakes of B and E vitamin supplements but disappeared rapidly after administration of 100–200 mg of ascorbic acid per day for about 1 week (G. N. Schrauzer, unpublished observations).

Schrauzer and Rhead (80) stated that ascorbic acid conditioning effects are not necessarily permanent, based on an 18-months observation period. The recently observed reappearance of symptoms of hypovitaminosis C indicates that the conditioning effects may be long lasting or even permanent in some if not all individuals who previously had been receiving large doses of vitamin C for extended periods. This caveat against megavitamin C dosage and therapy is necessary in the light of increased interest in preventive medicine of the general public, the easy accessibility of ascorbic acid in virtually unlimited quantities, and the sometimes unscrupulous exploitation of the vitamin C myths by distributors of health food supplements. The regular ingestion of large doses of vitamin C can only be described as an "unnatural" act and is certainly not without consequences. This is even known to megavitamin therapists, one of whom has recommended combating an apparent dependence on large doses of vitamin C by taking additional vitamins and minerals (3). The same writer also warns, "You know there's another danger. If a patient who's accustomed to high vitamin C intake is hospitalized or otherwise comes under the care of certain physicians, the physician may cut off the C. . .and do it just when the patient needs it most" (3). Systemic conditioning to vitamin C may be sufficiently widespread by now to require further research on the seriousness of the phenomenon. Major research needs are as follows:

1. Quantitative determination of vitamin C catabolism in human subjects during or after long-term vitamin C overdosage.
2. Continuous monitoring of urinary excretion and of blood ascorbate during withdrawal of vitamin C supplements.
3. Studies of the reversibility of the adaptation syndrome.
4. Effects of vitamin C overdosage on the metabolism of other vitamins, hormones, drugs, and trace minerals.
5. Assessment of secondary effects of long-term vitamin C excess during and after dosing, including emotional stability and intellectual performance.

Additional Effects of Massive Vitamin C Intake

The abuse of vitamin C at dosage levels reaching previously unimaginable extremes has created a need for more work in vitamin toxicology. Although hypervitaminoses have been studied before, the earlier work had mainly academic interest. It has now acquired considerable practical significance. Vitamin C, if taken alone in large quantities, may interfere with other vitamins and thus create a higher demand that cannot be met by diet alone. The joint intake of two or more vitamins in excessive quantities may create entirely new conditions with far-reaching consequences. Observations with vitamin C and vitamin B_{12} may be mentioned in this context. It has been reported (81, 86) by two independent observers to cause a reversible inhibition of sperm fluid production, an effect that should be investigated in greater detail. Thornton observed that vitamin C injected into chicks promoted the mobilization of bone materials and increased the excretion of phosphorus over a 4-day period (87). The animals were vitamin D–deficient and demonstrated decreased phosphate retention and changes in the dynamics of bone mineralization. Cultured chick tibiae demonstrated increased oxygen consumption after exposure to vitamin C.

Large doses of vitamin C administered to swine increase the excretion rate of hydroxyproline (88). This is indicative of an acceleration in collagen catabolism. Effects of vitamin C in massive doses on the metabolism of essential trace minerals are as yet largely unknown. However, vitamin C has been shown to exert a protective effect against the toxicity of certain heavy metals, notably cadmium, in Japanese quail (89). More research is necessary before firm conclusions about the value of vitamin C in heavy metal detoxification can be reached. It is also necessary to assess the trace mineral status of habitual vitamin C takers.

In discussing the safety of high ascorbic acid dosage, Barness (90) listed a number of potential factors, some of which have not been covered but which are now mentioned at least briefly.

1. Acidosis: Barness (90) does not regard acidosis to be a major problem. However, the much higher doses (100 g/day) that are now being propagated require consideration of the potential disturbances in electrolyte balance.
2. Oxaluria-oxalosis: the possibility of renal stone formation has been mentioned in the literature since a part of ingested ascorbic acid is metabolized to oxalate. A few possibly vitamin C–related cases have been observed (91).
3. Renal stones: persons with cystinuria, oxalosis, and hyperuricemia could form renal stones more easily after ascorbic acid overdosage. (So far, no case histories exist.)
4. Hyperglycemia-glycosuria: false laboratory findings suggesting the presence of sugar in urine when the substance present was ascorbate now show the necessity of more careful testing for glucose in diabetic patients.
5. Gastrointestinal disturbances: nausea, diarrhea, and abdominal cramps are frequently consequences of high vitamin C intakes. These effects appear to be harmless and can be avoided by complementing ascorbic acid with bicarbonate of sodium or ingesting the sodium salt of ascorbic acid.
6. Prothrombin: a patient with pulmonary embolism received Dicoumarol (an inhibitor of prothrombin). When vitamin C was given to treat a developing cold the effect of the drug was temporarily weakened.

7. Serum cholesterol: increased levels of serum cholesterol were noted in patients receiving large doses of vitamin C. The question of whether or not vitamin C overdosage may aggravate atherosclerosis requires further experimental study.
8. Vitamin B_{12}: Herbert and Jacob (92) noted that vitamin B_{12} may be destroyed by ascorbic acid under certain conditions. The problem is not universally appreciated but should be investigated further. Hines (93) observed low vitamin B_{12} levels in three patients that had been taking 0.5 g of ascorbic acid per day for extended periods.

Barness mentions, in addition, occasional fatigue after vitamin C overdosage in human subjects, as well as effects on body zinc and copper levels, especially in deficient patients. At least one instance of sterility after ascorbate ingestion has been reported, according to Barness, but no references are given (90).

Schneider et al. (94) observed that ascorbic acid aggravates the condition of children suffering from nephropathic cystinosis. Originally, treatment with ascorbic acid appeared promising on the basis of in vitro experiments with cultured skin fibroblasts from children afflicted with this inborn metabolic disease.

CONCLUSIONS AND OUTLOOK

Scientific research during the past 8 years has in general not confirmed the great hopes placed in the value of vitamin C as a drug useful against many diseases. The hypothesis (95, 96) according to which man is a genetically hypoascorbemic species provided the intellectual basis of this new trend in vitamin C usage, which has become one of the most persistent nutritional fads in history. The validity of the genetic hypothesis has been questioned by Jukes (97–99). The fact that many persons are ingesting vitamin C in amounts 100–1000 times the actual requirements is indicative of an inflation of the vitamin concept that is spreading to other vitamins as well. Present applications of vitamin E may be quoted as examples. To reverse these trends would require considerable efforts on various levels; obviously, better information and education of the general public in the nutritional sciences are necessary. Since it is unlikely that the consumption of vitamin C will rapidly drop to reasonable levels, all that can be done at present is to reiterate that no evidence has been forthcoming to justify any changes in the recommended dietary allowances for vitamin C since "scientific efforts have been consistently and successfully expended to obtain 'definite information' on the vitamin C requirements for human subjects" (98). [Amounts of ascorbic acid somewhat larger than those proposed in the Dietary Allowances may have a beneficial effect in populations exposed to certain toxic elements (see Underwood, this volume, pp. 225–226) — eds.].

REFERENCES

1. Pauling, L. (1970). Vitamin C and the Common Cold. W. H. Freeman, San Francisco.
2. Grafe, E. (1958). Ernährungs- und Stoffwechselerkrankungen und ihre Behandlung, p. 278. Springer-Verlag, Berlin.
3. Luberoff, B. J. (1978). Chemtech February: 76.
4. Recommended Dietary Allowances. (1974). Food and Nutrition Board, United States National Research Council, National Academy of Sciences, Washington, D. C.
5. Schmidt, A. M. (1973). Fed. Regist. 38:20717.
6. Food and Nutrition Board, United States National Research Council (1968). Recommended Dietary Allowances, Publ. No. 1694. National Academy of Sciences, Washington, D. C.
7. Bartley, W. H., Krebs, A., and O'Brien, J. R. P. (1953). Vitamin C requirement of human adults. Medical Research Council Special Report, Ser. No. 280. H. M. Stationery Office, London.
8. Jakovliev, N. (1961). The Nutrition of the Athlete. Physculture and Sport, Moscow.
9. Howald, H., Segesser, B., and Körner, W. F. (1975). Ann. N. Y. Acad. Sci. 258:458.
10. Grafe, E. (1958). Ernährungs- und Stoffwechselerkrankungen und ihre Behandlung, p. 279. Springer-Verlag, Berlin.
11. Hodges, R. E., Hood, J., Canham, J. E., Sauberlich, H. E., and Baker, E. M. (1971). Am. J. Clin. Nutr. 24:432.
12. Sauberlich, H. E. (1975). Ann. N. Y. Acad. Sci. 258:438.
13. Fragner, J. (1964). Vitamine Chemie und Biochemie, p. 448. VEB Gustav Fischer Verlag, Jena.
14. Kübler, W., and Gehler, J. (1971). Int. J. Am. Nutr. Res. 40:442.
15. Mašek, J., Hrubá, F., and Novák, M. (1958). Ernährungsforschung 3:425.
16. Lamden, M. P., and Chrystowski, G. A. (1954). Proc. Soc. Exp. Biol. Med. 85:190.
17. Atkins, G. L., Dean, B. M., Griffin, W. J., and Watts, R. W. E. (1964). J. Biol. Chem. 239:2975.
18. Korbsch, R. (1938). Med. Klin. 45:100.
19. Dahlberg, G., Engel, A., and Rydin, H. (1944). Acta Med. Scand. 119:540.
20. Tebrock, H. E., Arminio, J. J., and Johnston, J. H. (1956). JAMA 162:1227.
21. Bibile, S. W. (1967). Med. News January 20 Issue.
22. Walker, G. H., Bynoe, M. L., and Tyrrell, D. A. (1967). Br. Med. J. 1:603.
23. Vilter, R. W. (1967). In W. H. Sebrell and R. S. Harris (eds.), The Vitamins, Ed. 2, Vol. 1, p. 458. Academic Press, Inc., New York.
24. Ritzel, G. (1961). Helv. Med. Acta 1:63.
25. Glazebrook, A. J., and Thompson, S. (1942). J. Hyg. 42:1.
26. Cowan, D. W., Diehl, H. D., and Baker, A. B. (1942). JAMA 120:1268.
27. Lewis, T. L., Karlowski, T. R., Kapikian, A. Z., Lynch, J. M., Shaffer, G. W., George, D. A., and Chalmers, T. C. (1975). Ann. N. Y. Acad. Sci. 258:505.
28. Coulehan, J. L., Kapner, L., Eberhard, S., Taylor, F. H., and Rogers, K. D. (1975). Ann. N. Y. Acad. Sci. 258:513.
29. Anderson, T. W. (1975). Ann. N. Y. Acad. Sci. 258:498.
30. Crandon, J. H., Lund, C., and Dill, D. B. (1940). N. Engl. J. Med. 223:353.
31. Goldberg, J. H. (1971). N. Engl. J. Med. 285:59.
32. Vrana, M. (1971). N. Engl. J. Med. 285:59.

33. VanderKamp, H. (1966). Int. J. Neuropsychiatr. 2:204.
34. Herjanic, M., and Moss-Herjanic, B. L. (1967). J. Schizophrenia 1:257.
35. Milner, G. (1963). Br. J. Psychiatry 109:294.
36. Bauer, K. H. (1963). Das Krebsproblem, 2nd ed., p. 26. Springer-Verlag, Berlin.
37. Cameron, E., and Pauling, L. (1974). Chem. Biol. Interact. 9:273.
38. Cameron, E., and Pauling, L. (1976). Proc. Natl. Acad. Sci. USA 73:3685.
38a. Cameron, E., and Campbell, A. (1974). Chem. Biol. Interact. 9:285.
39. Alcantara, E. N., and Speckmann, E. W. (1977). Am. J. Clin. Nutr. 30:662.
40. Alcantara, E. N., and Speckmann, E. W. (1976). Am. J. Clin. Nutr. 29:1035.
41. Schlegel, J. U. (1975). Ann. N. Y. Acad. Sci. 258:432.
42. Schlegel, J. U., Pipkin, G. E., and Duke, G. A. (1969). Invest. Urol. 7:206.
43. Schlegel, J. U., Pipkin, G. E., and Schultz, G. N. (1970). J. Urol. 103:155.
44. Soloway, M. S., Cohen, S. M., and Dekernian, J. B. (1975). J. Urol. 113:483.
45. Brill, E., and Radonski, J. (1977). Res. Commun. Chem. Pathol. Pharmacol. 16:85.
46. Miller, T. R., and Sokoloff, B. (1955). Am. J. Roentgenol. 73:472.
47. Private communication to author by patient, April, 1978.
48. Karkar, S. C., Wilson, W. M., and Moriarty, M. J. (1977). Ir. J. Med. Sci. 146:289.
49. Barkhan, P., and Howard, A. N. (1958). Biochem. J. 70:163.
50. Sokoloff, B., and Eddy, W. H. (1953). Proc. Am. Assoc. Cancer Res. 1:54.
51. Andrews, J., and Brook, M. (1966). Lancet 1:1350.
52. Loh, H. S., and Wilson, C. M. (1971). Br. Med. J. 3:733.
53. Krassner, N., and Dymock, I. W. (1974). Br. J. Cancer 30:142.
54. Magliozzi, J. A. (1977). Br. J. Cancer 35:448.
55. Roberts, W. B., and Dalton, A. J. (1949). J. Natl. Cancer Inst. 10:53.
56. Kumar, M., and Axelrod, A. E. (1969). J. Nutr. 98:41.
57. Weisburger, J. H., and Raineri, R. (1975). Toxicol. Appl. Pharmacol. 78:387.
58. Weisburger, J. H. (1977). Lancet 2:607.
59. Mirvish, S. S., and Shubik, P. (1974). Nature 252:179.
60. Schrauzer, G. N., and Rhead, W. J., unpublished observations.
61. Demole, V. (1934). Biochem. J. 28:770.
62. Lang, K. (1965). Wiss. Veröff. Dtsch. Ges. Ernähr. 14:149 and references cited therein.
63. Campbell, G. D., Steinberg, M. H., and Bower, J. D. (1975). Ann. Intern. Med. 82:310.
64. Stewart, C. P., Learmonth, J. R., and Pollock, G. A. (1941). Lancet 818.
65. Radsma, W. (1957). Acta Physiol. Pharmacol. Neerl. 5:330.
66. Pedersen, J. M. (1941). Nature 148:84.
67. Pfannenstiel, W. (1938). Luftfahrtmediz. Abhandl. 2:234.
68. Pfannenstiel, W. (1965). Cited in L. K. Lang (1965). Wiss. Veröff. Dtsch. Ges. Ernähr. 14:155.
69. Doerholt, G. (1938). Luftfahrtmediz. Abhandl. 2(3/4):240.
70. Schrauzer, G. N., Ishmael, D., and Kiefer, G. W. (1975). Ann. N. Y. Acad. Sci. 258:377.
70a. Goldstein, M. I. (1971). JAMA 216:332.
71. Altmann, O. (1936). Z. Neur. Psych. 156:633.
72. Gagi, V. (1936). Cited in Seifried, O. (1943). Vitamine und Vitaminmangelkrankheiten bei Haustieren, p. 214. Enke-Verlag, Stuttgart.
73. Seifried, O. (1943). Vitamine und Vitaminmangelkrankheiten bei Haustieren, p. 214, and references cited therein. Enke-Verlag, Stuttgart.

74. Samborskaja, E. P. (1962). Biull. Eksp. Biol. Med. 54:110.
75. Samborskaja, E. P. (1964). Biull. Eksp. Biol. Med. 57:105.
76. Neuweiler, W. (1951). Int. J. Vitam. Nutr. Res. 22:392.
77. Mouriquand, G., and Edel, V. (1953). Compt. Rend. Soc. Biol. 147:1432.
78. Jakovliev, N. (1958). Ernährungsforschung 3:446. (Also (1958). Vopr. Pitan. 17:3.)
79. Gordonoff, T. (1960). Schweiz. Med. Wochenschr. 90:726.
80. Schrauzer, G. N., and Rhead, W. J. (1973). Int. J. Vitam. Nutr. Res. 43:201.
81. Rhead, W. J., and Schrauzer, G. N. (1971). Nutr. Rev. 29:262.
82. Wachholder, K. (1947). Klin. Wochenschr. 1947:806.
83. Sorensen, D. I., Devine, M. M., and Rivers, J. M. (1974). J. Nutr. 104(8):1041.
84. Cochrane, W. A. (1965). Can. Med. Assoc. J. 93:893.
85. Norkus, E. P., and Rosso, P. (1975). Ann. N. Y. Acad. Sci. 258:401.
86. Jakisch, P. F. (1971). Chem. Eng. News 49:86.
87. Thornton, P. A. (1970). J. Nutr. 100:1479.
88. Brown, R. G., Sharma, V. D., and Young, L. G. (1971). Can. J. Anim. Sci. 51:439.
89. Fox, S. M. R. (1975). Ann. N. Y. Acad. Sci. 258:144.
90. Barness, L. A. (1975). Ann. N. Y. Acad. Sci. 258:523.
91. Smith, L. H. (1978). N. Engl. J. Med. 298:856.
92. Herbert, V., and Jacob, E. (1974). JAMA 230:241.
93. Hines, J. B. (1975). JAMA 234:24.
94. Schneider, J. A., Schlesselman, J. J., Mendoza, S. A., Orloff, S., Godfrey, A. B., and Schulman, J. D. (1978). Pediatr. Res. 12:457.
95. Stone, I. (1966). Acta Genet. Med. Gemellol. 15:345.
96. Pauling, L. (1974). Proc. Natl. Acad. Sci. USA 67:1643.
97. Jukes, T. H., and King, J. L. (1975). J. Hum. Evol. 4:85.
98. Jukes, T. H. (1974). Proc. Natl. Acad. Sci. USA 71:1949.
99. Jukes, T. H. (1975). Proc. Natl. Acad. Sci. USA 72:4151.

International Review of Biochemistry
Biochemistry of Nutrition IA, Volume 27
Edited by A. Neuberger and T. H. Jukes
Copyright 1979   University Park Press   Baltimore

7
Dietary Fiber: Its Role in Diverticular Disease, Colon Cancer, and Coronary Heart Disease

J. A. STORY and D. KRITCHEVSKY

Purdue University, West Lafayette, Indiana, and The Wistar Institute of Anatomy and Biology, Philadelphia, Pennsylvania

Current interest in the role of dietary fiber in the etiology of disease originated with the epidemiological observations of Burkitt et al. (1). Interest in

This research was supported in part by the Indiana Agricultural Experiment Station (Paper #7246), Grants HL-03299 and HL-05209 from the United States Public Health Service, and a Research Career Award (HL-0734) from the National Heart, Lung and Blood Institute.

Table 1.   Large intestine cancer and diet changes in Connecticut males[a]

Diet component	Change in annual per capita consumption (1935-1965)	Correlation coefficient with large intestine cancer
Beef	+55%	+0.905
Meat, poultry, and fish	+35%	+0.941
Cereal	-30%	-0.974
Potatoes	-26%	-0.968

[a]From Leveille (7).

dietary fiber was not new and, in fact, a large body of evidence concerning the role of dietary fiber had been developed in the laboratory of Walker (2-4). Cleave (5) had also postulated that many of the diseases common in developed countries were due to overconsumption of refined carbohydrate.

Extensive popular interest in this relationship has resulted in frequent oversimplification and a group of claims for the benefits of increased consumption of dietary fiber that are, in large part, unfounded. The original hypothesis (1) involved the differences observed in the incidence of a large number of diseases in developing countries (e.g., rural Africa) and in modern Western countries (e.g., United States). The diseases mentioned included heart disease, appendicitis, diverticular disease, gallstones, varicose veins, hiatus hernia, hemorrhoids, and colon cancer; all were found in very low incidence (or were nonexistent) in Africa and in very high incidence in the Western world. Many differences exist between these two populations, one of which is the high dietary fiber intake of the African populations in question.

In contrast with the observations of Burkitt, Drasar and Irving (6) correlated breast and colon cancer with several dietary components. Best correlations were between total fat and animal fat, whereas very weak negative correlations were seen with dietary fiber. Leveille (7) reviewed cancer incidence and dietary habits in Connecticut males, a group with one of the highest colon cancer rates in the world. Consumption of meat had increased dramatically during the period examined (1935-1965), and consumption of cereals and potatoes had decreased. During the same period of time, colon cancer rates had increased by 35%. Very strong positive correlations were observed with beef and meat, poultry, and fish and very strong negative correlations with cereals and potatoes (Table 1).

Enstrom (8), however, observed that, when we consider the entire United States, colon cancer rates have not changed dramatically since 1946, while meat consumption has doubled (Table 2). Geographically, cancer rates in the United States are high in the Midwest and Northeast and low in the South (9), a fact for which dietary differences can offer little explanation.

The epidemiological evidence has been reviewed extensively by Trowell and various co-workers. The observations mentioned earlier concerning

Table 2. Beef consumption and colorectal cancer rates in the United States (1945–1970)[a]

Year	Beef consumption (lbs/wk/person)	Colorectal cancer rates (deaths/100,000)
1945	1.1	21
1955	1.4	20
1965	1.9	20
1970	2.2	19

[a]From Enstrom (8).

comparisons of African natives and Western populations indicated a drastic difference in fiber consumption (20 g/day versus 6 g/day, crude fiber) and in heart disease rates (10–12). In addition, Trowell observed increased death from coronary heart disease in English women that corresponded with decreased dietary fiber intake from 1931–1971 (11). During the period of food rationing during World War II (1939–1947) fat consumption declined, dietary fiber consumption increased, and deaths from coronary heart disease in the above group did not increase as they had in the period between 1931 and 1939. Between 1956 and 1966, Morris and his co-workers (11a) conducted a 7-day dietary survey in 337 London men. By 1976, there had been 45 cases of coronary disease in this group, 26 of which were fatal. Morris et al. found two dietary characteristics that correlated with a lower incidence of coronary disease — high energy intake and high dietary fiber intake, primarily from cereals.

These observations led to the current hypothesis concerning dietary fiber, i.e., that decreased consumption of dietary fiber is associated with increased incidence of a large variety of diseases, among the most prominent of which were diverticular disease, colon cancer, and coronary heart disease. This chapter clarifies the current concept of the involvement of dietary fiber in these diseases as evidenced by the experimental data available.

DEFINITION AND ANALYSIS

A major problem that still interferes with the development of sound data concerning dietary fiber has been the acceptance of a uniform definition of dietary fiber and agreement on the analytical techniques to be used for its analysis. Until recently, any work concerning human foods was forced to rely on crude fiber analysis. This analysis, developed first in the nineteenth century (13, 14), has little physiological basis and has been shown to recover variable and inconsistent quantities of the components of dietary fiber (15–17). The elimination of all use of crude fiber data is generally accepted by all those who do research on dietary fiber.

Dietary fiber is now usually defined as the material in our diet that is not digested by our digestive enzymes or by our gut microflora (10). This means that the major cell wall components of plants, cellulose, hemicellulose, lignin, pectins, and gums are the major components of dietary fiber. The specifics of the chemistry of dietary fiber have been expertly reviewed by Southgate (18) and by Cummings (19).

Analytical methods for dietary fiber have been available for some time but have been used primarily for forage analysis by ruminant physiologists. Application of this methodology has begun to produce fairly thorough lists of dietary fiber analysis of human foods (20, 21). The two methods that have emerged as most reliable and applicable are those of Southgate (17, 22) and of Van Soest (23, 24). Southgate's method involves systematic extraction and quantification of fiber components, whereas Van Soest uses detergents to fractionate cell wall components for analysis. Agreement between the two methods is quite good (25). More complete lists of human foods based on thorough and uniform method of analysis should be forthcoming and will be essential to an understanding of the role of dietary fiber in human nutrition.

At this stage in the development of dietary fiber research, methodology is sufficiently developed so that we can insist on a complete analysis of the components of any dietary fiber source. Relying on crude fiber or failing to mention the characteristics of a source of dietary fiber should not be acceptable. As is noted later, the composition of fiber or the particular component of fiber used has a dramatic effect on the physiological response.

PHYSICAL PROPERTIES OF DIETARY FIBER

There are three main physical properties of dietary fiber that are, in large part, responsible for the observed effects — water-holding capacity, adsorption of bile acids or other solutes, and interaction with intestinal microflora. These properties are not totally independent, and their relative magnitude varies greatly with source and composition of dietary fiber. It is the nature of these interactions that determines the physiological effect of a particular source of dietary fiber.

Water Holding

McConnell et al. (26) examined the ability of many common sources of dietary fiber in human diets to hold water. They found that many types of vegetables, including some fresh vegetables, absorbed significant amounts of water (Table 3). Cooking and particle size had little effect on water holding; however, composition of the fiber did seem to determine its absorptive capacity. High proportions of polysaccharides in the fiber were best correlated with high water-holding capacity. Lignin content was not related to absorption of water.

Adsorption

Some component of laboratory rations has long been recognized as having an influence on bile salt metabolism in rats. Portman (27) found increased

Table 3.   Water-holding capacity of vegetables[a]

Vegetable	G of water/ g of fresh vegetable	G of water/g of acetone (dry powder)
Bran	4.5	3.0
Mango	3.1	20.4
Carrot	2.1	23.4
Apple	1.8	12.1
Oatmeal	1.7	1.8
Green bean	1.0	8.1
Lettuce	1.0	23.7
Celery	0.9	19.2
Potato	0.5	2.0
Turnip	0.4	9.0

[a]From McConnell et al. (26).

excretion and a reduction in the half-life of cholic acid in rats fed commercial laboratory rations as compared with rats fed a semipurified diet. Some component of the grain in the commercial diets was found to be responsible for this change.

Eastwood and Boyd (28) found that significant quantities of bile salts were somehow bound to the insoluble contents of the small intestine of rats. Eastwood and Hamilton (29) later found that dry grain, a high fiber byproduct of the brewing industry, bound significant quantities of bile salts in vitro. They also postulated that this adsorption was hydrophobic in nature.

Kritchevsky and Story (30) found that many of the materials commonly used in animal diets bound sodium taurocholate in vitro, whereas others, such as highly purified cellulose, did not. All bile acids and bile salts are not adsorbed to the same extent by fiber and its components (31, 32), making generalizations from partial data somewhat questionable (Table 4). Many fiber-containing materials commonly found in both human and animal diets have been shown to adsorb bile salts (33–36).

Eastwood et al. (37) have developed a method for measuring adsorption in materials with widely varying water-holding capacity. Since solvent held by fiber would contain solute, water-holding capacity would greatly modify

Table 4.   Binding of bile acids and bile salts by various types of dietary fiber[a]

Bile acid or salt	Alfalfa (% bound)[b]	Bran (% bound)	Cellulose (% bound)
Cholic	19.9	10.2	3.0
Taurocholic	6.9	1.4	1.0
Glycocholic	11.5	3.8	1.2
Deoxycholic	10.4	5.4	0.2
Taurodeoxycholic	11.4	3.4	0.7
Glycodeoxycholic	27.8	7.8	4.7

[a]From Story and Kritchevsky (32).
[b]50 mg of fiber was incubated with 50 μmol of bile acid or salt in 5 ml phosphate buffer (pH 7.0) for 2 hr at 37°C.

Table 5. Bile acid adsorption after washing[a]

Dietary Fiber	Washes[b]	Deoxycholate adsorbed (%)	
		2.5 mM	5.0 mM
Carrot	None	80	80
	1	63	65
	2	40	32
Bran	None	51	40
	1	31	24
	2	28	20

[a]From Eastwood et al. (37).
[b]Washed for 16 h with phosphate buffer (pH 8.0) at 37°C.

observed bile salt-binding capacity. This method involves extensive washing after initial incubation, yielding a measure of adsorbed bile salts only (Table 5).

Intestinal Microflora

Evidence concerning the effects of dietary fiber on the bacterial populations of the intestines has been inhibited by a lack of information concerning the "normal" numbers and species present. In fact we do not have a complete compendium of the species present in the human gut, not a surprising fact when one considers the amount of work involved in completing such a task. Information concerning the effects of diet on our microflora has thus been limited to general observations of some species or groups of species and/or the ability of preconditioned bacteria to metabolize certain substrates.

Comparisons of populations from various parts of the world showed differences in some types of fecal bacteria (38). Diet, especially dietary fiber, was thought to be a major cause for the observed differences. Large differences were observed between people eating a mixed diet and those eating largely vegetarian diets. Moore et al. (39), however, found that changing to a vegetarian diet did not change the spectrum of fecal bacteria in teenaged girls. The proportions of various species can be altered to a certain extent by diet (39), but dramatic changes such as suggested by epidemiological data have not been demonstrated.

Functional changes in the bacteria residing in the gut can apparently be changed by diet. Cyclamate is metabolized to cyclohexylamine by microflora that have been exposed to dietary cyclamate (40, 41). Before exposure these bacteria are unable to make this conversion. Vegetarians have been reported to exhibit no differences in type or number of fecal bacteria when compared to people eating a mixed diet. Cultures of these bacteria do, however, display a much lower level of bile acid 7-dehydroxylase (40). Thus, functional changes in bacterial metabolism, either directly or by changes in relative number of organisms, seem to be an important consideration in the examination of the role of dietary fiber.

Table 6.   Use of bran in symptomatic relief of diverticular disease[a]

Symptom	Before bran	After bran		Bran not tolerated
		Relieved	Not relieved	
Dyspeptic	64	55	5	5
Painful diverticular disease	69	63	1	5
Bowel symptoms	38	33	1	4

[a]From Painter et al. (45).

In addition, fermentation of fiber by intestinal bacteria may play a significant role in the effects of fiber on the diseases in question (41). Unabsorbed carbohydrates, either digestible or nondigestible, can be fermented by intestinal bacteria, resulting in gas formation, volatile fatty acid production, and other reactions that accompany the above (secondary bile acid formation). All of these can play a role in determining the effects of dietary fiber.

DIETARY FIBER AND DISEASE

Diverticular Disease

Diverticular disease can be described as a condition in which increased intralumenal pressures result in an outpocketing of the mucosal layer of the large intestine through the muscle layers (42). As much as 40% of the population of developed countries have diverticula and up to 10% of these cases require surgery (43, 44). Dietary fiber intake has been epidemiologically linked with the incidence of diverticular disease (1).

Experimentation with increased levels of dietary fiber with patients having diverticular disease has indicated an improvement of symptoms and a relatively low rate of rejection of the bran regimen (45–48) (Table 6). Changes in the consistency of the fecal mass within the intestine resulting from increased water-holding capacity have the net effect of decreasing colonic pressures (47, 49, 50), resulting in the relief of symptoms. The change in water content also results in decreased transit time and increased fecal bulk (47, 49, 54). Fermentation of fiber by intestinal bacteria resulting in volatile fatty acids that would then act as osmotic agents and increase fecal bulk has also been suggested as a mechanism (41).

In spite of the effectiveness of high fiber foods in preventing or reversing the symptoms of diverticular disease, linking them etiologically is still only a hypothesis. Bran has beneficial effects, but tests involving other foods that are more palatable and more easily added to one's diet than bran must be carried out before recommendations concerning dietary fiber in general can be made.

Colon Cancer

The suggested mechanisms for the involvement of dietary fiber in altering the incidence of colon cancer include all the physical properties mentioned above. Hill (55) summarized these possible mechanisms as follows: 1) the increased water-holding capacity of dietary fiber may dilute carcinogens or cocarcinogens in the intestine below their carcinogenic threshold; 2) increased water content would also decrease transit time, thus decreasing the time of exposure of carcinogens to the intestinal lining; 3) fiber may adsorb carcinogens or cocarcinogens, making them unavailable for interaction with the intestinal mucosa; and 4) interactions of intestinal bacteria with fiber may result in an alteration of microfloral metabolism to decrease production of carcinogens or cocarcinogens.

The above hypotheses are based mainly on the implication of bile acids in development of colon cancer and alterations in bile acid metabolism by dietary fiber. Bile acids are produced by the liver from cholesterol and secreted via the bile into the intestine. The major primary (synthesized) bile acids in man are cholic and chenodeoxycholic acids. In the intestine the primary bile acids are converted to secondary bile acids by the intestinal microflora. Cholic acid is converted to deoxycholic acid and chenodeoxycholic acid to lithocholic acid. The involvement of bile acids in carcinogenesis has resulted from the conversion, in the laboratory, of deoxycholic acid to methylcholanthrene, a potent carcinogen (56). In addition, deoxycholic acid has also been shown to be carcinogenic when applied to mouse skin (57).

Reddy et al. (58) found that cancer patients had much higher concentrations of fecal bile acids than healthy controls. Concentrations of secondary bile acids were about 70% higher in the cancer patients. Hill et al. (59) have also reported increased concentrations of fecal bile acids in colon cancer patients, a larger percentage of which were secondary bile acids.

Further evidence supporting the role played by bile acids in colon cancer has come from animal experiments. Nigro and Campbell (60) have summarized a group of studies done in their laboratory. Cholestyramine, an anion-exchange resin that adsorbs bile acids, thus increasing their excretion, results in changes in number and location of chemically induced gastrointestinal tumors in rats (Table 7). Cholestyramine-fed animals had many more tumors in both large and small bowel and dramatically more in the distal portion when azoxymethane, 1,2-dimethylhydrazine, or methylazoxymethanol was used as a carcinogen. They subsequently found that bile acid levels of the intestinal tissue were increased by either the carcinogen or by cholestyramine, but that this effect was not additive. By surgically moving the entry point for bile to the distal portion of the small intestine, resulting in a doubling of fecal bile acid concentrations, they were also able to show significant increases in the incidence of chemically induced tumor.

Table 7.   Chemical carcinogenesis in rats fed cholestyramine[a]

| Location | Tumors per rat[b] | |
	Control	2% Cholestyramine
Small bowel		
Proximal	3.7	3.9
Distal	0.5	2.6
Large bowel		
Proximal	1.9	3.5
Distal	0.8	3.7

[a]From Nigro and Campbell (60).

[b]Ten rats per group.

Since epidemiology and animal models seem to indicate a strong relationship between colon cancer and fecal bile acid concentrations, does dietary fiber in fact alter bile acid concentrations in the feces? Results of several experiments reporting this sort of data are summarized in Table 8. It appears that, in order to achieve the desired increase in excretion with decrease in concentration of fecal bile acids, 28 g of bran per day are needed. Lesser quantities of bran, pectin, or bagasse result in no change or increases in bile acid concentrations. These studies were of relatively short duration and, of course, yield no evidence concerning actual colon cancer rates.

Recently animal studies have investigated the role of dietary fiber in experimental carcinogenesis. Watanabe et al. (66) found that alfalfa or wheat bran (15% of diet) did not alter incidence of colon tumors induced in rats by azoxymethane but that pectin did decrease tumor incidence. Bile acid concentrations were not reported. Clinton and Visek (67) found a decreased induction of intestinal arylhydrocarbon hydroxylase in response to benzo(a)pyrene fed with bran. This would indicate a decrease in exposure of the intestine to benzo(a)pyrene, possibly as a result of dilution or binding.

Many questions remain unanswered concerning the role of dietary fiber in carcinogenesis. What is the exact nature of the effect of bile acids on carcinogenesis? Bile acid concentration appears to be related to tumor incidence and fiber could play a pivotal role in determining concentrations. Water holding and adsorption must be carefully examined before both are judged as beneficial since, if adsorption is increased relative to water held, bile acid concentrations will increase. Fiber sources such as bran hold large quantities of water but adsorb very little bile acid and, thus, as has been shown, can decrease bile acid concentrations. Further examination of the availability of adsorbed bile acids is also needed. Are these bile acids less harmful in this sequestered state or, as appears to be the case with cholestyramine, is their concentration the only factor involved?

Other diet ingredients influence the amount of bile acids present in the intestine (55) and thus may alter the functional significance of the amount of fiber in the diet. Indeed, the interaction of fiber itself with the intestinal

Table 8.   Effects of dietary fiber on fecal sterol excretion in man

Dietary fiber (type and amount)	Duration (wks)	Fecal neutral steroid		Fecal acidic steroid		Reference
		Mg/g of dry feces (% change)	Mg/day (% change)	Mg/g of dry feces (% change)	Mg/day (% change)	
Bran (16 g/day)	3	NR[a]	NR	+20	+32	(61)
Bran (28 g/day)	3	NR	NR	-35	+40	(62)
Bran (36 g/day)	3	-55	+36	-57	+40	(63)
Bran (39 g/day)	3	0	0	-41	-2	(64)
Bagasse (10.5 g/day)	12	-41	-10	0	+50	(64)
Pectin (15 g/day)	3	-11	+16	+7	+40	(65)

[a]NR, not reported.

microflora may alter the spectrum of bile acids present in the intestine. All these factors must be considered when examining the role of fiber in carcinogenesis, since any factor that alters the concentration, spectrum, or exposure of bile acids to the intestine may alter our susceptibility to colon cancer and possibly all types of cancer.

Lipid Metabolism and Atherosclerosis

Investigation into the role of dietary fiber in lipid metabolism and atherosclerosis has not been confined to the recent past. As part of the examination of the differences in atherogenicity of fats of various saturation in rabbits, it was noted (68) that saturated fats, without cholesterol, were only more cholesteremic when fed with a semipurified diet (69, 70). When fed with commercial rabbit diets they caused little change in cholesterol levels or atherosclerosis. Kritchevsky and Tepper (71, 72) found that the small amount of unsaturated fat in commercial diets was not responsible for the alteration of effects and suggested that some other dietary component, e.g., fiber or other carbohydrates, was responsible.

Moore (73) observed an effect of fiber-containing substances as part of an atherogenic, cholesterol-free, semipurified diet. Wheat straw or wheat straw–peat (3:1) were found to be less atherogenic and less cholesteremic than cellulose or cellophane when added to a semipurified diet containing 20% butterfat.

Suggested mechanisms for the effect of dietary fiber have centered on steroid excretion. Horlick et al. (74) found that alfalfa, already known to be hypocholesteremic in rabbits, greatly increased neutral steroid excretion (75). They concluded that alfalfa was interfering with cholesterol absorption. Kritchevsky and co-workers (76, 77) made a similar observation in rats. Using isocaloric diets with either alfalfa or cellulose as fiber, they found that alfalfa resulted in decreased cholesterol absorption. Leveille and Sauberlich (78) reported a significant increase in bile acid excretion, but not in neutral sterols, in rats fed 1% cholesterol with pectin added. At an earlier date Lin et al. (79) had made similar observations concerning pectin.

Based on this information and the ability of many types of dietary fiber to adsorb bile acids, we formulated a possible mechanism for the hypocholesteremic effects of fiber (80, 81). Since fiber can bind bile salts, thus increasing their excretion rates, this would increase the amount of cholesterol needed for synthesis of bile acids. In addition, if bile salts are unavailable for interaction with cholesterol for micelle formation in this bound form, cholesterol absorption would be greatly reduced. The result would be a 2-fold drain on body cholesterol — increased bile acid synthesis and decreased absorption.

The magnitude of the change in cholesterol level would be related to the capacity of the fiber for bile salts and the efficiency of the feedback control of cholesterol synthesis. Neither of these factors can be considered inde-

Table 9.   The effect of pectin on serum cholesterol levels in man

Pectin (g/day)	Duration (days)	Serum cholesterol (% change)	Reference
15	20	−5	(94)
15	20	−5	(94)
6	66	0	(95)
12	52	0	(95)
10	28	−5	(96)
6	28	−4	(96)
36	14	−12	(97)
12	21	−9	(98)
15	21	−15	(65)

pendent of the other. For this reason the alteration of cholesterol levels with various types of dietary fiber has not yielded consistent results. Cellulose, a weak adsorbant of bile acids, is apparently ineffective in lowering cholesterol levels of rats or rabbits (82–85). Pectin and lignin have been shown to lower cholesterol levels in rats and rabbits (78, 79, 85–88). Other animal models such as chickens, baboons, and vervet monkeys have also been used with favorable results (89–91).

In man the changes in lipid metabolism resulting from increased dietary fiber have been less uniform. Bran apparently has little effect on serum lipid levels in man (92), in spite of its alteration of bile acid excretion. Recently, in a study involving several sources of dietary fiber (93), hard red spring wheat bran and soybean hulls were found to lower serum cholesterol in men by 18% and 14%, respectively, when 26 g/day were added to the diet.

In contrast, pectin has been shown to be very effective in lowering serum cholesterol levels in man when fed at rates of from 6 to 15 g/day for 14–66 days, as has been summarized in Table 9. Pectin seems to function by increasing excretion of bile acids, whereas little change in neutral steroid excretion has been observed (65). Guar gum has also proven fairly effective in lowering human serum cholesterol levels (95–97).

The exact role of dietary fiber in the nutritional influence on lipid metabolism and atherosclerosis cannot be as simply explained as would appear from the above data. As with colon cancer, all dietary ingredients interact to varying degrees, and the resultant effect cannot be predicted on the basis of individual effects of the components. For example, Kritchevsky et al. (99) found that the difference in cholesteremia and atherogenicity of protein source in rabbits can be completely altered by the addition of different sources of dietary fiber (Table 10).

All the components of our diet can influence lipid metabolism. The resultant effect on our susceptibility to atherosclerosis depends on the balance of these components and probably is not dramatically altered by changing only one component at a time. Thus, the amount and source of

Table 10. Interaction of dietary fiber and protein in experimental atherosclerosis in rabbits[a]

Protein source	Dietary fiber	Serum cholesterol (mg/dl)	Liver cholesterol (g/100 g)	Atheroma[b]	Aortic FC/EC[c]
Casein	Cellulose	402	0.81	1.81	5.25
Casein	Wheat straw	375	0.84	1.17	3.92
Casein	Alfalfa	193	0.73	0.70	1.81
Soya	Cellulose	248	0.93	1.50	5.57
Soya	Wheat straw	254	0.85	1.04	3.25
Soya	Alfalfa	159	0.77	0.88	2.38

[a]From Kritchevsky et al. (99).
[b]Aortic arch, 0–4 grade.
[c]Free cholesterol/ester cholesterol.

dietary fiber in our diets, just as with dietary lipid, may play a role in determining our atherosclerotic potential, but, as with any other factor, differences in dietary fiber cannot be the sole cause or cure of heart disease.

CONCLUSIONS

From this evidence it is obvious that dietary fiber plays an important role in our diet. Considering the past lack of interest in fibrous components of our diet, except where regularity of defecation was concerned, this is probably the most important outcome of the recent extreme interest in dietary fiber. As with all interests of this sort, all of the claims that have been made cannot be supported. Similarly, there are certain effects of dietary fiber that must be closely monitored to prevent possible ill effects of overconsumption of high fiber diets.

The increase in volatile gas production in the large intestine can be related to sigmoid volvulus, a twisting of the large intestine (100). Phytate, a component of many sources of fiber, binds divalent cations and can cause deficiency of such cations as a result of decreased bioavailability (101–105). Wheat bran and some other types of dietary fiber contain trypsin and chymotrypsin inhibitors that could influence digestion and hence availability of marginal diets (106–107). Recent reports have examined the effects of various sources of dietary fiber on the topography of the intestines (108). Both small and large intestines of alfalfa- and cholestyramine-fed animals showed evidence of breakdown in the epithelial barrier and cell destruction when examined by scanning electron microscopy. This sort of breakdown could partially explain the observed differences in experimental carcinogenesis mentioned earlier (60).

Dietary fiber research is in its infancy and, as a result, needs to be directed carefully. The exact roles in the etiology of the diseases mentioned here, as well as of others, need to be sought out systematically, since such vast differences in sources of dietary fiber and in the effects of its components exist. Generalizations cannot be made and the mechanisms apparently are complex.

Regardless of these complexities, dietary fiber may hold great potential for altering patterns of many diseases of epidemic proportions in the Western world. Researchers must examine the mechanisms involved in the role of fiber in these diseases, decide which of these are valid, and finally make realistic recommendations for changes in our diet.

REFERENCES

1. Burkitt, D. P., Walker, A. R. P., and Painter, N. S. (1974). JAMA 229:1068.
2. Walker, A. R. P., and Arvidson, U. B. (1954). J. Clin. Invest. 33:1366.
3. Walker, A. R. P., Mortimer, K. L., Kloppers, P. J., Botha, D., Grusin, H., and Seftel, H. C. (1961). Am. J. Clin. Nutr. 9:643.

4. Walker, A. R. P., and Walker, B. F. (1969). Br. Med. J. 3:238.
5. Cleave, T. L. (1956). J. R. Nav. Med. Serv. 42:55.
6. Drasar, B. S., and Irving, D. (1973). Br. J. Cancer 27:167.
7. Leveille, G. A. (1975). J. Anim. Sci. 41:723.
8. Enstrom, J. E. (1975). Br. J. Cancer 32:432.
9. Blot, W. J., Fraumeni, F. J., Jr., Stone, B. J., and McKay, F. W. (1976). J. Natl. Cancer Inst. 57:1225.
10. Trowell, H. (1972). Atherosclerosis 16:138.
11. Trowell, H. (1972). Am. J. Clin. Nutr. 25:926.
11a. Morris, J. N., Marr, J. W., and Clayton, D. G. (1977). Br. Med. J. 2:1307.
12. Trowell, H., Painter, N., and Burkitt, D. (1974). Am. J. Digest. Dis. 19:864.
13. Mangold, D. E. (1934). Nutr. Abstr. Rev. 3:647.
14. Horwitz, W. (1970). Official Methods of Analysis of the Association of Official Analytical Chemists, U.S.A., Ed. 11, p. 129. Association of Official Analytical Chemists, Washington, D. C.
15. Van Soest, P. J. (1973). Fed. Proc. 32:1804.
16. Van Soest, P. J., and McQueen, R. W. (1973). Proc. Nutr. Soc. 32:123.
17. Southgate, D. A. T. (1969). J. Sci. Food Agric. 20:331.
18. Southgate, D. A. T. (1976). In G. A. Spiller and R. J. Amen (eds.), Fiber in Human Nutrition, p. 31. Plenum Publishing Corp., New York.
19. Cummings, J. H. (1976). In G. A. Spiller and R. J. Amen (eds.), Fiber in Human Nutrition, p. 1. Plenum Publishing Corp., New York.
20. Southgate, D. A. T., Bailey, B., Collinson, E., and Walker, A. F. (1976). J. Human Nutr. 30:303.
21. Shipley, E. A. (1978). In G. A. Spiller (ed.), Topics in Dietary Fiber Research, p. 203. Plenum Publishing Corp., New York.
22. Southgate, D. A. T. (1969). J. Sci. Food Agric. 20:326.
23. Van Soest, P. J. (1963). J. Assoc. Off. Agric. Chem. 46:825.
24. Goering, H. K., and Van Soest, P. J. (1970). Forage Fiber Analyses. U. S. Department of Agriculture, Agricultural Handbook No. 379. United States Government Printing Office, Washington, D. C.
25. McConnell, A. A., and Eastwood, M. A. (1974). J. Sci. Food Agric. 25:1457.
26. McConnell, A. A., Eastwood, M. A., and Mitchell, W. D. (1974). J. Sci. Food Agric. 25:1457.
27. Portman, O. W. (1960). Am. J. Clin. Nutr. 8:462.
28. Eastwood, M. A., and Boyd, G. S. (1967). Biochim. Biophys. Acta 137:393.
29. Eastwood, M. A., and Hamilton, D. (1968). Biochim. Biophys. Acta 152:165.
30. Kritchevsky, D., and Story, J. A. (1974). J. Nutr. 104:458.
31. Kritchevsky, D., and Story, J. A. (1975). Am. J. Clin. Nutr. 28:305.
32. Story, J. A., and Kritchevsky, D. (1976). J. Nutr. 106:1292.
33. Birdner, H. J., and Kern, F., Jr. (1974). Gastroenterology 67:237.
34. Balmer, J., and Zilversmit, D. B. (1974). J. Nutr. 104:1319.
35. Story, J. A., and Kritchevsky, D. (1975). Nutr. Rep. Int. 11:161.
36. Kritchevsky, D., Story, J. A., and Walker, A. R. P. (1976). S. Afr. Med. J. 50:1831.
37. Eastwood, M. A., Anderson, R., Mitchell, W. D., Robertson, J., and Pocock, S. (1976). J. Nutr. 106:1429.
38. Hill, M. J., Crowther, J. S., Drasar, B. S., Hawksworth, G., Aries, V., and Williams, R. E. O. (1971). Lancet 1:95.
39. Moore, W. E. C., Cato, E. P., and Holdeman, L. V. (1969). J. Infect. Dis. 119:641.
40. Aries, V. C., Crowther, J. S., Drasar, B. S., Hill, M. J., and Ellis, F. R. (1971). J. Pathol. 103:54.

41. Hellendoorn, E. W. (1978). *In* G. A. Spiller (ed.), Topics in Dietary Fiber Research, p. 127. Plenum Publishing Corp., New York.
42. Price, A. B. (1975). Fiber Deficiency and Colonic Disorders, p. 101. Plenum Publishing Corp., New York.
43. Parks, T. G. (1974). Proceedings of the Fourth International Symposium on Gastrointestinal Mobility, p. 369. Mitchell Press, Vancouver.
44. Painter, N. S. (1969). *In* B. C. Morson (ed.), Diseases of the Colon, Rectum, and Anus, p. 201. Heineman, London.
45. Painter, N. S., Almeida, A. Z., and Colebourne, K. W. (1972). Br. Med. J. 1:137.
46. Plumley, P. F., and Francis, B. (1973). J. Am. Diet. Assoc. 63:527.
47. Findlay, J. M., Smith, A. N., Mitchell, W. D., Anderson, A. J. B., and Eastwood, M. A. (1974). Lancet 1:146.
48. Brodribb, A. J. M. (1977). Lancet 1:664.
49. Brodribb, A. J. M., and Humphreys, D. M. (1976). Br. Med. J. 1:424.
50. Hodgson, J. (1972). Br. Med. J. 3:729.
51. Kirwan, W. O., Smith, A. N., McConnell, A. A., and Eastwood, M. A. (1974). Br. Med. J. 4:187.
52. Connell, A. M., and Smith, C. L. (1974). Proceedings of the Fourth International Symposium on Gastrointestinal Mobility, p. 365. Mitchell Press, Vancouver.
53. Payler, D. K., Pomare, E. W., Heaton, K. W., and Harvey, R. F. (1975). Gut 16:209.
54. Connell, A. M. (1976). Am. J. Clin. Nutr. 29:1427.
55. Hill, J. J. (1976). *In* P. P. Nair and D. Kritchevsky (eds.), The Bile Acids, Vol. 3, p. 169. Plenum Publishing Corp., New York.
56. Wieland, H., and Dane, E. (1933). Hoppe Seylers Z. Physiol. Chem. 219:240.
57. Salaman, M. H., and Roe, F. J. C. (1956). Br. J. Cancer 10:363.
58. Reddy, B. S., Mastromarino, A., and Wynder, E. L. (1975). Cancer Res. 35:3403.
59. Hill, M. J., Drasar, B. S., Williams, R. E. O. (1975). Lancet 1:535.
60. Nigro, N. D., and Campbell, R. L. (1976). *In* P. P. Nair and D. Kritchevsky (eds.), The Bile Acids, Vol. 3, p. 155. Plenum Publishing Corp., New York.
61. Eastwood, M. A., Kirkpatrick, J. R., Mitchell, W. D., Bone, A., and Hamilton, T. (1973). Br. Med. J. 4:392.
62. Cummings, J. H., Hill, M. J., Jenkins, D. J. A., Pearson, J. R., and Wiggins, H. S. (1976). Am. J. Clin. Nutr. 29:1468.
63. Jenkins, D. J. A., Hill, M. S., and Cummings, J. H. (1975). Am. J. Clin. Nutr. 28:1408.
64. Baird, I., McLean, Walters, R. L., Davies, P. S., Hill, M. J., Drasar, B. S., and Southgate, D. A. T. (1977). Metabolism 26:117.
65. Kay, R. M., and Truswell, A. S. (1977). Am. J. Clin. Nutr. 30:171.
66. Watanabe, K., Reddy, B. S., and Kritchevsky, D. (1978). Fed. Proc. 37:262.
67. Clinton, S. K., and Visek, W. J. (1978). Fed. Proc. 37:263.
68. Kritchevsky, D. (1964). J. Atheroscler. Res. 4:103.
69. Lambert, G. F., Miller, J. P., Olsen, R. T., and Frost, D. V. (1958). Proc. Soc. Exp. Biol. Med. 97:544.
70. Malmros, H., and Wigand, G. (1959). Lancet 2:729.
71. Kritchevsky, D., and Tepper, S. A. (1965). Life Sci. 4:1467.
72. Kritchevsky, D., and Tepper, S. A. (1968). J. Atheroscler. Res. 8:357.
73. Moore, J. H. (1967). Br. J. Nutr. 21:207.
74. Horlick, L., Cookson, F. B., and Fedoroff, S. (1967). Circulation 36(suppl. II):18.

75. Cookson, F. B., Altschul, R., and Fedoroff, S. (1967). J. Atheroscler. Res. 7:69.
76. Kritchevsky, D., Casey, R. P., and Tepper, S. A. (1973). Nutr. Rep. Int. 7:61.
77. Kritchevsky, D., Tepper, S. A., and Story, J. A. (1974). Nutr. Rep. Int. 9:301.
78. Leveille, G. A., and Sauberlich, H. E. (1966). J. Nutr. 88:209.
79. Lin, T. M., Kim, K. S., Karveinen, E., and Ivy, A. C. (1957). Am. J. Physiol. 188:66.
80. Kritchevsky, D., Tepper, S. A., and Story, J. A. (1975). J. Food Sci. 40:8.
81. Story, J. A., and Kritchevsky, D. (1976). *In* G. A. Spiller and R. J. Amen (eds.), Fiber in Human Nutrition, p. 171. Plenum Publishing Corp., New York.
82. Wells, A. F., and Ershoff, B. H. (1961). J. Nutr. 74:87.
83. Kiriyama, S., Okazaki, Y., and Yoshida, A. (1969). J. Nutr. 97:382.
84. Tsai, A. C., Elias, J., Kelly, J. J., Lin, R. S. C., and Robson, J. R. K. (1976). J. Nutr. 106:118.
85. Hamilton, R. M. G., and Carroll, K. K. (1976). Atherosclerosis 24:47.
86. Berenson, L. M., Bhandaru, R. R., Radhakrishnamurthy, B., Sranivasan, S. B., and Berenson, G. S. (1975). Life Sci. 16:1533.
87. Judd, P. A., Kay, R. M., and Truswell, A. S. (1976). Proc. Nutr. Soc. 35:71A.
88. Story, J. A., Czarnecki, S. K., Baldino, A., and Kritchevsky, D. (1977). Fed. Proc. 36:1134.
89. Fisher, H., Soller, W. G., and Griminger, P. (1966). J. Atheroscler. Res. 6:292.
90. Kritchevsky, D., Davison, L. M., Shapiro, I. L., Kim, H. K., Kitagawa, M., Malhotra, S., Nair, P. P., Clarkson, T. B., Bersohn, I., and Winter, P. A. D. (1974). Am. J. Clin. Nutr. 27:29.
91. Kritchevsky, D., Davison, L. M., Kim, H. K., Krendel, D. A., Malhotra, S., Vander Watt, J. J., du Plessis, J. P., Winter, P. A. D., Ipp, T., Mendelsohn, D., and Berohn, I. (1977). Exp. Pathol. 26:28.
92. Truswell, A. S., and Kay, R. M. (1976). Lancet 1:367.
93. Munoz, J. M., Sanstead, H. H., Jacob, R. A., Logan, G. M., Jr., and Klevay, L. M. (1978). Fed. Proc. 37:755.
94. Keys, A., Grande, F., and Anderson, J. T. (1961). Proc. Soc. Exp. Biol. Med. 106:555.
95. Fahrenbach, M. J., Riccardi, B. A., Saunders, J. C., Louri, I. N., and Heider, J. G. (1965). Circulation 32(suppl. II):11.
96. Palmer, G. H., and Dixon, D. G. (1966). Am. J. Clin. Nutr. 18:437.
97. Jenkins, D. J. A., Leeds, A. R., Newton, C., and Cummings, J. H. (1975). Lancet 1:1116.
98. Durrington, P. N., Manning, A. P., Bolton, C. H., and Hartog, M. (1976). Lancet 2:394.
99. Kritchevsky, D., Tepper, S. A., Williams, D. E., and Story, J. A. (1977). Atherosclerosis 26:397.
100. Sutcliffe, M. M. L. (1968). Br. J. Surg. 55:903.
101. Reinhold, J. G., Parsa, A., Kariman, N., Hammick, J. W., and Ismail-Beigi, F. (1974). J. Nutr. 104:976.
102. Haghshenass, M., Mahlondji, M., Reinhold, J. G., and Mohammadi, N. (1972). Am. J. Clin. Nutr. 25:1143.
103. Reinhold, J. G., Nasr, K., Lahimgarzadeh, A., and Hedayati, H. (1973). Lancet 1:28.
104. Reinhold, J. G., Faradji, B., Abadi, P., and Ismail-Beigi, F. (1976). J. Nutr. 106:493.
105. Dobbs, R. J., and Baird, I. McL. (1977). Br. Med. J. I:1641.

106. Mistuanaga, T. (1974). J. Nutr. Sci. Vitaminol. 20:153.
107. Scheeman, B. O. (1977). Fed. Proc. 36:1118.
108. Cassidy, M. M., Grund, B., Lightfoot, F., Vahouny, G., Gallo, L., Kritchev-
     sky, D., Story, J., and Treadwell, C. (1978). Fed. Proc. 37:543.

International Review of Biochemistry
Biochemistry of Nutrition IA, Volume 27
Edited by A. Neuberger and T. H. Jukes
Copyright 1979   University Park Press   Baltimore

8
New Findings with Trace Elements: Including Effects of Processing on Supplies and Availability

E. J. UNDERWOOD

University of Western Australia, Nedlands, Western Australia

Fifteen trace elements are presently believed to be essential for animal life. The popular terms "trace elements" or "trace minerals" arose because the early workers were unable to determine their precise concentrations with the analytical methods then available and frequently referred to them as occurring in trace amounts. This designation has persisted despite the fact that most of them can now be estimated with great sensitivity and accuracy. The remarkable advances in analytical techniques that have made this possible have been major factors in stimulating and facilitating biological research with trace elements over the last two decades.

The 15 trace elements now accepted as essential for animals are iron, iodine, copper, manganese, zinc, cobalt, molybdenum, selenium, chromium, nickel, silicon, tin, fluorine, vanadium, and arsenic. Cadmium may also be essential for the rat, if suggestive preliminary evidence (1) is confirmed. Evidence for the essentiality of the last six of these — nickel, silicon, tin, fluorine, vanadium, and arsenic, often referred to as the "newer" trace elements — rests largely upon growth effects obtained mostly with laboratory species maintained on highly purified diets under environmental conditions in which atmospheric contamination is controlled (2). No specific physiological functions or involvement in particular enzymes systems have yet been identified for any of them except silicon (3). Nor, on present evidence, does it appear likely that the newer trace elements will be found to be of great practical significance to man or farm animals. However, selenium and chromium, which are now known to be of great nutritional importance to man and domestic livestock, were originally believed to be only of scientific interest. Already it has been suggested that silicate silicon may be the active agent in dietary fiber that affects the development of atherosclerosis and that lack of silicon may be an important etiological factor in this disease (4). High amounts of bound silicon are present in the arterial wall, especially in the intima, where it acts as a cross-linking agent, and also in certain kinds of dietary fiber that are active in preventing experimental models of atherosclerosis, reducing serum cholesterol and blood lipid levels, and binding bile acids in vitro.

A further group of trace elements, notably lead, cadmium, and mercury, may be classified as toxic elements because their biological significance is principally restricted to their toxic properties at low concentrations. Such a classification has limited usefulness and can be misleading because all elements are toxic if ingested or inhaled at high enough levels or for long enough periods. Moreover, the essential trace elements — copper, molybdenum, selenium and fluorine — are toxic to animals at naturally occurring levels in some parts of the world, and therefore need to be classified as essential elements or as toxic elements depending upon the circumstances.

Until 15 years ago only three trace elements were known to be associated with significant human health problems — iron and the two halogens iodine and fluorine. The classically recognized disease conditions related to them were anemia resulting from inadequate intakes of available iron and endemic goiter resulting from lack of environmental iodine. Also, mottled enamel of teeth and other manifestations of fluorosis had been related to above normal intakes of fluoride from the water supply in some areas, and the incidence of dental caries in man had been associated with inadequate fluoride intakes. Within recent years marginal or overt deficiencies of zinc and chromium have been observed in some human populations and a number of clinical disorders and genetic abnormalities have been related to trace element deficiencies, toxicities, or metabolic defects. These are discussed in later sections of this chapter.

Great progress has been made in the last two decades in our understanding of the mode and locus of action of the trace minerals. A range of metalloenzymes involving the trace metals has been identified and shown to participate in the basic biochemical processes of the cells and tissues. Environmental aspects of these elements, particularly of the heavy metals, have become of increasing concern because of the growing industrialization and urbanization of the Western world. Technological developments in food production and processing have presented further problems. These aspects are considered in the appropriate sections that follow.

MODE OF ACTION OF TRACE ELEMENTS

The only property that the essential trace elements have in common is that they occur and function in the tissues in low concentrations. Similar physicochemical properties bear little relation to physiological function. Even such chemically similar elements as nickel and cobalt function quite differently in living tissues. The normal ranges of tissue concentrations vary greatly in magnitude and are characteristic for each element. They are usually expressed as parts per million (μg/g) or parts per billion (ng/g). Certain elements that are nonessential on present evidence, such as bromine and rubidium, occur in foods and animal tissues in concentrations well above those of most of the essential trace minerals.

The characteristic concentrations of the essential trace elements in the tissues and fluids of the body, or of their functioning forms, must be maintained within narrow limits if the functional and structural integrity of the body is to be safeguarded and the growth, health, and fertility of the organism are to remain unimpaired. Continued ingestion of diets or continued exposure to environments that are deficient, imbalanced, or excessively high in a particular element induces changes in the levels or activities of that element in the body tissues and fluids so that they fall below, or rise above, the permissible limits. In these circumstances biochemical defects develop, physiological functions are affected, and structural disorders may arise in ways that differ with different elements, with the degree and duration of the dietary deficiency or toxicity, and with the age, species, sex, and activity of the organism. Such changes in tissue concentrations, especially in the blood, hair, and urine, provide valuable diagnostic criteria that have wide applicability in the detection of trace element disorders. For example, free thyroxine (T_4) assays of plasma can sharply differentiate hypothyroid and thyrotoxic patients from euthyroid individuals (5) (Table 1). The glutathione peroxidase (GSH-Px) level of chick plasma is directly related to the selenium level in the diet and to the effectiveness of selenium in the prevention of exudative diathesis (6). Also, signs of cobalt deficiency in ruminant animals begin to develop when the serum vitamin B_{12} level falls below 0.2 ng/ml (7, 8) or the level of cobalt in the rumen fluid falls below 0.5 ng/ml (9).

The trace elements act as catalysts in enzyme systems, some through weak ionic effects and some through specific associations known as metalloenzymes, in which the metal is firmly associated with the protein. In these cases there is a fixed number of metal atoms per molecule of protein, and these atoms cannot be removed without loss of activity. They usually cannot be replaced by any other metal; however, cobalt and cadmium can be substituted for the native zinc atoms in several zinc enzymes and the enzyme remains active (10). Some of the metal present in certain metalloenzymes is critical to their catalytic step, whereas the rest seems to serve primarily in preserving the protein structure (11). Further evidence that the protein-metal interactions not only enhance the catalytic activity of enzymes but may also increase the stability of the protein moiety to metabolic turnover has recently been obtained (12). Copper was shown to be a key regulator of lysyl oxidase activity in the aorta of chicks and a major determinant of the steady state levels of the enzyme in that tissue. Further understanding of the molecular mechanisms involved in the metalloenzymes and the nature of the metal-ion specificity has emerged from a study of the five known molybdenum enzymes — nitrogenase, nitrate reductase, aldehyde oxidase, xanthine oxidase, and sulfite oxidase (13). A simple molecular mechanism embodying coupled electron-proton transfer to and from the substrate, compatible with the coordination chemistry of molybdenum, was demonstrated for each of these enzymes with their diverse functions.

A large number of trace metal-enzyme associations have been identified, and in many cases their levels and activities have been related to manifestations of deficiency in the animal (14). Examples of such metalloenzymes, containing iron, copper, zinc, manganese, molybdenum, and selenium, are given in Table 2, illustrating the wide range of cellular activities in which the trace elements participate. Iron and copper enzymes have been recognized for some time, but most of the zinc metalloenzymes have only recently been discovered. In the 20 years after the 1940 discovery that carbonic anhydrase contains zinc, which is essential to its action (15), only five additional zinc metalloenzymes were identified, but between 1960 and 1975 the total number rose to about 24 (16). Critical reviews of the structure and function of zinc (16) and copper (17) metalloenzymes have recently appeared.

Individual metalloenzymes are not confined to single metals. For example, superoxide dismutase, which catalyzes the dismutation of the super-

Table 1.   Values (mean and standard deviation) for thyroid function tests in normal subjects and in patients with untreated primary thyroid disorders[a]

Group	PBI (μg/100 ml)	Resin uptake (% normal)	Free T4 index (T3/100 × PBI)	Free T4 concentration (μg/100 ml)	Free T4(%)
Hypothyroid (15)[b]	1.89 ± 0.69	72.5 ± 12.1	1.34 ± 0.51	1.71 ± 0.73	0.05 ± 0.01
Euthyroid (23)	5.33 ± 0.98	96.5 ± 10.2	5.09 ± 0.84	5.43 ± 0.99	0.07 ± 0.01
Hyperthyroid (15)	11.06 ± 2.40	131.4 ± 16.8	15.37 ± 3.90	19.01 ± 6.25	0.11 ± 0.02

[a]From Wellby and O'Halloran (5).
[b]Figures in brackets indicate number of subjects.

Table 2.   Important metalloenzymes

Metal	Enzyme	Function
Iron	Ferredoxin	Photosynthesis
	Succinate dehydrogenase	Aerobic oxidation of carbo-hydrates
	Cytochromes	Electron transfer
	Catalase	Protection against H_2O_2
Copper	Cytochrome oxidase	Principal terminal oxidase
	Lysyl oxidase	Lysine oxidation
	Tyrosinase	Melanin formation
	Ceruloplasmin	Iron utilization
	Uricase	Allantoin formation
	Superoxide dismutase (hemocuprein)	Dismutation of the superoxide anion free radical O_2^-
Zinc	Carbonic anhydrase	CO_2 formation: regulation of acidity
	Alcohol dehydrogenases	Alcohol metabolism
	Carboxypeptidases	Protein digestion
	Alkaline phosphatase	Hydrolysis of phosphate monoesters
	RNA polymerase	
	DNA polymerase	
	Thymidine kinase	Thymidine triphosphate formation
Manganese	Arginase	Urea formation
	Pyruvate carboxylase	Pyruvate metabolism
	Superoxide dismutase	Dismutation of the superoxide anion free radical
Molybdenum	Xanthine oxidase	Purine metabolism
	Sulfite oxidase	Sulfite oxidation
Selenium	Glutathione peroxidase	Removal of H_2O_2

oxide free radical according to the reaction $O_2^- + O_2^- + 2H^+ \rightarrow O_2 + H_2O_2$, may contain copper and zinc, or manganese instead of the copper and zinc. This enzyme was first isolated from bovine erythrocytes and was shown to be identical with the protein known as hemocuprein, erythrocuprein, or cerebrocuprein (18). The type of enzyme that contains copper and zinc (2 g of atoms of each metal per mole of protein) is located in the cell cytosol and has been isolated from a range of eukaryotic species (19). The superoxidase dismutase that contains manganese has been prepared from prokaryotes, whereas chicken liver contains both types, the manganoprotein in the mitochondria and the copper-zinc enzyme in the cytosol (20). Pathological disturbances in man or animals related to lack of superoxidase dismutase activity have not been demonstrated, although lower levels of this enzyme in the brains of copper-deficient neonatal rats than in controls have been reported (21).

By contrast, the tissue levels of the copper metalloenzyme lysyl oxidase are clearly related to the vascular defects that occur in chicks and pigs fed copper-deficient diets. The role of copper in the formation of aortic elastin (and collagen) has been stated in the following terms: "The primary biochemical lesion is a reduction in amine-oxidase activity of the aorta. This reduction in enzyme activity results, in turn, in a reduced capacity for oxidatively deaminating the epsilon-amino group of the lysine residues in elastin. The reduction in oxidative deamination results, in turn, in less lysine being converted to desmosine. The reduction in desmosine, which is the cross-linkage group of elastin, results in fewer cross-linkages in this protein, which in turn results in less elasticity of the aorta" (22). A detailed account of this relationship appears in the recent review by O'Dell, one of the original discoverers (17).

The earliest known metabolic defect in zinc deficiency is a decreased activity of thymidine kinase, the enzyme leading to thymidine triphosphate formation, a prerequisite for DNA synthesis and cell division (23). This and a number of other nucleotide polymerases, including DNA polymerase, are zinc metalloenzymes (16). Zinc therefore participates in fundamental metabolic steps critical to growth and development. Impaired activity of fetal thymidine kinase during embryonic morphogenesis probably explains the teratogenic effects of zinc deficiency (24). These gross malformations can even be related to regional differences in DNA synthesis in the body of zinc-deficient embryo rats and the particular vulnerability of the central nervous system (CNS) to prenatal zinc deprivation related to the finding that DNA synthesis in the head region, and especially in the CNS, is reduced more in zinc deficiency than it is in the rest of the body (25).

Clinical and pathological disorders arising from trace mineral deficiencies are known that cannot yet be explained in such convincing enzymatic or biochemical terms. Other physiologically significant metalloenzymes will no doubt be discovered and their particular loci and functions identified. The trace elements may also be found to participate in the structure and function of quite different compounds in the cells and tissues of the body, as has now been demonstrated for silicon. After the discovery of its essentiality for growth in chicks (26) and rats (27), silicon has been shown to be a vital cross-linking agent in connective tissue, with high concentrations in collagen (28), and involved in the mineralization process in bone (29). This element thus serves both a matrix or catalytic function and a structural function in bone development.

SOURCES OF TRACE ELEMENTS

The trace minerals occur in foods and dietaries from three main sources. They are present as *natural or inherent components,* absorbed and retained from the rocks, soils, and fertilizers on which the plants depend. These either pass directly to man and animals in the foods and feeds of vegetable origin consumed, or indirectly to man via the edible tissues and fluids of animals consuming the plants. The trace metals also occur in foods as *contaminants,* arising from exposure to atmospheric dusts and fumes, from the use of pesticides, fumigants, and feed additives, and from contact with metals in food storage, processing, and cooking. They may also be present as *deliberate additives,* either through direct incorporation into foods and beverages (as with iron and iodine in bread and flour, iodide or iodate in domestic salt, and fluoride in drinking water) or, more indirectly, through their adventitious presence in pigments, gels, stabilizers, and preservatives added to improve the color, flavor, keeping quality, or physical properties of the food.

Normally a high proportion of total daily trace metal intakes by man comes from their natural presence as inherent components of foods. The levels present in food of plant origin are primarily a reflection of the plant species and varieties and of the soil and fertilizer conditions under which the plants are grown. In an investigation of 17 grass species grown together on the same soil and sampled at the same time, the cobalt concentration was found to range from 0.05 to 0.14 μg/g, the copper from 4.5 to 21.1 μg/g, and the manganese from 96 to 815 μg/g on the dry basis. Intraspecies differences were highlighted by New Zealand investigations of pasture species. The total iodine levels of two strains of white clover were significantly different, and tenfold differences were observed among varieties of rye grass growing on similar soils (30).

The seeds of leguminous plants and the oil seeds are generally appreciably higher in most trace elements than are the cereal grains. Species differences among the cereal grains are small, with the exception of manganese. Thus wheat and oat grains are normally five times higher in manganese than maize or corn grain and some three times higher than barley (31, 32) or sorghum (33). Marked species differences in the manganese concentrations of the seeds of lupins (*Lupinus* spp.) also occur. Thus the seeds of *Lupinus albus* contained levels ranging from 817 to 3397 μg of manganese/g, or 10–15 times those of other lupin species growing on the same sites (33a).

These species differences in manganese content are profoundly important in the nutrition of poultry, but have no known significance in human dietaries. However, a metabolic antagonism between manganese and iron exists in which dietary manganese levels as low as 50 and 125 μg/g were found to adversely affect hemoglobin formation in pigs and rabbits (34). Abnormally high dietary intakes of manganese would therefore appear undesirable, especially in view of the precarious position in respect to available iron of many women during their fertile years. A further species difference of nutritional interest is the high molybdenum content of millet or sorghum grain (*Sorghum vulgare*) as compared with rice or wheat. In some parts of India where sorghum is a dietary staple molybdenum intakes up to 1.5 mg/

day can occur (35). No increase in uric acid excretion was apparent in individuals consuming such diets, but urinary copper excretion was markedly increased, presumably reflecting the well-established metabolic interaction between copper and molybdenum.

In a study of tomatoes and carrots, significant varietal differences were found in the concentrations of iron, manganese, zinc, and copper, but the range of variation was mostly only two- to fourfold (36). The effect of location on variation was greater than that of variety in this investigation and very much greater in earlier studies of vegetables (37, 38) and of fruits (39). These variations in trace mineral content arise primarily from differences in the available levels of the elements in the soil. This effect is particularly apparent with selenium, both on an inter- and an intranational basis. For example, samples of Swedish wheat were reported to contain 0.007–0.022 μg of selenium/g (40). The corresponding values for wheat samples from other countries were as follows: Argentina, 0.05; United States (hard winter), 0.37; United States (durum), 0.70; and Canada (Manitoba), 1.30 μg of selenium/g. The median selenium levels of wheats from the eastern United States were 0.05, as compared with 0.80 μg/g in wheats from South Dakota (41). Marked variation with locality is also evident with foods of animal origin, reflecting the intakes of selenium by the animal. For example, the mean levels for a low-selenium county in Oregon were 0.005 μg/g for milk and 0.050 μg/g for eggs (42). The corresponding values for these foods from two normal-selenium counties were 0.05–0.07 μg/g for milk and 0.4–0.5 μg/g for eggs, a tenfold difference in each case. Similar differences occur in the selenium levels in organ and muscle meats from animals on selenium-deficient and selenium-adequate diets.

The use of fertilizers designed to increase crop yields can markedly modify the trace mineral levels in the resulting crops. This was shown some years ago when the zinc concentration of wheat grown with the aid of a zinc-containing fertilizer averaged 32 μg/g, as compared with 16 μg/g for similar wheat grown on the same zinc-deficient soil without the fertilizer (44). More recently a marked increase has been observed in the zinc content of pea seeds when grown in water culture to which zinc sulfate was added (45). It was suggested that the nutritional value of legume seeds with respect to zinc content could be improved by applying zinc fertilizers "possibly in excess of requirements for optimal plant yields." This suggestion warrants further consideration in view of the marginal zinc deficiency apparent in some Western-style diets, as discussed under "Clinical Disorders Involving Zinc."

Fertilizer usage can also increase the levels of potentially harmful trace metals. Cadmium concentrations as high as 1 μg/g, or 10–20 times normal, have been produced in soybean seeds by the application of 144 metric tons/hectare of sewage sludge solids to the soil (46). Prolonged use of superphosphate containing 38–48 μg of cadmium/g can greatly increase the cadmium levels in pasture species, especially clovers (47). In a study of rice from 22 countries, marked regional differences in cadmium content were observed (48). The mean levels in the polished rice samples ranged from 0.002 and 0.008 $\mu g/g$ for Brazil and Iran to 0.03 and 0.06 $\mu g/g$ for Taiwan and Japan. Varietal differences may have contributed to this variation, but it is probably more a result of variations in soil type, fertilizers used, and the extent of pollution.

It is clear from the foregoing that trace element levels in foods vary considerably with their genetic constitution and with the environmental conditions under which they are grown or produced. This can be extremely important to grazing animals, in which many "area" problems, such as copper, cobalt, and selenium deficiencies and molybdenum, copper, and selenium toxicities, occur throughout the world (14). The relationship of man to the soil and geochemical environment is less direct because he is at the end of the food chain. Gross deficiencies or toxicities involving the trace minerals will therefore generally have been detected and corrected, or mainly so, earlier in the food chain in order to maintain the health and productivity of crops and stock. Also modern dietaries in the developed world contain a variety of types of food, obtained from ever-widening geographical sources. In this way mineral abnormalities in one type or source of food would tend to be ameliorated or offset by the consumption of foods of other types or from other sources. In addition, food processing technology imposes changes in the trace mineral composition and availability of foods in ways that further modify man's relationship to his geochemical environment.

For the bulk of mankind the food, rather than the water or the atmosphere, supplies a major proportion of trace element intakes. A high inverse correlation between the iodine content of the drinking water and the incidence of endemic goiter has long been known, but only some 10% of the total intakes of this element comes from the water supply, in goitrous and nongoitrous regions alike. In a study of the levels of 17 trace elements in the public water supplies in the United States, it was calculated that only 0.3-10.1% of the total daily intakes came from the water supply (49). Such conclusions do not necessarily apply in areas where the water supplies are not subject to comparable purification and control processes. Areas are known in which the drinking water is naturally and unusually high in arsenic, boron, fluorine, lithium, and strontium (see ref. 14).

The domestic treatment that the water receives can also affect its trace metal content, as has been shown with copper and lead. Some years ago a considerable increment in the copper content of soft water as compared with hard water from reservoir to homes with copper piping was reported (50). It was claimed that some soft waters, with their capacity to corrode metallic copper, could raise copper intakes by as much as 1.4 mg/day, as compared with only 0.05 mg/day from hard waters. In a more recent New Zealand study (51) it was calculated that if the beverages consumed by one individual were made up with soft water from the cold tap 0.4 mg/day would be contributed from this source alone and if from the hot tap 0.8 mg/day would be so supplied. This source of copper is substantial indeed as compared with the 1.0–1.2 mg/day obtained from the food in most Western-style diets, and could possibly be nutritionally significant since copper at high intakes is a metabolic antagonist of iron and zinc, which can be marginal in such diets.

The position with respect to lead and soft water is probably more serious, at least for children in some areas. In three groups of households in Glasgow, where the water is very soft, the mean lead levels in the cold tap water were as follows: houses with lead storage tank and piping, 1000 μg/liter; houses with no tank and lead piping in excess of 20 meters, 220 μg/liter; and houses with less than 20 meters of lead piping, 100 μg/liter (52). The mean blood levels of the inhabitants were significantly positively correlated with water lead content. In a further study of Glasgow soft water (53), significantly increased water lead levels were observed even in houses with copper pipes that had lead-soldered joints. Sources of lead of the magnitude reported could be deleterious to the health and well-being of children, because children absorb lead much more efficiently than adults and this absorption would probably be further increased where the children's diets are low or marginal in available iron, as they often are in poor families, since enhanced lead absorption occurs in iron-deficient, as compared with normal, animals (54, 55).

EFFECT OF PROCESSING ON TRACE ELEMENTS IN FOODS

An increasing proportion of the foods comprising modern diets is subjected to a variety of technological processes prior to consumption. These processes, which are designed to improve their safety, keeping quality, convenience, consumer appeal, and sometimes their nutritive value, can modify both the levels and the physiological availability of the trace elements that occur in the foods.

In the past treatments such as pasteurization, drying, and holding in metal containers could double the original iron (56) and copper (57) contents of milk. Changed technology, involving treatment in glass and stainless steel vessels, has reduced this form of contamination, but another, more hazardous kind of contamination of milk has been introduced in some areas. Where iodophor antiseptics are used in milking machines, storage vats, and tankers, the iodine content of milk can be markedly increased. This iodine passes into ice cream and confections containing milk products. In Tasmania, where iodophor bactericidal agents were used in dairies, the iodine level in milk ranged from 113 to 346 μg/liter, compared with 13–23 μg/liter in milk from areas where they were not used (58). Another halogen, fluorine, may also be of some nutritional concern. Commercial processing of vegetables with water containing 1 ppm of fluorine increased their fluorine levels by 0.34–0.75 μg/g on the fresh basis (59). In foods subjected to processing with fluoridated water and then reconstituted with similar water in the home there can be a multiplying effect. This has been shown for some infant foods (60, 61), but could occur with any foods so treated. A dry milk formula diluted 1 to 6 with 1 ppm of fluoridated water contained 1.3 mg of fluorine/liter, or more than 50 times the average fluorine level in breast milk. Such a multiplying effect did not pose a significant health hazard or a cosmetic problem such as teeth mottling (61), but concern has been expressed at the recent escalation of fluorine in the human food and beverage chain, revealed in several surveys. This increase probably reflects the increased consumption of fluoridated water–processed convenience foods and beverages to which water is added, especially in areas with fluoridated water (61a). It was further pointed out that the intakes recently recorded in nonfluoridated areas (i.e., 2 mg of fluorine/day or more) now match or exceed the level that was predicted for fluoridated communities.

Substantial losses of most trace minerals occur in the milling of wheat to white flour and in the refining of sugar. In a study of molasses and unrefined, brown, and highly refined sugar from several countries, the following mean levels of chromium were reported: 266 ± 58 ng/g for the molasses; 162 ± 36 ng/g for the unrefined sugar; 64 ± 5 ng/g for the brown sugar; and 20 ± 3 ng/g for the white sugar (62). It was pointed out that the high intake of refined sugar in typical United States diets not only contributed virtually no chromium, but could lead to a loss of body chromium through the chromium-depleting action of glucose (63). Comparable losses of other mineral elements in the refining process are evident from another study (64). The mean concentrations reported for Barbados brown sugar and granulated white sugar, respectively, were: iron, 49 and 0.1 μg/g; copper, 3 and 0.08 μg/g; silicon, 735 and 4 μg/g; vanadium, 400 and 2 ng/g; and iodine, 30 and 1 ng/g.

The losses that occur in the milling of wheat vary with the element and the degree of extraction of the flour — the lower the extraction the greater the losses. The milling of North American wheat to 72% extraction flour resulted in the following approximate percentage losses: cobalt, 88; manganese, 85; zinc, 78; iron, 75; copper, 68; molybdenum, 48; chromium, 40; and selenium, 16 (65). Essentially similar figures were reported in an earlier review (66), as shown in Figure 1. The relatively low levels of iron, zinc, and chromium remaining in white flour, compared with whole meal or higher extraction flour, are of some concern from the point of view of adequate supplies of these elements to man. However, the concurrent reduction in the mineral-binding fiber and phytate in the white bread increases the availability or absorbability of the remaining zinc and iron, partially compensating for the reduced total quantity present. This aspect is discussed in the next section of this chapter.

Silicon is another essential element that suffers substantial loss in the milling process. A level of 21 μg of silicon/g was recently recorded for 65%

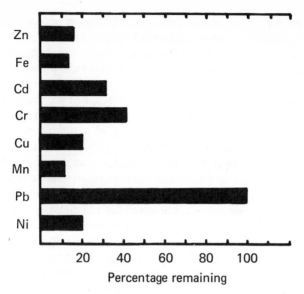

Figure 1.   Trace minerals remaining in white flour (hard wheat, 70% extraction). Reproduced from Gortner (66).

extraction white wheaten flour, as compared with 229–1720 μg/g in wheaten bran from three sources. The possible significance of this loss in relation to the development of atherosclerosis was mentioned above.

Losses of potentially toxic elements also occur in the milling of grain, although the data are limited and largely confined to lead and cadmium. Lead is not highly concentrated in the germ and branny layers of wheat, so that little is lost in the production of white flour (66, 67). The position is different with cadmium. For example, the following mean values were reported for Swedish wheat products: whole wheat, 0.05 μg of cadmium/g; white flour, 0.03 μg/g, and bran, 0.15 μg/g (68). For North American products the following values were given: hard wheat, 0.10 μg of cadmium/g; soft wheat, 0.07 μg/g; and white flour, 0.05 μg/g (67). The relatively high levels reported for white bread (0.16 and 0.19 μg/g, dry basis) suggest that sources other than flour were contributing cadmium to the bread. Cadmium is not lost in the polishing of rice, as judging by the comprehensive study of polished and unpolished rice (48) mentioned earlier. Mean levels of 0.03 μg/g were obtained for both types. Small losses of both zinc and copper were evident in the polished rice.

FORMS AND AVAILABILITY OF TRACE ELEMENTS IN FOODS

While the total amounts of the trace elements present in foods, as analyzed physicochemically, are clearly important in determining their adequacy or their safety, it is the amounts that can be absorbed and used by the animal that are of most concern. Physiological availability or potency is influenced by two main factors — the chemical form or combination in which the element is ingested and the ratio or proportion that the dietary concentration of that element bears to other elements or compounds with which it reacts metabolically.

Progress is now being made in our knowledge of the chemical forms in which many of the trace elements occur in foods and the relation of these forms to absorption and use. Cobalt occupies a unique position in this respect. Man and other nonruminant animals require their dietary cobalt to be supplied preformed as vitamin B_{12}. Their tissues are unable to incorporate cobalt into this vitamin and their intestinal flora are unable to achieve this vital transformation at a point in the digestive tract at which vitamin B_{12} can be absorbed. The cobalt status of human foods and dietaries is, therefore, of minor importance; it is their vitamin B_{12} status that is critical. Ruminants, by contrast, readily synthesize elemental or ionic cobalt into its physiologically active form, vitamin B_{12}, through the activities of their ruminal microflora. The cobalt, rather than the vitamin B_{12}, status of their diets is, therefore, critical.

For most other trace minerals man and animals enjoy an apparently complete capacity to produce the required physiologically active organic combinations from inorganic forms of the element after absorption from the diet. The position of chromium is intermediate between that of cobalt and that of other elements, as just described. Chromium occurs in foods to a varying extent in combination with a small organic molecule not yet fully characterized — the glucose tolerance factor or GTF. Chromium no doubt occurs in other unidentified chemical forms, but the GTF is better absorbed and is more potent in glucose metabolism than inorganic forms of the element (69). The value of a food as a source of chromium thus varies with its chromium content and with the extent to which this chromium is present as GTF or comparable readily absorbed and utilized forms. Great variation in the relative biological values of foods as a source of chromium has been demonstrated (70). Brewer's yeast is exceptionally high in physiologically active chromium.

Variations similarly exist among different chemical forms of selenium in their capacity to meet the needs of animals for this element and to induce toxic effects. In the early studies selenium compounds were divided into categories with respect to their potency against liver necrosis in rats (71). The first category included elemental selenium and certain compounds that are practically inactive because of poor absorption. Elemental selenium was later shown to be unavailable for the prevention of exudative diathesis in chicks (72). Compounds in the second category, which included most inorganic salts such as selenite and selenate and the selenium analogs of cysteine and methionine, were more or less equally protective against liver necrosis. More recent investigations have revealed significant differences within this category and even differences between the effectiveness of the same selenium compound in protecting against different manifestations of selenium deficiency. For example, selenomethionine is less effective than selenite in preventing exudative diathesis in chicks (6), but the reverse is true for the prevention of pancreatic fibrosis (73). In fact, selenomethionine was four times as effective for this purpose as either selenite or selenocystine. A distinct superiority of the selenium in most feeds of plant origin over that in animal products (various fish meals and bone meals) for the prevention of exudative diathesis is also apparent (72). These differences presumably stem largely from differences in the chemical forms in which the selenium is present, but neither the nature of the forms nor the reasons for the differing nutritional effectiveness are well understood.

The importance of chemical form in determining the availability of trace elements is further illustrated by recent investigations with zinc. The rat intestinal mucosa contains a low molecular weight, zinc-containing compound that plays a role in zinc absorption (74, 75). This finding has been confirmed for rats 16 days of age and older, and the compound has been shown to be similar to the zinc-binding ligand (ZBL) discovered in rat milk and human milk, but absent from cow's milk (76, 77). No such zinc-binding ligand is present in the mucosa of neonate rats from birth to 16 days of age (77). These important discoveries suggest that the ZBL of maternal milk enhances zinc absorption in the neonatal period before the development of intestinal mechanisms for zinc absorption and is the factor responsible for the therapeutic value of human milk in the treatment of the genetic disorder of zinc metabolism, acrodermatitis enteropathica (AE), by increasing zinc absorption. The latter point acquires particular significance when it is realized that cow's milk contains a higher average concentration of total zinc than human milk, but does not afford protection against AE.

Diets containing protein of plant seed origin require higher levels of zinc supplementation than those containing protein from animal sources. Such differences have been attributed to the presence or absence of phytates, which bind the zinc in a form from which it is not readily released or absorbed (78). This hypothesis is supported by the finding that the addition of phytic acid to egg albumin diets markedly reduced the retention of zinc by rats (79). Zinc absorption from combinations of zinc with phytic acid is increased by autoclaving (78), and fermentation with yeast greatly increases the availability of zinc in leavened whole meal bread (80). The latter effect was so much greater than could be accounted for by the action of yeast in destroying phytate that other factors were sought. Evidence has now been produced that a metal-binding effect of fiber is at least partly responsible for the depressed absorption of zinc from whole meal unleavened bread (81, 83). The production of flour of less than 90% extraction has consequently been proposed in order to lower the fiber intakes of rural populations of developing countries consuming predominantly unleavened bread (81). Even with leavened bread, a reduced fiber and phytate content can be important. Thus, in a recent study of Swedish breads made from 100% and 72% extraction flour, the absorption of zinc by human subjects was $8.2 \pm 0.6\%$ and $13.2 \pm 1.1\%$, respectively (82).

Evaluation of the forms and availability of iron in food has proved particularly difficult, partly because food iron absorption involves two different mechanisms, one for heme iron and one for nonheme iron, and partly because there is a composite effect of different iron forms and complexes on iron absorption from the whole diet. Heme iron compounds are well absorbed into the intestinal mucosa as the heme moiety without the necessity of release from conjugation. These compounds, as they occur in meat and fish, also significantly increase iron absorption from the total diet (85). Other animal products, such as milk and cheese, do not enhance the absorption of nonheme iron in this way (85), nor does the iron of egg yolk, which is itself poorly absorbed, enhance iron absorption, except when combined with sufficient ascorbic acid (86).

The absorption of nonheme food iron varies with the chemical form or combination in which it is ingested and with the nature of the rest of the diet, particularly the presence of chelates that can enhance or depress nonheme iron absorption. The presence of animal tissues (meat and fish) is also important. Progress in this area has been greatly facilitated by the development of an extrinsic tagging technique that enables nonheme iron absorption to be measured from a complete diet (87). The pronounced enhancing effect of ascorbic acid on iron absorption in man was demonstrated by such a technique, although a favorable effect of this vitamin, which both reduces and chelates iron, had previously been established in experimental animals. In a study of Venezuelan diets the inclusion of 150 g of papaya containing 66 mg of ascorbic acid increased iron absorption five times, and the addition of 60 mg of ascorbic acid to a meal of rice tripled iron absorption (88). The potent effect of ascorbic acid is shown further by a report on iron absorption by Indian women (89). The mean iron absorption from maize meal porridge was very low (3.8%), and was only 2.7% when tea was drunk with the meal. Addition of 50 or 100 mg of ascorbic acid to this porridge caused an approximate tenfold increase in iron absorption. When tea was present the increase was smaller — twofold with 50 mg and fivefold with 100 mg of ascorbic acid.

The synthetic chelate EDTA, which is added to some processed foods to prevent oxidative damage by free metals, by contrast, can seriously impair nonheme iron absorption. A 1:1 molar ratio EDTA to iron reduced this absorption in human subjects by 28%, and by approximately 50% when the ratio was increased to 2:1 (90). Apparently a soluble iron complex is formed at the low pH of the stomach that is insoluble at the high pH of the duodenum, the principal site of iron absorption. For women and young children, who are frequently in an unfavorable position in respect to iron status, and for those consuming predominantly vegetarian diets, it is clearly important that dietary intakes of substances such as EDTA that inhibit iron absorption should be reduced or eliminated and that intakes of those that enhance this absorption, such as ascorbic acid, should be increased.

The addition of sodium phytate reduces iron retention in rats (79) and in man (91), but the normal phytates in foods appear to have a limited effect on the absorption of iron in man (92, 93) or in chicks (94). Most of the iron in wheat consists of monoferric phytate, which is well absorbed by rats, with little difference in availability between the iron in ferrous ammonium sulfate and that in wheat and its milling fractions, bran, germ, and shorts (84). This suggests that iron is well absorbed by man from both white and whole meal flour and bread, but more definitive data are needed, especially in view of the prevalence of iron deficiency anemia in some rural populations consuming large amounts of unleavened whole meal bread. This suggests that iron binding by fiber is occurring concurrently with the zinc binding (81), a contention that is supported by the finding that the consumption of a fibrous cereal (rolled oats) depresses iron absorption and that this effect is not due to phytate (95).

INTERACTIONS AMONG THE TRACE ELEMENTS

Metabolic interactions among the trace elements that affect their absorption, excretion, and use, and therefore minimum needs and maximum tolerances of animals, are powerful and pervasive. A "true" or basic minimum requirement can be conceived as one in which all the dietary conditions affecting the element in this way are at an optimum. These conditions are rarely achieved in practice and a series of minimum requirements exist, depending on the extent to which interacting elements or compounds are present or absent from the diet. Similarly, a series of "safe" dietary levels of potentially toxic elements exist, depending on the extent to which other elements or compounds that affect their absorption, retention, or metabolic behavior are present in the diet. For example, field conditions actually exist in which sheep and cattle, at the same or closely similar levels of dietary copper, suffer from either copper deficiency or chronic copper poisoning, depending on the extent of the concurrent intakes of molybdenum and sulfur (14). Metabolic interactions of this and other types have been the subject of two recent comprehensive reviews (96, 97). Coverage here is confined to examples illustrating the importance and diversity of these interactions.

The significance of trace mineral interactions was highlighted by the discovery, over 20 years ago, that a three-way interaction exists between copper, molybdenum, and sulfate and that the ability of molybdenum to limit copper retention in the sheep can only be expressed in the presence of adequate inorganic sulfate (98). This classic finding has been amply confirmed and extended to other species (14), although total dietary sulfur rather than inorganic sulfate is now known to be the more useful measurement in the context of the copper-molybdenum-sulfate nexus (96). The primary site of this complex interaction is probably in the gut, with three essential steps postulated as follows: 1) reduction in the rumen of sulfate to sulfide; 2) reaction of this sulfide to form thiomolybdate; and 3) reaction of the thiomolybdate with copper to give the highly insoluble copper thiomolybdate, $CuMoS_4$ (99). The concept of the formation of thiomolybdate and the tight complexing of this ion with copper is supported by other studies (96, 100), but a metabolic interference with copper by molybdenum and sulfur is not confined to the gastrointestinal tract. Adverse effects on the use of copper at many essential sites and abnormal copper-binding proteins in the tissues, in response to molybdenum, have been demonstrated (100, 101). The precise significance of these changes is unknown, but is under investigation (100).

It should be appreciated that relatively low levels of dietary molybdenum (1 μg/g or less) can affect copper retention, at least in sheep and guinea pigs (96). Significant increases in urinary copper excretion from a relatively small increment in dietary molybdenum have also been observed in man (35). At a molybdenum intake of 160 μg/day, urinary excretion of copper was 24 μg/day; at 540 μg of molybdenum/day it was 42 μg/day; and at 1540 μg of molybdenum/day it increased to 77 μg/day. The molybdenum appeared to have induced tissue copper mobilization, because there were no corresponding increases in fecal copper. These findings raise the possibility of a molybdenum-induced copper deficiency arising in populations dependent upon sorghum as a dietary staple, since the higher dietary molybdenum intakes were obtained from high molybdenum samples of sorghum grain.

A mutual metabolic antagonism between selenium and mercury and between selenium and cadmium occurs in animals. The first evidence for this came from studies showing that selenite protects against the renal necrosis and mortality produced in rats by injected mercuric chloride and against the testicular necrosis similarly produced by cadmium chloride (102). Dietary selenium also exerts a protective effect against the chronic toxic effects of ingested inorganic and methyl mercury compounds (103, 105). Conversely, the toxic effects of ingested selenium are partially alleviated by dietary additions of mercuric chloride and of phenylmercuriacetate (105). The biochemical mechanisms involved in these interactions have not yet been identified, although it is known that selenium does not increase mercury excretion. In fact, there appears to be an increase in mercury retention and a redistribution of retained mercury, resulting in a diversion to possibly less sensitive sites. It is also known that the protection given by mercury against selenium poisoning is not dependent upon either element being in the inorganic form (105).

How far the above findings can be applied to man remains to be determined, but they suggest that the danger from mercury in fish, such as tuna, would be lessened by its naturally high selenium content and the maximum ''safe'' dietary levels of mercury would be influenced by the dietary intakes of selenium. Similarly, the optimal or desirable intakes of selenium by man should be influenced by the extent of his exposure to mercury. Selenium-mercury interactions have acquired further interest from the discovery that there is a coaccumulation or increment of these two elements in the tissues of several species. This occurs in an approximate 1:1 molar ratio in tuna (103), marine mammals (105a), and men following exposure to high levels of inorganic mercury from mines (105b). The coaccumulation is particularly evident in the liver and brain, and appears to be a natural or autoprotective phenomenon. It occurs whether the mercury is present in the methyl or inorganic form, and whether the diet is relatively abundant in selenium or not. In the marine mammals studied (seals, dolphins, and porpoises) very little of the large amounts of mercury present in the tissues were in the methylated form (105c). It was therefore suggested that these animals are able to detoxify the methylmercury obtained from the fish on which they feed by a specific mechanism involving selenium (105b). The nature of any such mechanism has yet to be determined.

Trace metal interactions are to be expected among elements that share common chemical parameters and compete for common metabolic sites (106). This is particularly apparent with zinc, cadmium, iron, and copper at the absorptive level. Thus, zinc absorption is depressed by copper (107), high zinc intakes depress copper absorption (108), and copper absorption is increased in zinc deficiency (109). A well-defined competition for transport across the intestinal wall has been demonstrated between cadmium and zinc, cadmium and mercury, and cadmium and copper (110). Cadmium also depresses iron uptake in chicks (111) and quail (112). Decreased concentrations of cadmium in the liver and kidneys of quail result from dietary supplements of zinc, manganese, and copper above the dietary requirements of each metal (112). This occurs when the dietary cadmium levels are relatively high (10, 20, and 40 μg/g) and the levels of zinc, copper, and manganese are also high, and when the dietary cadmium levels are lower and the excesses of the interacting metals more modest. It seems that cadmium shares a common or similar absorptive mechanism with these divalent metals and that competition within this mechanism is largely responsible for the mutual antagonism among them.

Of further interest in this connection is the finding that the severe iron deficiency anemia characteristic of cadmium toxicity in quail can be prevented by ferrous iron, or by ascorbic acid through its beneficial effect on iron absorption (113, 114). This suggests that persons consuming diets limited in ascorbic acid, iron, zinc, and copper may be more susceptible to the adverse effects of cadmium and that workers exposed to high levels of cadmium might benefit from supplements of ascorbic acid, zinc, copper, and iron II at levels appreciably but not massively higher than the generally recognized requirements (114). Furthermore, ascorbic acid must now be regarded as a critical dietary component both in respect to iron nutriture in man and in respect to increased exposure to cadmium. The metabolic antagonism between cadmium and zinc further suggests that marginal or overt zinc deficiency, already evident in some human populations, would be aggravated by above normal intakes of cadmium and, conversely, above normal intakes of zinc would be expected to afford some protection against above normal intakes of cadmium.

In the preceding paragraphs referring to interactions among the heavy metals, attention has mostly been restricted to competitive absorption. Protection against heavy metal toxicity can also occur through interactions within the cells and tissues, after absorption has taken place. Thus the retention of cadmium in the liver and kidneys is related to its selective storage or sequestration in the protein thionein. Metallothionein (MT) was originally discovered in equine renal cortex to contain 5.9% cadmium and 2.2% zinc and to be uniquely high in sulfhydryl groups (115). MT from the livers of cadmium-pretreated rats was later shown to contain 7 g of atoms of metal ions per 12,000 g of protein and to have a zinc-to-cadmium ratio of 1:1.4 (116), but the metal components can vary greatly in type and amount according to circumstances. Thus, cadmium-binding proteins occur throughout the body that form associative complexes with copper and mercury, as well as zinc, and can contain up to 11% of total metal.

MT was first believed to serve a detoxification function for cadmium (117) and to reduce the toxicity of Hg^{2+} and other divalent cations involved in zinc metabolism. Increases in liver zinc are associated with an increase in the amount of this element appearing in MT or MT-like forms, and almost the whole of liver zinc can be accounted for as MT when the zinc content of the rat's diet is increased to high levels (119). This fact led to the suggestion that MT serves as a storage protein for zinc, analogous to ferritin for iron, and functions as a temporary storage for this metal (and/or copper) prior to the use of these metals for essential functions (120). More recent data indicate that MT is more involved in accumulation of excessive zinc than in storage of the metal for later use (121), and may function also in body defense against such agents as disease, infections, and environmental stresses, all of which induce disturbances in the metabolism of various trace metals (122).

CLINICAL DISORDERS INVOLVING COPPER

Copper deficiency has been implicated in the etiology of several different clinical syndromes in the human infant. In the first of these, anemia, hypoproteinemia, and low serum iron and copper levels are present, and combined iron and copper therapy is necessary to promote complete recovery (123). Copper deficiency was subsequently reported in untreated malnourished infants (124), in small premature infants (125), and in malnourished infants on total parenteral nutrition (126). A further syndrome affects malnourished infants being rehabilitated on high calorie, low copper diets and exhibiting anemia, marked neutropenia, chronic or recurrent diarrhea, scurvy-like bones changes, and hypocupremia, all of which are responsive to copper therapy (127, 128). Later studies with infants have disclosed two effects of copper deficiency on iron metabolism (129). The first, occurring early, is an adverse effect on iron absorption or mobilization, probably due to a loss of ferroxidase activity. The second and later effect of copper deficiency is inadequate erythropoiesis, even in the presence of abundant iron stores.

A further clinical disorder in infants involving copper is Menke's kinky hair syndrome, characterized by subnormal levels of copper in blood, liver, and hair, progressive mental deterioration, hypothermia, defective keratinization of hair, metaphyseal lesions, and degenerative changes in aortic elastin (130). This disease is not due to copper deficiency, but arises from an X-linked defect in copper transport from the intestinal mucosa cell to the blood (131). The precise disturbance in copper absorption has not yet been delineated and parenteral copper therapy is ineffective. It seems that a widespread cellular defect, i.e., in tissues additional to the intestinal mucosa, prevents copper usage both in Menke's syndrome and in mutant mottled mice (132). The demonstration of a primary defect in copper absorption from the mucosa in X-linked mottled mutant mice (133) has provided a useful experimental animal for further studies of the biochemical defect or defects of this disorder. These aspects have been thoroughly discussed in a very recent review (134).

Wilson's disease (hepatolenticular or hepatocerebral degeneration) arises from an inborn error of copper metabolism that affects copper homeostasis. The abnormality is inherited as an autosomal recessive character occurring in either sex, but is rare because both parents must carry the abnormal gene. The pattern of inheritance of this disease, its clinical and pathological features, and its treatment and biochemical bases have recently been reviewed (135). The genetic abnormality leads to excessive accumulation of copper in the liver, kidneys, brain, and cornea, together with low serum ceruloplasmin levels, high levels of serum copper not bound to ceruloplasmin, increased urinary copper, and decreased fecal copper. The biochemical mechanism or mechanisms primarily involved in this metabolic abnormality remain to be determined, although the synthesis of an abnormal protein with a high affinity for copper is clearly important. Such a compound, copper thionein, has recently been prepared from the livers of Wilson's disease sufferers and has been shown to have a copper binding constant four times as great as that of the protein from control subjects (136). The authors explain the probable role of this abnormal protein as follows: "The increased binding affinity of the temporary storage protein in the hepatocyte of Wilson's disease patients probably shifts the normal equilibrium of the hepatic Cu pool, which results in both depressed biliary Cu excretion and decreased incorporation of Cu into caeruloplasmin. As the disease progresses, the binding sites on the storage protein become saturated and the excess metal is ingested by the hepatic lysosomes. Saturation of the hepatic Cu-binding sites results in a decreased uptake of the metal with a concomitant elevation in plasma Cu not bound to caeruloplasmin. Whether the increased deposition of copper in extrahepatic tissues results from the elevated non-caeruloplasmin Cu or from the presence of the protein in these organs is not known'' (136).

Wilson's disease was invariably progressive and fatal until 1951, when a decoppering chelating agent was introduced (137). With the advent of penicillamine (β,β-dimethylcysteine) all overt manifestations of the disease could be prevented and an apparently normal life span for sufferers became possible (138). One gram of penicillamine per day is the optimal dosage for most patients and results in a markedly increased output of urinary copper (132). Signs of zinc deficiency, including severe parakeratosis, have been observed in one patient so treated, but the lesions were reversed by oral zinc therapy (139). Any antipyridoxine effect from the penicillamine can be compensated for by a pyridoxine supplement at the rate of 25 mg/day (135).

CLINICAL DISORDERS INVOLVING ZINC

A wide range of zinc-responsive pathological conditions has been observed in animals and man since zinc was first shown to be a dietary essential for rats over 40 years ago (140). The critical role that zinc plays in DNA synthesis and nucleic acid and protein metabolism, as described earlier, means that all systems of the body suffer in zinc deficiency, particularly when the cells of particular systems are rapidly dividing, growing, or synthesizing. Growth and reproduction would thus be especially affected by lack of zinc.

The primary features of the conditioned zinc deficiency syndrome in adolescent males in Egypt are growth failure and hypogonadism (141). Later studies in Iran revealed a similar syndrome in females (142) and zinc-responsive growth failure and delayed sexual maturation in schoolboys (143). Total zinc intakes in these circumstances appear to be adequate. The zinc deficiency is conditioned by poor availability of the zinc and excessive zinc losses. The poor absorption results from the high fiber and phytate present in the unleavened whole meal bread that forms the staple diet and the high zinc losses from the high environmental temperatures causing large sweat losses and, in some areas, from schistosomiasis.

Zinc deficiency, manifested by poor growth and appetite, impaired taste acuity (hypogeusia), and low hair zinc levels, appears to be quite common in otherwise normal infants and children in the United States (144). Certain infant diets low in zinc can be growth limiting for male infants (145), and the diets consumed by some preschool children from low-income families are lacking in available zinc, as evidenced by subnormal hair and

Table 3.   Possible causes of conditioned zinc deficiency[a]

Conditioning factors	Mechanisms
Dietary phytate, fiber, EDTA, poly-phosphates, clay, and laundry starch	Chelation of zinc
Alcohol	Increased urinary excretion of zinc
Pancreative insufficiency	Steatorrhea, lack of binding factor
Gastrectomy (partial or total)	Steatorrhea, achlorohydria
Diverticuli or blind loop	Steatorrhea, bacterial utilization
Intestinal mucosal disease	Steatorrhea, uxudation, increased secretions, mucosal block
Cirrhosis of the liver	Increased urinary loss
Other liver diseases	Steatorrhea
Renal failure	Anorexia
Malabsorption syndrome	Intestinal loss of zinc
Nephrotic syndrome	Proteinuria
Renal tubular disease	Failure of tubular reabsorption of zinc
Dialysis	Removal of zinc in dialysate
Hemolytic anemias	Urinary excretion of RBC zinc
Neoplastic disease	Anorexia, catabolism
Psoriasis	Loss of skin cells
Burns	Exudation, catabolism
Parasitic infection	Chronic blood loss, steatorrhea
Iatrogenic	
Antimetabolite drugs	Catabolism
Antianabolic drugs	Nonanabolism
Chelating drugs	Increased urinary excretion of zinc
Parenteral alimentation	Failure to add zinc to i.v. fluids
Surgical trauma	Catabolism
Genetic and congenital defects	
Hemolytic anemias	Urinary excretion of RBC zinc
Pancreatic defect	Lack of zinc binding factor (?)
Intestinal defect	Mucosal block
Renal tubular defect	Failure of tubular reabsorption of zinc
Diabetes mellitus	Increased urinary excretion of zinc
Congenital absence of the thymus gland	Unknown
Mongolism	Unknown
Acrodermatitis enteropathica	Possibly impaired intestinal absorption of zinc
Inflammation	
Infectious disease	Mobilization of zinc by LEM and subsequent urinary excretion
Collagen disease	Catabolism
Tissue necrosis	Catabolism
Pregnancy	Fetal uptake of zinc

[a]From Sandstead et al. (150).

plasma zinc levels and low growth percentiles (146). Individuals on such diets are at particular risk from marginal or inadequate zinc nutrition, because the best dietary sources of this metal are the more expensive foods, especially meats (147). However, hypogeusia responsive to oral zinc therapy is not confined to children from low-income families. Hypogeusia and dysgeusia (disordered taste or pica) is not uncommon in adults and can respond to dietary zinc supplementation (148, 149).

Various other clinical disorders occur in man as a consequence of either poor absorption or excessive losses of zinc or both together (150) (see Table 3). These include severe trauma (151), chronic renal disease (152), alcoholism and/or cirrhosis (153), and proteinuria or aminoaciduria (154), all of which involve high urinary zinc excretion. Inflammatory diseases of the bowel and malabsorption syndrome result in decreased zinc uptake (150), and patients with chronic or inflammatory infectious disease display disturbances in zinc metabolism (155). Zinc may also be indirectly involved in celiac disease. The disease can be triggered by early weaning, which could be related to the loss of the zinc-binding ligand present in breast milk that promotes zinc absorption.

Plasma zinc levels in women fall in late pregnancy (156–158). Mean values of 60, 56, and 48 μg of zinc/100 ml were reported in these studies, as compared with a normal adult level close to 100 μg/100 ml. Recent Swedish investigations indicate that this decline can be clinically significant (159). Women with abnormal deliveries and/or abnormally developed infants had significantly lower serum zinc concentrations during pregnancy than those with mature infants by normal delivery. Eight infants from the 234 gravidae studied revealed congenital malformations, and five of these infants came from mothers with the lowest serum zinc levels recorded. Of 20 other gravidae with serum zinc levels below 11.5 μmol/liter (75 μg of zinc/100 ml), five had dysmature infants. By contrast, seven of these mothers who received oral zinc therapy (90 mg of Zn^{2+} daily as zinc sulfate) had normal deliveries. Of a further group of 33 gravidae with refractory anemia, 31 had low or very low serum zinc levels. Twenty-one women from this group developed complications during labor, some with excessive bleeding, or gave birth to immature, dysmature, or, in one case, malformed infants, and/or were not delivered at normal term. These results are strikingly similar to those obtained with zinc-deficient pregnant rats (160–163). They suggest that low serum zinc concentrations during human pregnancy can be indicators of a zinc deficiency that increases maternal morbidity and involves a high risk to the fetus. They suggest further that any factors that impair zinc absorption, such as disease or drugs and the consumption of low protein, high phytate and fiber diets, place pregnant women at particular risk.

Alopecia and gross skin lesions have been a conspicuous feature of zinc deficiency in experimental animals since the original demonstration of this deficiency in rats (140) and in pigs (164). An association between subnormal plasma or serum zinc concentrations and skin disorders has also been observed in man. In one study of eight patients with indolent ulcers the mean serum zinc level was 58 ± 15 μg/100 ml, as compared with 96 ± 12 in controls (165). In 20 out of 23 paraplegic patients with pressure sores, fasting plasma zinc levels were low (166), and improved rate of healing from oral zinc therapy has been demonstrated in patients with leg ulcers (167) and gastric ulcers (168). Zinc deficiency was identified in 16 patients with impaired wound healing after major operations and severe burns with accompanying zincuria (151). The addition of supplementary zinc resulted in improved wound healing clinically, concomitantly with increases in the zinc concentration within the epithelium and granulation tissue of the wounds. However, no such benefits from zinc have been obtained in other studies with man (169, 170), and the position with normally nourished experimental animals is conflicting. In zinc-deficient animals the evidence is unequivocal that the rate of wound healing is impaired and that it is accelerated by supplemental zinc (14). The enhancement of wound healing that can occur from zinc may be due to a heightened metabolic demand for this element for collagen synthesis in the process of tissue repair, with an increase in collagen synthesis and cross-linking explaining gains in wound tensile strength (171). A drastic reduction in cystine incorporation into skin protein in zinc-deficient rats has now been reported (172). The importance of this lies in the exceptionally high cystine content of the keratins of the epidermal layer of the skin and also of hair.

The most severe and clear-cut clinical disorder in man caused by zinc deficiency is the autosomal recessive inherited disease acrodermatitis enteropathica (AE). This disease begins in infancy, often coincident with the change from breast milk to cow's milk, and is characterized by dermatitis, alopecia, and severe diarrhea. Without treatment a relentless progression of severe malnutrition, poor growth and development, intercurrent infections, and death within 3 years is usual. With adequate oral zinc treatment clinical remission is rapid and complete, and plasma and hair zinc and urinary zinc excretion rise to normal values (173, 174). The disease is caused by an intestinal mucosal abnormality that impairs zinc absorption and that is returned to normal after oral zinc therapy (175). Congenital malformations in infants from patients with AE have been recorded (176), comparable with those that appear in embryos and pups from zinc-deficient pregnant rats (160, 161). The high frequency of monilial and bacterial infections in this disease points to a breakdown in host defense mechanisms. This has now been shown to be caused by a zinc-responsive defect in chemotaxis of neutrophils and monocytes (177). It is apparent that studies of this rare disease are revealing new areas of knowledge on the nutritional physiology of zinc in man and are pointing the way to further avenues of research with this element.

CHROMIUM DEFICIENCY

Impaired glucose tolerance in rats fed certain diets was first observed in 1957 (178). It was postulated that the condition was caused by a deficiency of a new dietary agent designated the glucose tolerance factor (GTF). The active component was then shown to be trivalent chromium and various trivalent chromium compounds were found to be effective in restoring tolerance to injected glucose (179). Other systems involving carbohydrate metabolism respond to chromium plus insulin (180), and chromium deficiency in experimental animals is further characterized by impaired growth and longevity and by disturbances in lipid and protein metabolism (69).

In severe chromium deficiency a syndrome that resembles diabetes mellitus, with fasting hyperglycemia and glycosuria, occurs in rats, and can rapidly be reversed when 2 or 5 ppm of chromium are supplied in the drinking water (181). A decreased sensitivity of peripheral tissue to insulin appears to be the primary biochemical lesion in chromium deficiency. In chromium-deficient systems the response to doses of insulin is significantly inferior and higher doses of the hormone are required to elicit metabolic responses similar to those of chromium-sufficient controls. On the other hand, in the absence of insulin these responses do not differ from those of controls. Chromium is therefore not an insulin-like agent but is a "true potentiator of the action of the hormone" (182). Glucose tolerance factor, which is presumably the physiologically active form of chromium, has not been fully characterized, but is under active investigation. A compound containing chromium, nicotinic acid, and glutathione and exhibiting significant biological activity has now been synthesized (183).

In some parts of the world (184, 185), but not in others (186), the severe impairment of glucose tolerance characteristic of kwashiorkor, or protein-calorie malnutrition, can rapidly be improved by oral chromium therapy. A single dose of chromium as $CrCl_3$ increased the glucose removal rates of the infants from 0.6–1.2%/min to 2.9%/min (185), and the effect of the single dose lasted from 8 to 40 days (184). Responses to chromium in glucose tolerance are slow and delayed in elderly and middle-aged subjects as compared with the rapid results obtained with infants. Thus, four out of six maturity-onset diabetics displayed improved glucose tolerance when given 180–1000 μg of chromium daily for 4 months (188). No such improvement in 10 adult diabetics was observed when they were given 150 μg of chromium daily for 16 weeks (189).

It is apparent that some infants and adults are ingesting sufficient chromium to maintain normal glucose utilization and that some are not. The minimum human requirement for chromium that is compatible with long-term health and well-being cannot yet be given because of inadequate knowledge of the forms and availability of this metal in foods, as discussed under "Forms and Availability of Trace Elements in Foods." However, dietary chromium intakes by man are known to be reduced as the amounts and proportions of refined carbohydrates consumed are increased. A daily intake of 20–500 μg of chromium, depending on the chemical nature of the chromium in individual foods, would be needed to compensate for a urinary loss of 5 μg of chromium/day (190). Many individuals excrete more than 5 μg/day and insulin-dependent diabetics much more (191). A strong negative correlation between urinary chromium excretion and the efficiency of glucose utilization has been demonstrated in Turkish children (192). It seems that urinary chromium excretion is closely related to glucose metabolism and can be a useful indicator of the chromium status of population groups.

The levels of chromium in hair provide a further index of the chromium status of groups, although absolute levels indicative of chromium deficiency in the individual remain to be defined. In premature newborn infants and those with evidence of retarded intrauterine growth, the mean hair chromium concentrations are below normal, as are those of insulin-dependent diabetic children and parous women (191, 193). A mean of 750 ng of chromium/g was reported for the hair of 10 nulliparous women and of 220 ng/g for that of 11 parous women (193). These findings suggest that dietary chromium intakes were inadequate to maintain tissue chromium stores during pregnancy.

The most striking evidence of severe isolated chromium deficiency in man comes from a subject on prolonged total parenteral nutrition (194). The patient exhibited weight loss, impaired glucose tolerance, peripheral neuropathy, and subnormal blood and hair chromium concentrations, all of which responded to oral chromium therapy.

SELENIUM AND VITAMIN E

Selenium is necessary for growth and fertility in animals and for the prevention of a range of disease conditions that show a variable response to vitamin E. These are liver necrosis in rats and other species, exudative diathesis and pancreatic fibrosis in poultry, hepatosis dietetica in pigs, and nutritional muscular dystrophy (white muscle disease, WMD) in lambs, calves, and other species. In the early Oregon experiments, vitamin E fed to pregnant ewes was ineffective in alleviating WMD in their lambs, although selenium was subsequently found to be highly effective (195). Recent evidence indicates that the vitamin preparation used in those experiments was poorly absorbed and that vitamin E, as well as selenium, affords considerable protection against the disease (196). The resorption sterility in rats and encephalomalacia in chicks that occur in vitamin E–deficient diets do not respond to selenium. On the other hand, the selenium-responsive unthriftiness in sheep and cattle and the seasonal infertility in ewes due to high embryonic mortality that occur in parts of New Zealand cannot be prevented by either vitamin E or the antioxidant, ethoxyquin (197, 198).

The relationship between selenium and vitamin E is still imperfectly understood. Selenium is clearly required for growth, even in the presence of adequate vitamin E. Chicks consuming a diet containing only 0.005 μg/g of selenium or less exhibited poor growth and high mortality even when 200

$\mu g/g$ of D-α-tocopherol were added (199). Higher tocopherol levels prevented mortality, but even with 1000 $\mu g/g$ growth was inferior to that obtained with selenium and without tocopherol. Comparable findings with rats indicate that selenium does not function merely as a substitute for vitamin E (200). However, selenium influences the metabolism of vitamin E. Poor absorption of this vitamin has been observed in selenium-deficient chicks (201), and selenium-deficient rats metabolized vitamin E more rapidly than selenium-supplemented ones (202). These findings suggest that selenium deficiency increases the requirements for vitamin E, possibly as a consequence of the greater metabolic rate of selenium-deficient rats, as indicated by greater oxidation of glucose and more rapid turnover of fatty acids (203).

The discovery that glutathione peroxidase (GSH-Px) is a selenium-containing enzyme (204) with an activity in the blood and tissues directly related to the selenium level in the diet gave a new dimension to studies of the mode of action of selenium and its relationship to vitamin E. GSH-Px catalyzes the removal of H_2O_2 according to the following coupled reaction:

$$\begin{array}{ccc} 2GSH + H_2O_2 & \underline{\hspace{1cm} GSH\text{-}Px \hspace{1cm}} & GSSG + H_2O \\ GSSG + NADPH & glutathione\ reductase & 2GSH + NADP^+ \end{array}$$

Selenium and vitamin E both protect biological membranes from oxidative degradation. The most acceptable hypothesis is that selenium functions as a component of cytosolic GSH-Px, which reduces peroxides, and vitamin E functions as a lipid-soluble antioxidant in the membrane (6). The GSH-Px is therefore of primary importance, acting to destroy peroxides before they can attack the cellular membranes, whereas vitamin E acts within the membrane itself in preventing the chain-reactive autoxidation of the membrane lipids. Either of these two mechanisms can be effective in some circumstances. For example, exudative diathesis (ED) in chicks can be prevented completely either by selenium or vitamin E, presumably by the two different mechanisms that have been postulated. The effectiveness of vitamin E against ED is not a result of a simple oxidative action, because the antioxidant ethoxyquin, which will substitute for this vitamin in the prevention of encephalomalacia in chicks and WMD in lambs (196), has no preventive effect on the incidence or severity of ED in vitamin E and selenium-deficient chicks (6).

Recent studies of lead poisoning in rats provide a further example of the differing mechanism of action of these two nutrients. Vitamin E deficiency increases the splenomegaly, anemia, and red cell fragility of lead-poisoned rats (205), whereas selenium deficiency has no such enhancing effect on their susceptibility to the hemolytic effect of lead (206). Similarly, the appreciable protection afforded by vitamin E and by the synthetic antioxidant, N,N'-diphenyl-p-phenylenediamine (DPPD) (207), against these effects of lead, particularly the mechanical fragility of the red cells, is not shared by selenium. These observations suggest that lead exerts its deleterious effect in the interior hydrophobic region of the red cell membrane where the lipid-soluble antioxidants can penetrate, whereas selenium as part of GSH-Px is confined mainly to the aqueous phase of the cell, since the enzyme occurs largely in the cytoplasm (206).

Evidence is accumulating that selenium serves additional functions in the tissues unrelated to GSH-Px. It has been proposed that selenium and particularly selenide have a role in the electron transfer functions associated with the mitochondria and smooth endoplasmic reticulum (208). A seleno-protein that is not present in these tissues in the selenium-deficient animal and resembles cytochrome c in some of its properties has been isolated from the heart and muscle of lambs given adequate selenium (209). It was suggested that this compound could be involved in the prevention of WMD (210). A nonselenium-containing glutathione peroxidase (glutathione: cumene hydroperoxide oxidoreductase, Cum-Px), which preferentially destroys organic peroxides, has been demonstrated in rat liver (211), and data have been produced that suggest that this enzyme could be involved in the protection of liver and kidney against WMD, but not in the protection given by selenium and vitamin E against heart and muscle damage (212). Selenium may be involved further in the metabolism of sulfhydryl groups (213, 214), glutamate (215), and succinate (216).

Conclusive evidence of naturally occurring selenium deficiency or selenium toxicity affecting the health of human populations has not been produced. In parts of the Great Plains of North America, where severe selenosis of livestock occurs, surveys of families living in the area revealed no symptoms clearly pathognomonic of selenium poisoning. A higher tolerance to this element by man as compared with domesticated animals seems unlikely. The explanation probably lies in differences in dietary habits — the consumption by man of foods from nonseleniferous areas and the losses of selenium that occur in the cooking of meat and vegetables and the milling of wheat to white flour. At the other end of the selenium scale, in parts of Oregon, and in New Zealand where selenium deficiency in livestock is widespread, clear-cut signs of marginal or overt selenium deficiency in man are similarly absent. Again this is probably due to the proportion of foods in human dietaries that now come from wide geographical sources and for other reasons discussed under "Sources of Trace Elements." However, whole blood selenium levels of normal New Zealand people are low and those of visitors to that country decline to the low range of New Zealand residents within 3–9 months (217). This finding has recently been confirmed and a high correlation found between the selenium concentrations and the activities of GSH-Px in the blood of New Zealanders (218) (Figure 2). The authors consider that some groups may be "at risk."

Epidemiological studies have tentatively linked dietary selenium status with two public health problems in man. The first is the higher prevalence of dental caries in children from high selenium areas in the United States than in

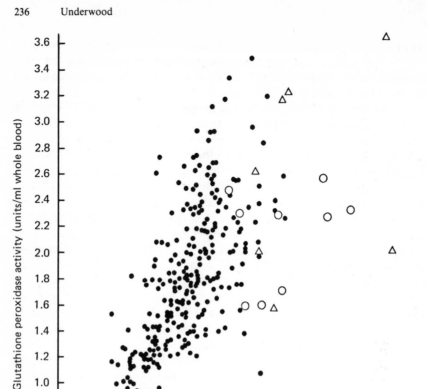

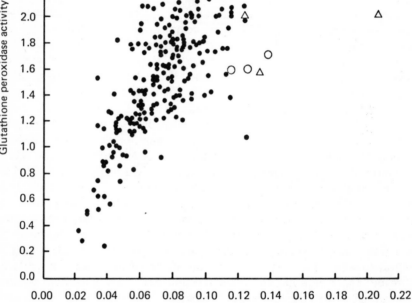

Figure 2.   Selenium concentrations and glutathione peroxidase activities expressed in units/ml of whole blood of 264 New Zealand residents (●), nine New Zealand residents returned from overseas visits (△), and seven new settlers to New Zealand (△). Reproduced from Thomson et al. (218).

those from low selenium areas (42, 219, 220). The second is the high inverse correlation demonstrated between blood selenium levels and human cancer death rates, also in the United States (221, 222). These findings received support from later studies comparing age-adjusted cancer mortality rates and published female breast cancer mortality rates with the median levels of selenium in grains and forages of different areas (223). On the basis of these studies it would be logical to conclude that human cancer incidence and mortality could be lowered by appropriate dietary selenium supplementation in low selenium areas. However, correlations do not necessarily imply causal relationships, and neoplasia is not observed among the various lesions attributed to selenium deficiency in animals. In addition, there is no evidence that New Zealand residents, with their known low selenium status, have an unusually high incidence of total cancer or breast cancer.

REFERENCES

1. Schwarz, K., and Spallholz, J. (1976). Fed. Proc. 35 (abstr.):255.
2. Smith, J. C., and Schwarz, K. (1967). J. Nutr. 93:182.
3. Nielsen, F. H. (1976). *In* A. S. Prasad (ed.), Trace Elements in Human Health and Disease, Vol. II, p. 379. Academic Press, Inc., New York.
4. Schwarz, K. (1977). Lancet 1:454.
5. Wellby, M., and O'Halloran, M. W. (1966). Br. Med. J. 2:668.
6. Noguchi, T., Cantor, A. H., and Scott, M. L. (1973). J. Nutr. 103:1502.
7. Dawbarn, M. C., Hine, D. C., and Smith, J. (1957). Aust. J. Exp. Biol. Med. Sci. 35:273.
8. Andrews, E. D., and Stephenson, B. J. (1966). N. Z. J. Agric. Res. 9:491.
9. Smith, R. M., and Marston, H. R. (1970). Br. J. Nutr. 24:857, 879.
10. Vallee, B. L. (1971). *In* W. Mertz and W. E. Cornatzer (eds.), Newer Trace Elements in Nutrition, p. 33. Marcel Dekker, New York.
11. Vallee, B. L. (1974). *In* W. G. Hoekstra et al. (eds.), Trace Element Metabolism in Animals, Vol. 2, p. 5. University Park Press, Baltimore.
12. Harris, E. D. (1976). Proc. Natl. Acad. Sci. USA 73:371.
13. Stiefel, E. J. (1973). Proc. Natl. Acad. Sci. USA 70:988.
14. Underwood, E. J. (1977). Trace Elements in Human and Animal Nutrition, Ed. 4. Academic Press, Inc., New York.
15. Keilin, D., and Mann, J. (1940). Biochem. J. 34:1163.
16. Riordan, J. F., and Vallee, B. L. (1976). *In* A. S. Prasad (ed.), Trace Elements in Human Health and Disease, Vol. I, p. 227. Academic Press, Inc., New York.
17. O'Dell, B. L. (1976). *In* A. S. Prasad (ed.), Trace Elements in Human Health and Disease, Vol. I, p. 391. Academic Press, Inc., New York.
18. McCord, J. M., and Fridovich, I. (1969). J. Biol. Chem. 244:6049.
19. Carrico, R. J., and Deutsch, H. F. (1970). J. Biol. Chem. 245:723.
20. Weisiger, R. A., and Fridovich, I. (1973). J. Biol. Chem. 248:3582.
21. Prohaska, J. R., and Wells, W. W. (1974). J. Neurochem. 23:91.
22. Hill, C. H., Starcher, B., and Kim, C. (1968). Fed. Proc. 26:129.
23. Prasad, A. S., and Oberleas, D. (1974). J. Lab. Clin. Med. 83:634.
24. Dreosti, I. E., and Hurley, L. C. (1975). Proc. Soc. Exp. Biol. Med. 150:161.
25. Eckhert, C. D., and Hurley, L. C. (1977). J. Nutr. 107:855.
26. Carlisle, E. M. (1972). Science 178:619.
27. Schwarz, K., and Milne, D. B. (1972). Nature 239:333.
28. Schwarz, K. (1973). Proc. Natl. Acad. Sci. USA 70:1608.
29. Carlisle, E. M. (1974). Fed. Proc. 33:1758.
30. Johnson, J. M., and Butler, G. W. (1957). Physiol. Plant. 10:100.
31. Schaible, P. J., Bandemer, S. L., and Davidson, J. A. (1938). Michigan Agric. Exp. Station Tech. Bull. No. 159.
32. Underwood, E. J., Robinson, T. J., and Curnow, D. H. (1947). J. Dept. Agric. W. Aust. 24:259.

33. Gartner, R. W. J., and Twist, J. O. (1968). Aust. J. Exp. Agric. Anim. Husbandry 8:210.
33a. Gladstones, J. S., and Drover, D. P. (1962). Aust. J. Exp. Agric. Anim. Husbandry 2:46.
34. Matrone, G., Hartman, R. H., and Clawson, A. J. (1959). J. Nutr. 67:309.
35. Deosthale, Y. G., and Gopalan, C. (1974). Br. J. Nutr. 31:351.
36. Leveille, G. A., Bedford, C. L., Kraut, C. W., and Lee, Y. C. (1974). Fed. Proc. 33:2264.
37. Hopkins, H., and Eisen, J. (1959). J. Agric. Food Chem. 7:633.
38. Warren, H. V., Delavault, R. E., Fletcher, K., and Wilks, F. (1971). *In* D. D. Hemphill (ed.), Trace Substances in Environmental Health, Vol. IV, p. 94. University of Missouri, Columbia.
39. Zook, E. G., and Lehmann, J. (1968). J. Am. Diet. Assoc. 52:68.
40. Lindberg, P. (1968). Acta Vet. Scand. 9(suppl.):23.
41. Scott, M. L., and Thompson, J. N. (1971). Poultry Sci. 50:1742.
42. Hadjimarkos, D. M. (1969). Caries Res. 3:14.
43. Ku, P. K., Ely, W. T., Groce, A. W., and Ullrey, D. E. (1972). J. Anim. Sci. 34:208.
44. Underwood, E. J. (1962). Proceedings of the 12th World Poultry Congress, Sydney, Australia, 1962, p. 216.
45. Welch, R. R., House, W. A., and Allaway, W. H. (1974). J. Nutr. 104:733.
46. Jones, R. L., Hinesly, T. D., and Ziegler, E. L. (1973). J. Environ. Qual. 2:351.
47. Williams, C. H., and David, D. J. (1973). Aust. J. Soil Res. 11:43.
48. Masironi, R., Koirtyohann, S. R., and Pierce, J. O. (1977). Sci. Total Environ. 7:27.
49. Hadjimarkos, D. M. (1967). J. Pediatr. 70:967.
50. Schroeder, H. A., Nason, A. P., Tipton, I. H., and Balassa, J. J. (1966). J. Chron. Dis. 19:1007.
51. Robinson, M. F., McKenzie, J. M., Thompson, C. D., and van Riij, A. L. (1973). Br. J. Nutr. 30:195.
52. Goldberg, A. (1974). Environ. Health Perspect. 7:103.
53. Moore, M. P. (1977). Sci. Total Environ. 7:109.
54. Six, K. M., and Goyer, R. A. (1972). J. Lab. Clin. Med. 79:128.
55. Ragan, H. A. (1977). J. Lab. Clin. Med. 90:700.
56. Feulillen, Y. M., and Plumier, M. (1952). Acta Pediat. 41:138.
57. Davies, W. L. (1936). The Chemistry of Milk. Chapman and Hall, London.
58. Connolly, R. J. (1971). Med. J. Aust. 1:1268.
59. Marier, J. R., and Rose, D. (1966). J. Food Sci. 31:941.
60. Ericsson, Y., and Ribelius, V. (1971). Caries Res. 5:78.
61. Farkas, C. S., and Farkas, E. J. (1974). Sci. Total Environ. 2:399.
61a. Marier, J. R. (1977). Sci. Total Environ. 8:253.
62. Masironi, R., Wolf, W., and Mertz, W. (1973). W. H. O. Bull. 49:322.
63. Glinsmann, W. H., Feldman, F. J., and Mertz, W. (1966). Science 152:1243.
64. Hamilton, E. I., and Minski, M. J. (1972–73). Sci. Total Environ. 1:375.
65. Nesheim, R. O. (1974). Fed. Proc. 33:2267.
66. Gortner, W. A. (1972). Food Technol. Aust. 24:504.
67. Zook, E. G., Greene, F. E., and Morris, E. R. (1970). Cereal Chem. 47:720.
68. Linman, L., Andersson, A., Nilsson, K. O., Lind, B., Kjellstrom, T., and Friberg, L. (1973). Arch. Environ. Health 27:45.
69. Mertz, W. (1969). Physiol. Rev. 49:163.
70. Toepfer, E. W., Mertz, W., Roginski, E. E., and Polansky, M. M. (1973). Agric. Food Chem. 21:69.

71. Schwarz, K., and Foltz, C. M. (1958). J. Biol. Chem. 233:245.
72. Cantor, A. H., Scott, M. L., and Noguchi, T. (1975). J. Nutr. 105:96.
73. Cantor, A. H., Langevin, M. L., Noguchi, T., and Scott, M. L. (1975). J. Nutr. 105:106.
74. Van Campen, D. R., and Kowalski, T. J. (1971). Proc. Soc. Exp. Biol. Med. 136:294.
75. Hahn, C., and Evans, G. W. (1973). Proc. Soc. Exp. Biol. Med. 144:793.
76. Eckhert, C. D., Sloan, M. V., Duncan, J. R., and Hurley, L. S. (1976). Science 195:789.
77. Hurley, L. S., Duncan, J. R., Sloan, M. V., and Eckhert, C. D. (1977). Proc. Natl. Acad. Sci. USA 74:3547.
78. O'Dell, B. L., and Savage, J. E. (1960). Proc. Soc. Exp. Biol. Med. 103:304.
79. Davies, N. T., and Nightingale, R. (1975). Br. J. Nutr. 34:243.
80. Reinhold, J. G., Parsa, A., Karimian, N., Hammick, J. W., and Ismael-Beigi, F. (1974). J. Nutr. 104:976.
81. Reinhold, J. G., Faradji, B., Abadi, P., and Ismael-Beigi, F. (1976). In A. S. Prasad (ed.), Trace Elements in Human Health and Disease, Vol. I, p. 163. Academic Press, Inc., New York.
82. Sandström, B., Arvidsson, B., and Cederblad, A. (1978). In M. Kirchgessner (ed.), Trace Element Metabolism in Man and Animals, Vol. 3, p. 129. Arbeitsgemeinschaft für Tierenahrungs forschung, Weihenstephan.
83. Ismael-Beigi, F., Reinhold, J. G., Faraji, B., and Abadi, P. (1977). J. Nutr. 107:510.
84. Morris, E. R., and Ellis, R. (1976). J. Nutr. 106:753.
85. Cook, J. D. (1977). Fed. Proc. 36:2028.
86. Morris, E. R., and Greene, F. E. (1972). J. Nutr. 102:901.
87. Cook, J. D., Layrisse, M., and Martinez-Torres, C. (1972). J. Clin. Invest. 51:805.
88. Layrisse, M., Martinez-Torres, C., and Gonzalez, M. (1974). Am. J. Clin. Nutr. 27:152.
89. Derman, D., Sayers, M., Lynch, S. R., Charlton, R. W., Bothwell, T. H., and Mayet, F. (1977). Br. J. Nutr. 38:261.
90. Cook, J. D., and Monsen, E. R. (1976). Am. J. Clin. Nutr. 29:614.
91. Hussain, R., and Patwardhan, V. N. (1959). Indian J. Med. Res. 47:676.
92. Walker, A. R. P., Fox, F. W., and Irving, J. T. (1948). Biochem. J. 42:452.
93. Callender, S. T., and Warner, G. T. (1970). Lancet 1:546.
94. Davis, P. N., Norris, L. C., and Kratzer, F. H. (1968). J. Nutr. 94:407.
95. Sharpe, L. M., Peacock, W. C., Cooke, R., and Harris, R. S. (1950). J. Nutr. 41:433.
96. Suttle, N. F. (1975). In D. J. D. Nicholas and A. R. Egan (eds.), Trace Elements in Soil-Plant-Animal Systems, p. 271. Academic Press, Inc., New York.
97. Underwood, E. J. (1977). In F. W. Oehme (ed.), Heavy Metals in the Environment. Dekker, New York.
98. Dick, A. T. (1954). Aust. J. Agric. Res. 5:511.
99. Dick, A. T., Dewey, D. W., and Gawthorne, J. M. (1975). J. Agric. Sci. 85:567.
100. Mills, C. F., Bremner, I., El-Gallad, T. T., Dalgarno, A. C., and Young, B. W. (1978). In M. Kirchgessner (ed.), Trace Element Metabolism in Man and Animals, Vol. III, p. 150. Arbeitsgemeinschaft für Tierernahrungsforschung, Weihenstephan.
101. Smith, B. S. W., and Wright, H. (1975). J. Comp. Pathol. 85:299.
102. Parizek, J., Benes, I., Ostadalova, I., Babicky, A., Benes, J., and Pitha, J. (1969). In D. Barltrop and W. L. Butland (eds.), Mineral Metabolism in

Paediatrics. Blackwell, Oxford.
103. Ganther, H. E., Gondie, C., Sunde, M. L., Kopecky, M. J., Wagner, P., Hoh, S., and Hoekstra, W. G. (1972). Science 175:1122.
104. Potter, S., and Matrone, G. (1974). J. Nutr. 104:638.
105. Hill, C. H. (1974). J. Nutr. 104:593.
105a. Koeman, J. H., van der Ven, W. S. M., de Goeij, J. J. M., Tjioe, P. S., and van Haaften, J. L. (1975). Sci. Total Environ. 3:279.
105b. Kosta, L., Byrne, A. R., and Zelenko, V. (1975). Nature 254:238.
105c. Koeman, J. H., Peeters, W. H. M., Kondstaal-Hob, C. H. M., Tjioe, P. S., and de Goeij, J. J. M. (1973). Nature 245:385.
106. Hill, C. H. (1976). In A. S. Prasad (ed.), Trace Elements in Human Health and Disease, Vol. II, p. 281. Academic Press, Inc., New York.
107. Van Campen, D. R. (1969). J. Nutr. 97:104.
108. Van Campen, D. R., and Scaife, P. U. (1967). J. Nutr. 91:473.
109. Schwarz, F. J., and Kirchgessner, M. (1974). Int. J. Vitam. Nutr. Res. 44:258.
110. Van Campen, D. R. (1966). J. Nutr. 88:125.
111. Freeland, J. H., and Cousins, R. J. (1973). Nutr. Rep. Int. 8:337.
112. Fox, M. R. S. (1976). In A. S. Prasad (ed.), Trace Elements in Human Health and Disease, Vol. II, p. 401. Academic Press, Inc., New York.
113. Fox, M. R. S., and Fry, B. E., Jr. (1970). Science 169:989.
114. Fox, M. R. S., Fry, B. E., Jr., Harland, B. F., Schertel, M. E., and Weeks, C. E. (1971). J. Nutr. 101:1295.
115. Margoshes, M., and Vallee, B. L. (1957). J. Am. Chem. Soc. 79:4813.
116. Weser, U., Rupp, H., Donay, F., Linnermann, F., Voelter, W., Voetsch, W., and Jung, G. (1973). Eur. J. Biochem. 39:127.
117. Winge, D., Krasno, J., and Colucci, A. V. (1973). In W. G. Hoekstra et al. (eds.), Trace Element Metabolism in Animals, Vol. 2, p. 500. University Park Press, Baltimore.
118. Shaikh, Z. A., Coleman, R. L., and Lucis, O. J. (1973). In D. D. Hemphill (ed.), Trace Substances in Environmental Health, Vol. VII, p. 313. University of Missouri, Columbia, Missouri.
119. Chen, R. W., Eakin, K. J., and Whanger, P. D. (1974). Nutr. Rep. Int. 4:195.
120. Bremner, I., and Davies, N. T. (1973). Rep. Rowett Inst. 29:126.
121. Chen, R. W., Vasey, E. J., and Whanger, P. D. (1977). J. Nutr. 107:805.
122. Oh, S. H., Deagen, J. T., Whanger, P. D., and Weswig, P. H. (1978). Am. J. Physiol. 234:E282.
123. Schubert, W. K., and Lahey, M. E. (1959). Pediatrics 24:710. Johns Hopkins Med. J. 126:34.
124. Holtzman, N. A., Charache, P., Cordano, A., and Graham, G. G. (1970). Johns Hopkins Med. J. 126:34.
125. al-Rashid, R. A., and Spangler, J. (1971). N. Engl. J. Med. 285:841.
126. Karpel, J. T., and Peden, V. H. (1972). J. Pediatr. 80:32.
127. Cordano, A., Baertl, J. M., and Graham, G. G. (1964). Pediatrics 34:324.
128. Graham, G. G., and Cordano, A. (1969). Johns Hopkins Med. J. 124:139.
129. Graham, G. G., and Cordano, A. (1976). In A. S. Prasad (ed.), Trace Elements in Human Health and Disease, Vol. I, p. 363. Academic Press, Inc., New York.
130. Danks, D. M., Campbell, P. E., Mayne, V., and Cartwright, E. (1972). Pediatrics 50:188.
131. Danks, D. M., Stevens, B. J., Campbell, P. E., Gillespie, J. M., Walker-Smith, J., Blomfield, J., and Turner, B. (1972). Lancet 1:1100.
132. Danks, D. M., Camakaris, J., and Stevens, B. J. (1978). In M. Kirchgessner (ed.), Trace Element Metabolism in Man and Animals, Vol. 3, P. 401. Arbeitsgemeinschaft für Tierernahrungseforschung, Weihenstephan.

133. Hunt, D. M. (1974). Nature 249:852.
134. Danks, D. M. (1977). Inorg. Perspect. Biol. Med. 1:73.
135. Scheinberg, H., and Sternlieb, I. (1976). *In* A. S. Prasad (ed.), Trace Elements in Human Health and Disease, Vol. I, p. 415. Academic Press, Inc., New York.
136. Evans, G. W., Dubois, R. S., and Hambidge, K. M. (1973). Science 181:1175.
137. Cumings, J. N. (1951). Brain 74:10.
138. Walshe, J. M. (1956). Am. J. Med. 21:487.
139. Klingberg, W. G., Prasad, A. S., and Oberleas, D. (1976). *In* A. S. Prasad (ed.), Trace Elements in Human Health and Disease, Vol. I, p. 51. Academic Press, Inc., New York.
140. Todd, W. R., Elvehjem, C. A., and Hart, E. B. (1934). Am. J. Physiol. 107:146.
141. Prasad, A. S., Miale, A., Farid, Z., Sandstead, H. H., and Schulert, A. R. (1963). J. Lab. Clin. Med. 61:537.
142. Halsted, J. A., Ronaghy, H. A., Abadi, P., Haghshenass, M., Amirhakeni, G. H., Barakot, R. M., and Reinhold, J. G. (1972). Am. J. Med. 53:277.
143. Ronaghy, H. S., Reinhold, J. G., Mahloudi, M., Ghavami, P., Fox, M. R. S., and Halsted, J. A. (1974). Am. J. Clin. Nutr. 27:112.
144. Hambidge, K. M., Hambidge, C., Jacobs, M., and Baum, J. D. (1972). Pediatr. Res. 6:868.
145. Walravens, P. A., and Hambidge, K. M. (1975). Pediatr. Res. 9(abstr.):310.
146. Hambidge, K. M., Walravens, P. A., Brown, R. M., Webster, J., White, S., Anthony, M., and Roth, M. L. (1976). Am. J. Clin. Nutr. 29:734.
147. Sandstead, H. H. (1973). Am. J. Clin. Nutr. 26:1251.
148. Schechter, P. J., Friedwald, W. T., Bronzert, D. A., Raff, M. S., and Henkin, R. I. (1972). Int. Rev. Neurobiol. 1(suppl.):125.
149. Henkin, R. I., Schechter, P. J., Hoye, R., and Mattern, C. F. T. (1971). JAMA 217:434.
150. Sandstead, H. H., Vo-Khactu, K. P., and Solomons, N. (1976). *In* A. S. Prasad (ed.), Trace Elements in Human Health and Disease, Vol. I, p. 33. Academic Press, Inc., New York.
151. Henzel, J. H., DeWeese, M. S., and Lichti, E. L. (1970). Arch. Surg. 100:349.
152. Mansouri, K., Halsted, J. A., and Gombos, E. A. (1970). Arch. Int. Med. 125:88.
153. Sullivan, J. F., and Hearney, R. O. (1970). Am. J. Clin. Nutr. 23:170.
154. Henkin, R. I. (1974). Adv. Exp. Med. Biol. 14:299.
155. Pekarek, R. S., and Beisel, W. R. (1975). Proceedings of the IX International Congress of Nutrition, Mexico City, Vol. 2, p. 193. Karger, Basel.
156. Halsted, J. A., Hackley, B. M., and Smith, J. C. (1968). Obstet. Gynecol. 44:666.
157. Hambidge, K. M., and Droegemueller, W. (1974). Obstet. Gynecol. 44:666.
158. Henkin, R. I., Marshall, J. R., and Meret, S. (1971). Am. J. Obstet. Gynecol. 110:131.
159. Jameson, S. (1976). Acta Med. Scand. 593(suppl. 4):89.
160. Hurley, L. S., and Swenerton, H. (1966). Proc. Soc. Exp. Biol. Med. 123:692.
161. Hurley, L. S., Gowan, J., and Swenerton, H. (1971). Teratology 4:199.
162. Apgar, J. (1968). Am. J. Physiol. 215:160, 1478.
163. Apgar, J. (1972). J. Nutr. 102:343.
164. Tucker, H. F., and Salmon, W. D. (1955). Proc. Soc. Exp. Biol. Med. 88:613.
165. Halsted, J. A., and Smith, J. C. (1970). Lancet 1:322.
166. Burr, R. G. (1973). J. Clin. Pathol. 26:773.
167. Hallbook, T., and Lanner, E. (1972). Lancet 2:786.
168. Frommer, D. J. (1975). Med. J. Aust. 2:793.

169. Barcia, P. J. (1970). Ann. Surg. 172:1048.
170. Myers, M. B., and Cherry, G. (1970). Am. J. Surg. 120:77.
171. McClain, P. E., Wiley, E. R., Beecher, G. R., Anthony, W. L., and Hsu, J. M. (1973). Biochim. Biophys. Acta 304:457.
172. Hsu, J. M. (1976). In A. S. Prasad (ed.), Trace Elements in Human Health and Disease, Vol. I, p. 295. Academic Press, Inc., New York.
173. Moynahan, E. J. (1974). Lancet 2:399.
174. Neldner, K. H., and Hambidge, K. M. (1975). New Engl. J. Med. 292:879.
175. Kelly, R., Davidson, G. P., Townley, R. R. W., and Campbell, P. E. (1976). Arch. Dis. Child. 51:219.
176. Hambidge, K. M., Neldner, K. H., and Walravens, P. A. (1975). Lancet 1:577.
177. Weston, W. L., Huff, J. C., Humbert, J. R., Hambidge, K. M., Neldner, K. H., and Walravens, P. A. (1977). Arch. Dermatol. 113:422.
178. Schwarz, K., and Mertz, W. (1957). Arch. Biochem. Biophys. 72:515.
179. Schwarz, K., and Mertz, W. (1959). Arch. Biochem. Biophys. 85:292.
180. Mertz, W., Roginski, E. E., and Schroeder, H. A. (1965). J. Nutr. 86:107.
181. Schroeder, H. A. (1966). J. Nutr. 88:439.
182. Mertz, W. (1974). Proc. Nutr. Soc. 33:307.
183. Anderson, R. A., Polansky, M. M., Brantner, J. H., and Roginski, E. E. (1978). In M. Kirchgessner (ed.), Trace Element Metabolism in Man and Animals, Vol. 3, p. 269. Arbeitsgemeinschaft für Tierernahrungseforschung, Weihenstephan.
184. Gürson, C. T., and Saner, G. (1971). Am. J. Clin. Nutr. 24:1313.
185. Hopkins, L. L., Ransome-Kuti, O., and Majaj, A. S. (1968). Am. J. Clin. Nutr. 21:203.
186. Carter, J. P., Kattab, A., Abd-al Hadi, K. A., Davis, J. T., Gholmy, A. E., and Patwardhan, V. N. (1968). Am. J. Clin. Nutr. 21:195.
187. Glinsmann, W. H., and Mertz, W. (1966). Metabolism 15:510.
188. Levine, R. A., Streeten, D. H. P., and Doisy, R. J. (1968). Metabolism 17:114.
189. Sherman, L., Glennon, J. A., Brech, W. J., Klomberg, G. H., and Gordon, E. S. (1968). Metabolism 17:439.
190. Trace Elements in Human Nutrition. (1973). W. H. O. Tech. Rep. Ser. 532.
191. Hambidge, K. M. (1971). In W. Mertz and W. E. Cornatzer (eds.), Newer Trace Elements in Nutrition, p. 169. Marcel Dekker, New York.
192. Saner, G., Wolf, W. R., and Gürson, C. T. (1974). Fed. Proc. 33:660.
193. Hambidge, K. M., and Rodgerson, D. O. (1969). Am. J. Obstet. Gynecol. 103:320.
194. Jeejeebhoy, K. N., Shu, R., Marliss, E. B., Greenburg, G. R., and Bruce-Robertson, A. (1975). Clin. Res. 23:636A.
195. Muth, O. H., Oldfield, J. E., Remmert, L. F., and Schubert, J. R. (1958). Science 128:1090.
196. Whanger, P. D., Weswig, P. H., Oldfield, J. E., Cheeke, P. R., and Schmitz, J. A. (1976). Nutr. Rep. Int. 13:159.
197. Hartley, W. J. (1967). In O. H. Muth (ed.), Selenium in Biomedicine, p. 79. Avi Publishing Company, Westport, Connecticut.
198. Hartley, W. J. (1963). Proc. N. Z. Soc. Anim. Prod. 23:20.
199. Thompson, J. N., and Scott, M. L. (1969). J. Nutr. 97:335.
200. McCoy, K. E. M., and Weswig, P. H. (1969). J. Nutr. 98:383.
201. Thompson, J. N., and Scott, M. L. (1970). J. Nutr. 100:797.
202. Fischer, W. C., and Whanger, P. D. (1977). J. Nutr. Sci. Vitaminol. 23:273.
203. Fischer, W. C., and Whanger, P. D. (1977). J. Nutr. 107:1493.
204. Rotruck, J. T., Hoekstra, W. C., Pope, A. L., Ganther, H. E., Swanson, A., and Hafeman, D. (1973). Science 179:588.

205. Levander, O. A., Morris, V. C., Higgs, D. J., and Ferretti, R. J. (1975). J. Nutr. 105:1481.
206. Levander, O. A., Morris, V. C., and Ferretti, R. J. (1977). J. Nutr. 107:378.
207. Levander, O. A., Morris, V. C., and Ferretti, R. J. (1977). J. Nutr. 107:363.
208. Diplock, A. T. (1974). Proc. Nutr. Soc. 33:315.
209. Whanger, P. D., Pederson, N. D., and Weswig, P. H. (1973). Biochem. Biophys. Res. Commun. 53:1031.
210. Pederson, N. D., Whanger, P. H., Weswig, P. H., and Muth, O. H. (1972). Bioinorg. Chem. 2:33.
211. Lawrence, R. A., and Burk, R. F. (1976). Biochem. Biophys. Res. Commun. 71:952.
212. Black, R. S., Tripp, M. J., Whanger, P. D., and Weswig, P. H. (1977). Bioinorg. Chem. 8:161.
213. Broderius, M. A., Whanger, P. D., and Weswig, P. H. (1973). J. Nutr. 103:336.
214. Sprinkler, L. H., Harr, J. R., Newberne, P. N., Whanger, P. D., and Weswig, P. H. (1971). Nutr. Rep. Int. 4:335.
215. Whanger, P. D. (1973). Biochem. Med. 7:316.
216. Bull, R. C., and Oldfield, J. E. (1967). J. Nutr. 91:237.
217. Griffiths, N. M., and Thompson, C. D. (1974). N. Z. Med. J. 80:199.
218. Thomson, C. D., Rea, H. M., Doesburg, V. M., and Robinson, M. F. (1977). Br. J. Nutr. 37:457.
219. Hadjimarkos, D. M. (1973). *In* D. D. Hemphill (ed.), Trace Substances in Environmental Health, Vol. VII, p. 25. Columbia, Missouri.
220. Ludwig, T. G., and Bibby, B. G. (1969). Caries Res. 3:32.
221. Shamberger, R. J., and Frost, D. V. (1969). Can. Med. Assoc. J. 100:682.
222. Shamberger, R. J., Tytko, S., and Willis, R. E. (1974). *In* D. D. Hemphill (ed.), Trace Substances in Environmental Health, Vol. VII, p. 35. University of Missouri, Columbia, Missouri.
223. Schrauzer, G. N., White, D. A., and Schneider, D. J. (1977). Bioinorg. Chem. 7:23, 35.

International Review of Biochemistry
Biochemistry of Nutrition IA, Volume 27
Edited by A. Neuberger and T. H. Jukes
Copyright 1979   University Park Press   Baltimore

9
Atherosclerosis as Related to Diet

H. TUNSTALL PEDOE and G. ROSE

St. Mary's Hospital Medical School, London, England, and London School of
Hygiene and Tropical Medicine, London, England.

In industrialized countries diseases with an atherosclerotic basis now cause more deaths than any other condition. Although many of these deaths are in the elderly, atherosclerotic diseases still lead all others in loss-of-life expectation during the economically active period of life. Incidence rates are now starting to rise also in countries of the developing world, especially in their cities; unless causes are identified and preventive measures instituted, the scale of the problem will undoubtedly grow. It is the aim of this chapter to assess how far one can disentangle specific nutritional causes from among the tangled complex that distinguishes the Western way of life, and to assess their relevance to preventive policy.

Inevitably the evidence is largely indirect. Experiments in laboratory animals long ago identified mechanisms whereby dietary manipulations, especially in fat content, might induce arterial disease. This makes dietary theories of causation in man plausible but it cannot prove them, especially since the animal models have generally failed to reproduce the typical human sequence of coronary atherosclerosis, thrombosis, and myocardial infarction.

In man it is unacceptable to conduct exposure experiments. "Abatement studies" should be possible in which the investigator tests the effect on naturally occurring disease of a controlled reduction in the level of exposure to a hypothesized cause. In practice, however, even these studies present serious problems. The number of subjects needs to be very large, and their adherence to prescribed dietary advice may be poor. Atherosclerosis is a chronic process and the period needed to demonstrate the effects of slowing or regression could well be a matter of decades; but the drop-out of subjects makes it hard to continue a controlled trial for longer than about 5 years. Finally, the critical period for the development of disease might be relatively early in life, and in that case trials of abatement of exposure in middle age or later could come too late to demonstrate benefits. For these reasons abatement trials in this field have been few and unsatisfactory, and it seems unlikely that there will be any further major attempts of this kind to test nutritional theories of causation.

This serious deficiency in the evidence results substantially from our inability to measure atherosclerosis as an end point except either after death or in that highly select group of patients whose illnesses justify hazardous and invasive investigations. Population-based studies are forced to depend for their end points on major illnesses or deaths, which happen only late in the course of atherosclerosis and, during the duration of a particular study, to only a minority of subjects. The whole situation would change dramatically if techniques could be developed (for example, with the use of ultrasound) that would permit the noninvasive measurement of atherosclerotic plaque and stenosis. Trials might then be expected to give results from relatively small numbers and perhaps within a much shorter period of time. Efforts to develop such techniques should be given high priority in the field of atherosclerosis research.

Table 1.   Cardiac pathology in men 45–59 years old dying from non-cardiovascular causes and coming to necropsy: apparent changes over a 45-year period[a]

Pathology	Deaths (%)	
	1908–1913 (N = 530)	1954–1956 (N = 1394)
Ischemic myocardial fibrosis	1.3	4.4
Coronary artery stenosis/occlusion	5.0	15.1
Severe coronary atherosclerosis	47	66

[a]From Morris and Crawford (1).

In the meantime, the evidence on causation in man is scientifically inferior, being largely observational rather than experimental, and depending on only an indirect assessment of the process that is to be elucidated. In such a field controversy is inevitable, and any conclusions must be provisional rather than dogmatic. At the same time the public health problem is large and pressing. Decisions on preventive policy must be taken, albeit based on probabilities and not certainties. Certainty is unattainable and seems likely to remain so.

INTERNATIONAL DISTRIBUTION

Relation of CHD to Atherosclerosis

The principal clinical consequences of atherosclerosis are coronary heart disease (CHD), cerebral infarction, and ischemia in the legs (intermittent claudication or gangrene). The latter is the least common of the three, and of itself it rarely causes death; for these reasons it is the least well documented. The relation of cerebral infarction to atherosclerosis is not straightforward, and clinically the condition is hard to distinguish from stroke caused by hypertension. The distribution of atherosclerosis has therefore often been equated with the distribution of CHD, and particularly (since this is best documented) with mortality therefrom. This assumption is not necessarily correct, since the clinical effects of coronary atherosclerosis depend also on factors influencing thrombosis, and perhaps on the underlying anatomy of the coronary arterial tree and its anastomoses. Thus it is possible, for example, that dietary or other factors might alter a population's incidence of CHD by their effect on thrombotic mechanisms rather than on the severity of atherosclerosis. A restrospective study of routine necropsy records in Britain over a period of nearly half a century (1) showed that there had been a large increase in the frequency of ischemic myocardial fibrosis and stenosis of coronary arteries, but a seemingly much smaller increase in atherosclerosis (Table 1). In the absence of standardized methods of measurement and reporting, the quantitative interpretation of such historical data must be cautious; probably the most than can be concluded is that severe atherosclerosis is not a new disease. This view recently received dramatic support from the findings in a mummified female corpse in China, believed to be 2100 years old (2). There were indications from the stomach contents that the woman had just eaten, and so presumably she had died suddenly; dissection revealed severe coronary atherosclerosis (she also had gall stones).

The difficulties of standardizing the measurement of atherosclerosis were effectively overcome in the International Atherosclerosis Project (3). Hearts were collected from necropsies on accidental and other noncardiovascular deaths, preserved, and shipped to a central laboratory in New Orleans, Louisiana, for standardized quantitative measurements. In Figure 1 the findings from various participating countries are related to the corresponding national CHD mortality rates. Irregularities are to be expected, particularly since the postmortem samples were not strictly representative of their parent populations. Nevertheless, the overall correlation is unlikely to have been due to chance, and one may infer that international differences in CHD mortality tend to reflect at least in part corresponding differences in the severity of atherosclerosis.

Distribution of CHD Mortality

Few developing countries have been able to institute adequate mortality registration systems and population censuses, and reliable mortality rates are mostly available only for industrialized countries. Table 2 shows, nevertheless, a sevenfold range, despite the fact that with respect to affluence and industrialization there is little difference between the bottom of the table (Japan) and the top (Finland and the United States). Clearly, an urbanized and industrialized way of life is not by itself a sufficient explanation of these enormous variations in CHD mortality.

Factors known to influence the incidence of atherosclerosis and its related diseases include hypertension, cigarette smoking, and physical inactivity. However, hypertension is known to be more prevalent in Japan than in the countries at the top of the table; cigarette consumption rates correlate poorly with national rates for CHD; and the highest CHD rates in the world occur in Eastern Finland among farmers and lumberjacks renowned for their high level of physical activity. So although these factors probably all contribute to international differences, they do not seem to be the major determinants. Nor are the differences predominantly ethnic in origin, according to the evidence from groups that have migrated from countries with lower CHD rates to those with high rates (Italians to Australia, Polynesians to New Zealand, Japanese to the United States). In such instances the migrants have tended within a few years to acquire the higher rates of their country of adoption.

From these observations it is concluded that the big international differences in the frequency of CHD reflect corresponding differences in the distribution of the environmental causes of atherosclerosis. From the animal

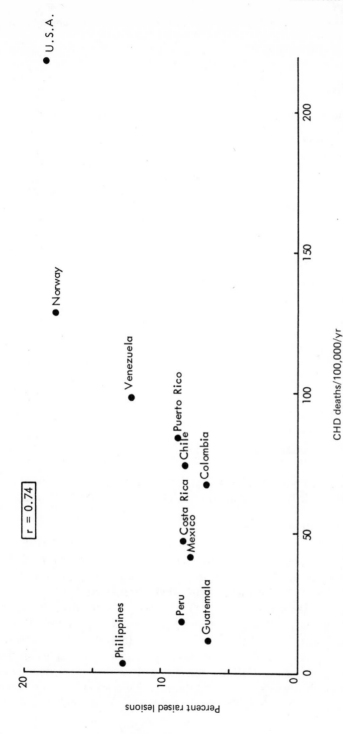

Figure 1.   Relationship between extent of atherosclerosis (area of raised lesions as percent of intimal area) and mortality from CHD (ICD, 8th revision, A.83) in 11 countries (men and women, ages 25–64 years, age adjusted).

Table 2. Mortality from coronary heart disease in 25 countries among men aged 35–74 years[a]

Country	Deaths/100,000/year
Finland	755
United States	677
Australia	669
United Kingdom	608
Scotland	744
Northern Ireland	701
England and Wales	583
Canada	564
Israel	523
Denmark	504
Czechoslovakia	501
Norway	491
Sweden	485
Netherlands	414
Trinidad and Tobago	409
Belgium	397
German Federal Republic	382
Puerto Rico	295
Italy	261
Switzerland	237
Poland	226
Yugoslavia	177
Greece	176
France	174
Spain	161
Hong Kong	107
Mexico	102
Japan	95

[a]1973 or nearest available year; ICD, 8th revision, code A.83; rates age-adjusted to population of England and Wales.

evidence, and from the inability of other coronary risk factors to account for the differences, it is reasonable to search for correlations with diet.

Dietary Correlations

Much of the literature on this subject has been concerned only with testing one specific hypothesis — that a high intake of saturated fat causes CHD. It is well, however, to first look more openmindedly at the evidence to see whether in fact it fits this theory better than alternatives.

Table 3 is taken from a W. H. O. analysis (4), using data that are now some 20–30 years old. There are strong associations at the national level between CHD mortality and the mean per capita intake of total calories and each of the main nutrients. The findings do not, however, distinguish clearly between the positive associations with fat (total or saturated), sucrose, and total calories on the one hand, and the negative association with complex carbohydrates on the other. The results may be taken as supporting the view

Table 3. Mortality from coronary heart disease in 25 countries as related to mean per capita intake of calories and nutrients (1940's–1950's)[a]

	Correlation coefficient		
	Men (45–54 yr)	Men (55–64 yr)	Both sexes (all ages)
Calories	+ 0.70	+ 0.75	+ 0.81
Complex carbohydrates	− 0.62	− 0.62	− 0.63
Sucrose	+ 0.62	+ 0.65	+ 0.75
Protein	+ 0.23	+ 0.26	+ 0.31
Total fat	+ 0.62	+ 0.63	+ 0.70
Unsaturated fat	+ 0.69	+ 0.73	+ 0.70

[a]From Masironi (4).

that some dietary factor or factors seem likely to be involved, but in terms of particular nutrients it is only possible to say that total protein appears to be less important than other major nutrients or total calories.

In a more recent analysis Knox (5) used dietary data for 20 countries (mainly European) from statistics of the Organization for Economic Cooperation and Development. He looked at total nutrients and at a variety of individual foods in relation to CHD and other mortality rates. Some of his results are given in Table 4. Again the correlations are strikingly high, but they are not uniquely strong for CHD, nor does any one foodstuff or group stand out clearly from the others. Knox concludes, after extensive multivariate analysis, that "no specific foodstuff, no foodstuff group, and none of the main calorie-providing nutrients can be resolved on the basis of these data as a primary determinant of death rates from ischaemic heart disease." In other words, routine international statistics lend general support to the belief that nutrition may be causally important, but they are too crude, and

Table 4. Mortality from various causes in 20 countries in 1970 as related to per capita intake of individual foodstuffs[a]

	Correlation coefficient			
Foodstuff	CHD	Cerebrovascular accidents	Breast cancer	Colon cancer
Sugar	+ 0.74	− 0.42	+ 0.82	+ 0.67
Milk	+ 0.71	− 0.09	+ 0.41	+ 0.23
Beef	+ 0.71	− 0.41	+ 0.66	+ 0.75
Eggs	+ 0.61	− 0.41	+ 0.72	+ 0.88
Butter	+ 0.57	− 0.05	+ 0.41	+ 0.27
Mutton	− 0.04	+ 0.20	− 0.26	− 0.05
Fish	− 0.28	+ 0.22	− 0.44	− 0.37
Cheese	− 0.35	− 0.55	− 0.04	− 0.20
Wheat	− 0.54	+ 0.26	− 0.68	− 0.54
Wine	− 0.62	+ 0.24	− 0.34	+ 0.03
Vegetables	− 0.64	+ 0.38	− 0.53	− 0.16
Fruit	− 0.71	+ 0.30	− 0.44	− 0.37

[a]From Knox (5).

the intercorrelations are too complex, to indicate one class of nutrients over the others. For that purpose more refined data are necessary.

THE DIETARY FAT THEORY

Although the greatest volume of research on the dietary fat theory of atherogenesis was carried out in the period after the Second World War, its roots go back to the early years of the twentieth century, to three separate discoveries. At a time when atherosclerosis was attributed to a variety of causes such as toxins or trauma and when other researchers had notably failed to mimic the disease in experimental animals, Anitschkov and his colleagues produced atheroma-like deposits of cholesterol in the arterial wall of rabbits fed a nonherbivorous diet of meat, milk, and eggs. By 1913 these workers had realized that is was not the animal protein that caused these lesions but the lipids (6). Atheromatous plaques had long been known to contain cholesterol, and it became apparent when the measurement of serum cholesterol levels (now often done on plasma) was introduced into clinical medicine that those conditions in which cholesterol levels were often unusually elevated, such as diabetes mellitus, predisposed the patient to premature atherosclerosis. However, de Langen in 1916 had observed that Javanese who ate a traditional diet that contained little fat or cholesterol had lower serum cholesterol levels than their countrymen who had adopted European diets (7). It seemed that serum cholesterol levels could be influenced by disease and by intrinsic metabolic differences but were also subject to dietary modification.

These three separate early discoveries, which constitute the essence of the dietary fat theory, can be summarized as follows:

Dietary fat ⟶ Atherosclerosis
(from experiments on animals)

Dietary fat ⟶ Serum lipids
(from comparisons of population groups)

Serum lipids ⟶ Atherosclerosis
(from clinical observations)

Over the following 50 years these statements have remained essentially unaltered except for increasing sophistication in the understanding and quantification of which dietary and serum lipids are involved. Further evidence for the associations, now widely believed to be causal, has been obtained from epidemiological studies both of differences between communities and of individual differences within groups, from experiments lasting weeks in metabolic wards, from large scale dietary trials involving hundreds of subjects for many years, and from animal experiments. Anitschkov's discoveries have given rise to a branch of experimental pathology. This last source of data is discussed briefly first and then each of the above statements in turn is discussed in relation to man.

Animal Experiments

The advantages of an animal model of atherosclerosis are considerable. In man lesions may take decades to appear and they can only be inspected with permission at death, surgery, or, in silhouette, by angiography. In contrast, the life span of most experimental animals and the time taken to develop lesions are considerably shorter, drastic changes in diet that would be unacceptable in man can be made, and progress of lesions can be followed by killing and examining samples of the study population. Atheroma-like lesions have now been produced in a great variety of warm-blooded animals, both birds and mammals, in omnivores, carnivores, and herbivores (8).

However, there is some doubt as to the applicability of these models to man. Species differ in their susceptibility and tissue responses to lipid deposition and in the dietary constituents necessary to produce it. Experiments have been criticized because the diets used have sometimes been extreme and the serum lipid levels obtained well outside the human range, because the fatty deposits produced tend to be located in the aorta and not the coronary arteries, and because they are more reminiscent of the fatty streaks seen in children than the histologically complex plaques seen in adults that lead to stenosis of the artery, ulceration, and thrombosis.

Many of these objections have been overcome by using animals that are more similar to man, such as the rhesus monkey, and by using less extreme diets for longer periods. In many species it has not only proved possible to demonstrate the development of atheroma-like lesions, but it has also been shown that discontinuation of the atherogenic diet leads, after some time, to regression of the fatty deposits (9). For example, Armstrong induced stenosing atheromatous coronary artery lesions in rhesus monkeys fed a serum cholesterol–elevating, high fat diet for 17 months and showed that a diet low in fat or one rich in linolenic acid caused regression of the lesions, with reabsorption of lipid and restoration of the lumen over 40 months (10). In a related species (cynomolgus monkeys) more prone to produce a fibrous reaction in induced atheromatous plaques, he and his colleagues have produced suggestive evidence that this may regress as well.

Despite the dietary, metabolic, and anatomical differences between man and other animals, the animal model of atherosclerosis is important because its findings are essentially compatible with the dietary fat theory in man and it has failed to produce evidence in serious conflict with that theory and in support of alternatives. It has been found repeatedly that a diet containing substantial quantities of saturated fat or cholesterol or both is a necessary prerequisite for the production of atheromatous lesions and in many species it is a sufficient cause. Similarly, the evidence that quite well established stenosing lesions in animals may regress under dietary control with a reduction in serum lipid levels is grounds for greater optimism in the treatment of human patients than if this had proved impossible.

Dietary Fat and Atherosclerosis in Man

Evidence that the risk of development of atherosclerosis correlates with the quantity and quality of dietary fat has been looked for in national statistics collected for other purposes, in comparative surveys of communities in different countries in which incidence of disease and diet have been measured more directly, and in studies of individuals to look for associations between their diet and coronary risk.

Although the incidence of atherosclerotic diseases is said to vary widely throughout the world, as do the constituents of human diets, the only routinely collected statistics on the former that can be compared are the age-specific or age-standardized mortality rates from coronary heart disease and these are available only for Europe, North America, and a few other countries; most of Asia and Africa and much of South America cannot provide them. Diagnostic criteria, the completeness of data, and the frequency of postmortem confirmation of cause of death vary widely from country to country. On the other hand consumption figures for different foodstuffs ignore wastage, maldistribution, and seasonal variations in diet. These inaccuracies are bound to weaken correlations calculated from these data, as will any modifying effects on mortality rates of other nondietary causal factors. The correlations achieved depend in part on which countries are admitted to the analyses and on whether simultaneous comparisons are made between mortality rates and consumption (5, 11) or whether these rates are related to consumption figures for previous decades (12, 13).

The results of these international correlations are largely compatible with the dietary fat theory, but tend also to corroborate alternative hypotheses that may have been generated from them. Thus Knox's (5) findings are seen to support the dietary fat theory if quoted selectively (see Table 4). The correlation coefficients between coronary heart disease mortality rates and consumption of certain foodstuffs are 0.69 for total animal fat, 0.57 for total fat, 0.61 for eggs, 0.57 for butter, 0.71 for milk, and 0.71 for beef, all good evidence for the theory, but less impressive when 0.74 for total animal protein and 0.74 for sugar are included. Knox's data were from 17 countries in Europe plus Canada, the United States, and, for some analyses, Japan.

In contrast to Knox's very guarded conclusions that the data revealed no specific primary determinant of death rates, Segall (11) analyzed virtually the same data and obtained correlation coefficients that agreed well with those of Knox. However, his conclusion was that a correlation coefficient of 0.72 for milk and milk products (excluding butter) suggested that milk was probably a coronary health hazard and consumption should be markedly reduced.

Another form of correlation can be obtained within one country between the secular or time trend of coronary heart disease mortality rates and the trends in foodstuff consumption. Although studies of diet in the early years of this century have been attempted (14) these can only be regarded as estimates and subject to error, as are coronary heart disease mortality rates. However, in some European countries coronary death rates are said to have leveled off or even fallen slightly during wartime austerity in the 1940s; since then most European countries have experienced a rapid increase in male rates (15) at the same time that there has been an increase in the proportion of food energy obtained from fat, particularly animal fat, and a reduction in carbohydrate consumption (16), so that these are strongly correlated. However, individual dietary components may give bizarre results in such an analysis (13). In England and Wales from 1950 to 1967 milk consumption fell while consumption of butter rose, so that milk consumption is negatively associated and butter consumption positively associated with male coronary heart disease mortality (in contrast to international comparisons and Segall's conclusions). To confuse the interpretations even further, there have been times when male and female coronary heart disease mortality rate trends appear to have been going in opposite directions (15); female rates do not appear to have risen as much since 1950. Analysis of short time periods might produce contradictory results for men and women. If diet is responsible for the trends there must be other confounding factors operating selectively in the two sexes.

Routinely collected statistics, therefore, are limited by the quality of the data, the relatively few countries for which they are available, the multiple comparisons that can be made, and the high degree of correlation (in the richer, statistics-producing countries) between different dietary constituents whose effects it is hoped to distinguish, such as fat, animal protein, and sugar.

In the International Atherosclerosis Project (3) an attempt was made to measure the amount of atherosclerosis in 15 different populations — nine in South America, two in the Caribbean, and one each in New Orleans, Louisiana, the Philippines, Durban, South Africa, and Oslo, Norway — with the use of a highly standardized method of postmortem examination. The results of these scoring systems were used to rank the populations by severity of atherosclerosis and this was correlated with rankings of amounts of different dietary constituents by using locally available information rather than special analyses (17). This study, therefore, overcame some of the difficulties inherent in international comparisons of incidence of atherosclerosis, although perhaps not those of diet, and was able to encompass countries often excluded from analysis of mortality statistics because of the incompleteness of data. The degree of atherosclerosis correlated well with the proportion of food energy obtained from fat ($r = 0.67$) and with animal protein consumption; but correlations with sugar were substantially lower ($r = 0.32$) and with the percentage of total fat from animal fat were negligible ($r < 0.1$). This particular study included a number of South American countries, in which much sugar and little fat are eaten, so that their effects appear to have been dissociated better than they are in European studies, in which there is a high degree of correlation.

The most energetic international researcher of the dietary fat theory has been Ancel Keys, who rounded off a number of preliminary investigations with colleagues in different countries with the Seven Countries Study (18, 19). In this study attempts were made to standardize both measurements of coronary heart disease incidence and the measurement of dietary intake and other risk factors. Although it was hoped to test the theory in different communities, these could not be chosen at random since local physicians, other personnel, facilities, and follow-up were essential. Finland and Japan were chosen as representing the extremes of known coronary heart disease mortality rates; American railwaymen were used as a reference group from the country with the oldest established coronary problem; Holland in the 1950s was said to have less coronary disease than its alleged high fat diet entitled it to, and Italy, Greece, and Yugoslavia were added. Other countries were left out because of local difficulties. Where possible, two or more populations with contrasting characteristics were chosen in each country and in each population several hundred men, ages 40–59, were examined for manifestations of coronary heart disease and for coronary risk factors. Those free of the disease were followed for 10 years for evidence of coronary heart disease and death, with detailed re-examination at 5 years.

The assessment of diet in the Seven Countries Study was done by taking sample members of each group and weighing all foods eaten for a week at a time. Consumption of different constituents was calculated from food tables and by chemical analysis of duplicates that were deep frozen, mixed, and homogenized with aliquots, then lyophilized and analyzed in central laboratories for lipids, protein, carbohydrate, and fatty acid composition. Sampling throughout the year allowed for seasonal changes in diet and the changing make-up of foodstuffs.

At the 5-year point it was possible to relate coronary heart disease incidence in the disease-free men in each cohort to the mean diet. The results showed a statistically significant correlation coefficient of 0.84 between coronary heart disease deaths and infarcts on the one hand and the percentage of food energy obtained from saturated fatty acids on the other. Other dietary correlations failed to reach the 5% level of significance ($r = 0.55$) for 13 cohorts included in this analysis: for example, percentage of food energy from total fat ($r = 0.40$); correlation between all coronary heart disease incidence and percentage of food energy from protein ($r = 0.14$) and monoene fatty acids ($r = -0.42$); and calories per kg of body weight ($r = 0.04$). Dietary cholesterol was not estimated in all countries and sucrose was reported separately (20) and is discussed later.

The Seven Countries Study, by standardized methods of recording coronary incidence and diet, achieved higher correlations for saturated fats than those obtained from national statistics. An r value of 0.84 would account for nearly 71% of the variance in incidence between cohorts. In addition the study showed that diet appeared to vary between cohorts more than other factors that were assessed. However, the number of cohorts was of necessity limited and 12 of them were from Europe, nine of these from southern Europe (five from Yugoslavia). While it is conceivable that this particular choice of countries might have produced better correlation coefficients for saturated fatty acids that others, the cohorts were not all chosen with fore-knowledge of what diet and incidence would be. Within countries, groups with contrasting diets or incidence were chosen and the Dutch, whose results fitted the theory, were included because it was thought that they might not.

An example of the difficulties created for the dietary fat theory by the absence of good data from many parts of the world is the work of Malhotra on railwaymen from the Indian subcontinent (21–23). He claimed that retro-spective analysis of medical records showed a sevenfold increase in coronary rates from the north to the south of India, although animal fat and particu-larly fermented milk played a major role in the northern diet, whereas south-erners eat far less fat and dairy products but more seed oils. He suggested that the fermentation, the churning of curd, and the use of turmeric for cooking in the north change the fats and lead to a predominance of short chain fatty acids and small fat globules that are absorbed and metabolized differently as a result. It has been suggested that fermentation of milk by the Masai may alter its dietary effects (24). These suggestions would imply that the preparation of foodstuffs is as important as their constitution and that broad correlations of consumption with disease incidence are bound to be imperfect.

Within communities attempts to correlate differences between in-dividuals in their fat consumption with coronary risk have been unsuccessful (25). Possible explanations are considered in the next section, since a similar problem arises with individual serum cholesterol levels.

Dietary Fat and Serum Lipids

After the original observation by de Langen that the Javanese on traditional low fat diets had lower mean serum cholesterol levels than those adopting fatty Westernized diets, it was assumed for many years that it was the total fat in the diet that determined the cholesterol level. However, Groen et al. in 1952 showed that not all fats had the same effect (26) and since then a large volume of work and considerable controversy have centered on the issues of which dietary fats influence cholesterol levels, whether cholesterol in the diet is of any importance, and whether other dietary constituents are relevant. These issues have been of interest to and debated by not only researchers and clinicians but representatives of the foodstuff producers and distributors. They have been oversimplified both for the purposes of polemic and for health education so that, for example, cholesterol-lowering and low cholesterol diets are commonly confused. In order to clarify subsequent discussion, the nature of dietary fats is described briefly (27, 28).

Although the more complex lipids are found in cell walls, the bulk of stored and ingested fat consists of triglycerides. There are a considerable number of fatty acids found in nature, but most dietary triglycerides consist of different proportions of the same small number. Different foodstuffs have characteristic fatty acid compositions but never one triglyceride only; they usually have a mixture of acids of different chain length and degree of saturation. Vegetable oils, particularly those from seeds, tend to be relatively unsaturated, as do fish oils, which contain long chain polyunsaturated fatty acids. Animal fats, on the other hand, are relatively more saturated. Although the quality of animal fats is partly determined by the fats in their diets (29), ruminant animals, such as cows, have bacteria in the rumen that break down the cellulose in the cud and hydrogenate the vegetable oils, saturating the fatty acids and isomerizing some of the remaining double bond linkages from the cis to the trans form (30). Both of these processes increase the hardness and raise the melting point of the fat. This process is copied by the food industry in the manufacture of margarines and shortenings. Vegetable oils and marine oils are hydrogenated to improve palatability, handling, and storage, but in the process considerable quantities of the abnormal transisomers of unsaturated acids are formed, as well as long chain saturated fatty acids.

Animal fats tend to be more saturated, but naturally contain large quantities of monounsaturated fatty acid. Not all vegetable fats are polyunsaturated. Coconut oil is very saturated and other vegetable fats may have been hydrogenated before sale.

Although cholesterol has been identified in plants, it is only found in any quantity in animal products (31), particularly in offal such as liver and kidney, in shellfish, and in eggs. Plants contain related sterols. A diet high in saturated fat is likely to contain quantities of cholesterol, whereas a low saturated fat, high polyunsaturated fat diet is likely to contain much less.

Work on the dietary determinants of serum (or now more commonly plasma) cholesterol levels has been done by following these levels in groups of volunteers while they are fed on a succession of different diets made up either from original foodstuffs (32) or from synthetic liquid formula diets (33). The experiments are costly and difficult for several reasons: because of the between-individual and within-individual variability of serum cholesterol levels, necessitating several subjects and many readings for each experiment; because the subjects need to be in energy balance, so that diets must be individually tailored; because dietary effects on the serum cholesterol level take 3 weeks or so to stabilize; and because a latin square or cross-over design is ideally followed.

Table 5.   Some of the more common dietary straight chain fatty acids[a]

Saturated	Monounsaturated	Polyunsaturated
$(C_{6:0}$ Caproic) traces		
$C_{8:0}$ Caprylic		
$C_{10:0}$ Capric	$C_{10:0}$ Decenoic ⎫	Variants with
$C_{12:0}$ Lauric	$C_{12:1}$ Dodecenoic ⎬	double bond between
$C_{14:0}$ Myristic	$C_{14:1}$ Tetradecenoic ⎭	different carbon atoms
$C_{16:1}$ Palmitic	$C_{16:1}$ Palmitoleic	
$C_{18:0}$ Stearic	$C_{18:1}$ cis-Oleic	$C_{18:2}$ Linoleic[b]
	trans-Elaidic	
$(C_{20:0}$ Arachidic) traces	$C_{20:1}$ Eicosenoic	$C_{18:3}$ Linolenic
	$C_{22:1}$ cis-Erucic	$C_{20:3}$ Arachidonic[b]
	trans-Brassidic	C_{22} ⎫
		C_{24} ⎬ various, in
		C_{26} ⎭ fish oils

[a]From Documenta Geigy (39).
[b]Essential fatty acids.

Keys and his colleagues attempted to produce a predictive formula that would account for the findings of a large number of experiments of others as well as their own (34–36). They suggested that the proportion of food energy obtained from saturated fatty acids was the major dietary determinant of cholesterol level, tending to push it up; dietary cholesterol had an additional small positive effect that diminished as the amount increased; polyunsaturated fatty acids, on the other hand, depressed cholesterol levels; and monounsaturated fatty acids and other dietary constituents had a neutral effect. These statements contradicted a number of previous beliefs, including some of their own, such as that total fats determined cholesterol, or that it was the source of the fat and the accompanying protein or the iodine number (a measure of both mono- and polyunsaturated components) that mattered; they also gave an important but not central role to the polyunsaturated or essential fatty acids (37, 38) (Table 5) (39). As originally stated, their predictive formula for the effect of a change of diet on mean serum cholesterol levels was:

$$\Delta Chol = 1.5\Delta Z + 1.35(2\Delta S - \Delta P)$$

where $\Delta Chol$ was the serum cholesterol change in mg/100 ml [multiply by 0.026 to convert to mmol/liter (S.I. Units)], ΔZ was the square root of the change in cholesterol intake in mg/day, ΔS was the change in percentage of food energy from saturated fatty acids, and ΔP was the change in percentage of food energy from polyunsaturated fatty acids.

This formula was subsequently found not to explain the effects of some dietary manipulations and it was suggested that only the saturated fatty acids with 12–16 carbon atoms — lauric, myristic, and palmitic — raised cholesterol levels; the shorter ones and stearic acid had a neutral effect on cholesterol but in the short term raised serum triglycerides (40–42). The Minnesota group therefore revised their predictive formula to:

$$\Delta\text{Chol} = 1.5\Delta Z + 1.2(2\Delta S^{\text{l}} - \Delta P)$$

where S^{l} was 12–16-carbon saturated fatty acids. (Although the revised formula is more accurate there are few situations in which the original formula is misleading, so that both can be used.)

These formulas have not been universally accepted. The importance of dietary cholesterol is still controversial, perhaps because the effects on plasma levels of added dietary cholesterol in different individuals vary from none at all to gross elevation (43, 44). Cholesterol-lowering effects are still being claimed for certain vegetable products such as soya protein (45), for dietary fiber (discussed later), and even for separated milk (46). The Minnesota doctrine has provoked one notable diatribe (47) to which the group has replied (48, 49), but at present their formulas account for the findings of large numbers of carefully conducted and controlled experiments, and the predictions are said to hold true not only for 3 weeks but over many months (50).

The above formulas are grossly compatible with the findings of the Seven Countries Study and other comparisons of ethnic groups on different diets (e.g., in Africa (51, 52)). In the former there was a good correlation ($r = 0.89$) between mean serum cholesterol levels in 14 groups of men and the percentage of food energy obtained from saturated fatty acids. Differences in polyunsaturated fat intake and cholesterol intake between the cohorts were too small to have much predictive value. However, the differences between mean serum cholesterol levels in the groups studied were greater than those predicted by the formulas, suggesting either that a lifetime of exposure to a diet exaggerates differences observed in 3-week experiments, or that there were other factors not included in the formulas that were having an additional effect. These could be complex carbohydrates found in vegetables, some of which have some cholesterol-lowering effect (19).

Although the mean serum cholesterol levels of groups can be correlated with their average diet there has been a signal failure to do the same for individuals within groups. Most studies range from showing an insignificantly poor degree of correlation between dietary saturated fat, total fat, or cholesterol consumption and serum cholesterol to showing no degree of correlation at all (19, 53–55). The lack of correlation between individual diets and serum cholesterol and individual diet and coronary risk is unfortunate for the dietary fat theory, but there is no shortage of explanations (19, 49, 56, 57).

Single cholesterol estimations are a poor indicator of a subject's mean cholesterol. With a coefficient of variation for repeated measurements in one person of 11.6% it is possible to state from a single measurement only that there is a 95% probability that his or her mean value is within ±23% of that reading, an enormous range in relation to the coefficient of variation of readings from different subjects, which at 18.6% is not much greater than that within subjects (58). Thus a single cholesterol estimation may result in a false estimate of the subject's mean serum cholesterol level; i.e., the decision that it is higher or lower than the group mean may be wrong. The same variability within the individual applies to dietary measurement, which is subject to certain special errors related to the accuracy of recall, the assessment of quantity, the effect on the subject of knowing that he or she is under observation, the validity of the food tables, or analyses used to calculate constituents, and also to a very large sampling error occasioned by the day-to-day changes in some dietary constituents that may make the sampling period unrepresentative of the true mean diet. Depending on the constituent concerned, a more or less protracted period of observation is needed to characterize an individual with any accuracy as having a high, medium, or low dietary intake (59–62).

Another explanation offered for this lack of correlation is that within one culture diets tend to be homogeneous and it is difficult to deviate appreciably from the average diet, but cholesterol values vary considerably between individuals on the same diet because of genetic factors. Evidence for genetic control of serum cholesterol comes from the Mendelian inheritance of conditions such as familial hypercholesterolemia and from some family studies, but a recently published comparison of identical and nonidentical twins suggests that little of the person-to-person variability in serum cholesterol is inherited, which means that most of it is unexplained (63).

Much of the random error in cholesterol and dietary measurement should be diminished by increasing the number of subjects, but unfortunately the larger the population studied the less accurate the method of measurement tends to be and also the shorter the period of observation. All these factors would explain a poor correlation; the failure of some studies to demonstrate any correlation at all remains an embarrassment. This failure does not mean that cholesterol is unaffected by diet. Even a crude questionnaire is readily able to identify a correlation between change in dietary fat and consequent change in serum cholesterol. The Minnesota group found that individual cholesterol change as a result of diet change was reasonably predictable (36). Gross differences in diets, such as those between vegetarians and nonvegetarians in the same society, are reflected in major differences in cholesterol levels (64–66) and repeated measurements of diets and serum cholesterol levels in Antarctica did lead to a correlation (67). There is no evidence that the effect on cholesterol level of diet change wears off with time (50), so that failure of habitual diet within a group to be reflected in cholesterol levels remains a conundrum. Between groups, the effect of diet is so marked that there is very little overlap of cholesterol levels between the Japanese and the East Finns in the Seven Countries Study, the mean levels being so far apart (68).

Although the lipid under observation has usually been the serum cholesterol, recent interest in different components of the circulating cholesterol and in the triglycerides as predictors of coronary heart disease has caused interest in their dietary control. The high density lipoprotein α-cholesterol appears to vary less between populations and to be less affected by diet than the β-cholesterol (57, 69). Triglycerides in the serum are elevated for several months when carbohydrates are used to replace fats in the diet, but they are low in populations that consume high carbohydrate diets all the time (50). However, as discussed below, their relevance to atherosclerosis may not be very great.

Serum Lipids and Atherosclerosis

The relationship of atherosclerosis to raised serum cholesterol levels was found first by clinical observation, then by formal comparison of diseased cases with controls, and finally by large scale measurement and follow-up of initially healthy populations, relating cholesterol levels at the start to subsequent risk of atherosclerosis; the best known example of this has been the Framingham study (70).

In all large scale prospective studies the risk of development of coronary heart disease has been convincingly related to serum (or plasma) cholesterol (19, 71, 72). Risk is also influenced by many other factors, both known and unknown; hence the predictive value of the cholesterol level for a particular individual is not very high. The cholesterol level has the advantage of having a slow time course for change, so that it is unaffected by recent meals and can be measured without fasting. In the last 10 years serum triglycerides have also been implicated by some workers as independently predictive (73), although others regard their independent contribution to risk assessment as insignificant or possibly only relevant at very high levels (74, 75). More recently an older observation that high density lipoprotein cholesterol or α-cholesterol is inversely correlated with risk has been revived and vigorously explored (76–80). Although comprising only about 20% of the total circulating cholesterol, the high density lipoprotein cholesterol has been found to have three times the predictive value of the remainder. This component shows no correlation with the total cholesterol, which explains why total cholesterol level can correlate with coronary risk, whereas a subcomponent is inversely correlated with it.

The older observations on serum cholesterol levels as a risk factor were often confused by the poor quality of standardization of cholesterol estimation, now greatly improved (81). Although high density lipoprotein cholesterol appears to be important in relation to coronary risk, it will not be possible, until its measurement has been equally well standardized and observations have been made of its variation within and between groups and the effects of dietary and other manipulations on it, to know whether it or the rest of the circulating cholesterol are more under environmental control.

The fact that it has several subcomponents may make both standardization of measurement and reporting difficult to achieve.

Returning to our original three statements on the dietary fat theory, these can be restated as follows:

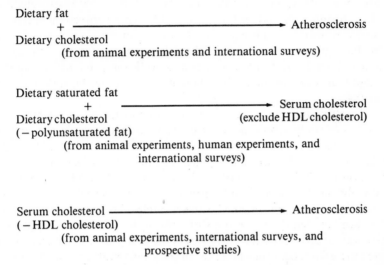

Dietary fat
+ ————————————————→ Atherosclerosis
Dietary cholesterol
(from animal experiments and international surveys)

Dietary saturated fat
+ ———————————→ Serum cholesterol
Dietary cholesterol   (exclude HDL cholesterol)
(−polyunsaturated fat)
(from animal experiments, human experiments, and
international surveys)

Serum cholesterol ———————————→ Atherosclerosis
(−HDL cholesterol)
(from animal experiments, international surveys, and
prospective studies)

These statements have given rise to a number of dietary trials and these are considered next.

Dietary Trials

If the effect of diet on atherosclerosis is mediated by elevated serum cholesterol levels, then cholesterol-lowering diets should lead to a lessened incidence of atherosclerosis. Trials of this prediction have been carried out either to prevent recurrences of coronary heart attacks in survivors (so-called secondary prevention) or to prevent them from occurring at all in healthy persons (primary prevention) (82). The secondary prevention trials have been easier to carry out because the number of subjects needed to generate a given number of events is smaller and the subjects are already under medical supervision.

Secondary Prevention Trials A number of such trials have been mounted, of which three large randomized controlled trials are described. Other trials have been done but have often been too small or used controls chosen in an unsatisfactory manner.

In three hospitals in London 264 male survivors of recent first episodes of myocardial infarction, less than 65 years of age, were randomly allocated either to a low fat diet (calculated at 40 g daily intake of fat) without any addition to polyunsaturated fat intake or to a usual diet (i.e., normal or occasionally weight reducing). The diets produced a sustained difference of 7–10% in mean cholesterol levels between the two groups over 4 years, during which time the recurrence rate for coronary heart attacks in the two groups was identical (83).

In a later study in the same hospitals of 393 men, those randomized to a treatment diet were given a diet containing 35 g of fat daily plus at least 43 g of soya bean oil (or, if poorly tolerated, corn oil). As might be expected from the Keys formula, the induced cholesterol difference between the special and normal diet groups in this experiment was considerably greater — initially 22%, but subsiding somewhat as the follow-up progressed, although remaining above 12%. Again there was no significant difference in relapse or mortality rates over the period of follow-up, which ranged from 2 to nearly 7 years (84).

These findings and those from two smaller British studies contrast with a number of studies showing positive results, of which the largest and best designed was done in Oslo, a place where cholesterol levels tend to be particularly high (85). In this study 412 men who had suffered a first myocardial infarction 1 or 2 years previously and who were aged 30–64 years were randomly allocated to special and normal diets. The special diet was low in animal fat but was supplemented with vegetable oil so that there was a mean difference between the two groups of 14% in the serum cholesterol levels. There was no difference in recurrences in the first year, but a difference appeared thereafter, being most marked in those below 60 years of age, with initially high cholesterol levels and no residual signs and symptoms from the first attack. The number of sudden deaths was the same in both groups (27) but there were 10 reinfarction deaths and 24 persons with nonfatal recurrences in the special diet group versus 23 reinfarction deaths and 31 persons with nonfatal recurrences in the normal diet group, giving a difference in cardiovascular mortality at 5 years of 7%.

These results suggest that, if cholesterol-lowering diets have an effect after infarction, it is on those who are younger, have a high cholesterol level, and have survived 1 or 2 years after the infarct without severe damage to the heart. Even then the effects of a diet change appear to be delayed.

Primary Prevention Trials   Fewer controlled primary prevention trials of diet have been attempted because of the numbers needed and the difficulty of securing compliance to diet change in healthy, free-living individuals. The first generation of trials was done in inmates of institutions.

In the Los Angeles Veterans Administration study (86) 846 middle-aged and elderly men (60% of them 60–69 years old) were randomly assigned to two diets, each with similar proportions of total fat, but the treatment diet contained about half as much dietary cholesterol, far less saturated fat, and four times the amount of polyunsaturated fatty acids as the control diet. A mean serum cholesterol difference of about 13% was achieved. Follow-up continued for up to 8 years, but few participants were in the trial for that long. Some results are given in Table 6. Most cardiovascular endpoint events, including death, were less common in the treatment group. However,

Table 6.   Los Angeles Veterans Administration Study: deaths[a]

Cause of death	Special diet	Normal diet
Acute atherosclerotic	39	60
Other atherosclerotic and mixed	18	21
Other causes	85	71
Uncertain	32	25
All causes	174	177

[a]From Dayton et al. (86).

the potential effect on mortality was largely canceled out by deaths from other causes, so that the total number of deaths in the two groups were virtually the same.

The second major institutional study was done in mental hospitals in Finland (87), a high coronary mortality country. In this study the two hospitals rather than the individual inmates were allocated to different dietary regimes for 6 years, from 1959 to 1965, when a cross-over took place, and they exchanged dietary regimes until 1971. Again the fats in the normal or control diet were replaced with polyunsaturated fatty acid–containing substitutes — soybean oil, reinforced skimmed milk, soft margarine, etc. A mean serum cholesterol difference of 12–18% was achieved and a difference in the fatty acid constituents of the adipose tissue in subjects from the two hospitals was found by using needle biopsy. The results (Table 7) show an apparent effect on male cardiovascular mortality that comes through in the all-causes mortality. In the women there was less effect on cardiovascular mortality and all-causes mortality was higher in the treatment group.

The design, conclusions, and interpretation of these trials have been the subject of criticism, as has the Anti-Coronary Club of New York, in which participants were poorly matched with controls, but positive results from the "prudent diet" were reported (88). In the mental hospitals, differences in age and admission and discharge policies plus knowledge of the allocation unit involved could have influenced results, for example (89). In the Los Angeles study the men were rather old and, although much of the management was done "blind," numbers were too small for many of the results to

Table 7.   Finnish Mental Hospital Study[a]

Mortality rates (per 1000 person years)	Special diet	Normal diet
Men (median age c. 50 yrs)		
Coronary heart disease	6.6	14.1
All causes	34.8	39.5
Women (median age c. 55 yrs)		
Coronary heart disease	5.2	7.9
All causes	30.9	29.0

[a]From Miettinen et al. (87).

reach statistical significance. The excess of noncardiovascular deaths in this trial in the treatment group raised the possibility that the treatment regime could even be harmful. However, pooling of results from several trials failed to provide evidence that polyunsaturated fatty acids caused cancer, as was feared (90).

During the 1960s a second generation of dietary trials was planned to overcome some of the weaknesses of earlier trials; in particular the possibility of double-blind mass field trials among free-living men was considered. Feasibility tests showed that it was possible to provide contrasting diets that resulted in differences in mean cholesterol levels of between 10% and 18%. However, the cost of providing these diets so that neither the subject nor the medical assessor knew the allocation was considerable. Participants in the trial were found to have become generally health conscious and a lot of them gave up smoking. Only a minority of those invited actually participated in the trial, and the incidence rate of coronary heart disease in the controls, who were on a normal diet, was only half that which was expected. It was estimated that a trial with considerably more than 100,000 participants would be needed to demonstrate a 20% reduction in incidence over 4–5 years and the idea was eventually abandoned (91). It seems unlikely that it will ever be revived.

Recent Developments in Trials of Coronary Heart Disease Prevention   Recent interest has swung away from testing the dietary fat theory in isolation, especially in view of the formidable problems just described, and toward simply proving that coronary heart disease is preventable. The interaction of smoking, hypertension, and perhaps lack of exercise with cholesterol level in prediction of coronary heart disease suggests that a combined assault on all these factors — multiple risk factor intervention — stands the best chance of success. The potential benefit from a small reduction in cholesterol levels alone may not be much (92). A reduction to the mean level in Japan does not appear feasible. There has in any case been a move away from the more drastic diets that involve the addition or substitution of large quantities of polyunsaturated fatty acids, although these lead to a large fall in mean serum cholesterol levels. Despite the prophets of doom (93, 94), there is little evidence that polyunsaturated fatty acids are harmful, but there are no known large healthy human populations that subsist on large quantities of them naturally. Adoption of such a diet would be sailing into unknown seas with unknown hazards; it is better to adopt a diet that is known to be compatible with good health and longevity, such as that of the Greek islands in the Seven Countries Study (19). In the multifactorial trials that are in progress, it is usual to suggest a reduction in total fat consumption and moderation in cholesterol-containing foodstuffs, with replacement of lost food energy by cereals and vegetables and vegetable oils being used only when the need for fat is inescapable — for spreads and cooking, for example. The mean serum cholesterol differences from controls in trials such as these in free-living populations tend to be lower than in the old unifactorial trials, nearer 5% (95–97). Since several risk factors are being changed at the same time, the contribution of the diet change to any observed effect on incidence will be difficult to assess, so that these will be trials involving diet rather than dietary trials.

OTHER NUTRITIONAL FACTORS

A number of other dietary constituents have been blamed for atherosclerosis and these factors are now considered. It will be appreciated that there is such a high degree of correlation both positive and negative between different dietary constituents that some hypotheses are in parallel with or mirror images of others.

Variants of the Dietary Fat Theory

A number of factors that correlate with high consumption of saturated fats have been blamed in their place. Hydrogenation of vegetable and marine oils in the manufacture of margarines and shortenings gives rise to some abnormally long chain saturated fatty acids and also to conversion of some unsaturated fatty acids to the abnormal transisomer (e.g., oleic to elaidic acid; see Table 5), which has different properties and is broken down more slowly. Thomas (98) has correlated consumption of these artificially hydrogenated fats in the United Kingdom with regional variation in coronary heart disease mortality, sex differences, social class differences, and time trends. Experiments in man have shown some cholesterol-raising effect of elaidic acid (although oleic acid has a neutral effect) (28). However, some isomerization of cis to trans acids also occurs in the ruminant stomach, so that man has been exposed to trans acids in the past in cow's milk, although not in such large amounts.

Manufactured fats also contain supplements of vitamin D and high consumption of fats correlates with high consumption of fat-soluble vitamins. One case control study in Norway has shown that myocardial infarction victims had eaten significantly more vitamin D than controls and there is evidence from animal studies that excess of vitamin D causes vascular damage and therefore may predispose to atherosclerosis (99, 100). Since childhood rickets is still seen among children of Asian immigrants in Britain, the decision on whether or not to supplement foods with vitamin D has arguments now on both sides.

The suggestion that atherosclerosis might be caused by deficiency of essential polyunsaturated fatty acids, first made by Sinclair (38), has been restated by Crawford (101). From studies of wild and domesticated bovids, he has suggested that the domestication of animals for meat and milk usually leads to gross infiltration of the carcass with "rubbish" saturated fats and a decline in the content of essential polyunsaturated fatty acids, which may therefore be deficient in cow's milk fed to human babies at a stage when their arteries are growing. These interesting observations have not so far been supplemented by good evidence that the levels of polyunsaturated fatty acids in babies fed cow's milk are pathologically low, although the future coronary heart disease rates of Dutch children who are fed on a maize oil–based formula will be of interest (29).

Finally, the suggestion has arisen that atherosclerosis has a basis in immune reactions. People in countries with high consumption of saturated fat tend to rely heavily on dairy foods and drink cow's milk even in infancy. The latter has been held responsible for allergic diseases such as eczema in children, and it has been claimed that production of antibodies to cow's milk in adults might lead to damage to blood vessels from immune complexes and to atherosclerosis. Early demonstrations of antibodies to cow's milk in myocardial infarction (102, 103) and theoretical arguments for an immune basis (104) have not been substantiated. Later studies that employ more sophisticated techniques have proved negative (105, 106).

Obesity and Calories

Obesity has long been popularly associated with risk of coronary heart disease, and some data from Framingham show a good correlation (70. 107). However, the correlation is far stronger for the development of angina pectoris of effort than for major coronary episodes or death. In British civil servants, extreme overweight appears to matter but lesser degrees do not (72). Keys has suggested that obesity has no independent predictive effect once the major coronary risk factors (blood pressure, cholesterol, and smoking) have been taken into account, and his observations have been repeated elsewhere (108–110). This might suggest that obesity is unimportant as a risk factor, but this conclusion is disputed by a report from Framingham (111) that suggests that subjects who lose weight show large and presumably beneficial falls in blood lipids and blood pressure. It is not clear, however, whether these effects occur only during negative energy balance or continue when weight is stabilized, since they are far more marked than the gradient of risk factors with weight observed in a group. During a period of weight loss cholesterol may fall, and blood pressure may fall as a result of reduced salt intake. Obesity correlates quite well with serum triglyceride levels, but the need to reduce these is controversial.

In the past it has also been assumed that coronary risk correlates with food energy intake, so that big eaters were at high coronary risk. International statistics suggest a correlation between coronary heart disease mortality and mean calorie (or MJ) intake (see Table 3). Within groups, however, the reverse may be true. Most subjects are neither gaining nor losing weight to any extent, so that over a period of time they are in energy balance. Food energy must then equal energy expenditure and those who are physically active need to consume more food. If physical activity is to any extent protective (112) then high energy consumption should correlate with diminished risk, as has recently been found by Morris and his colleagues (25). Physical activity also correlates with a lean body build so that energy consumption per kg of body weight is inversely related to measures of obesity such as skinfold thickness (19). The popular confusion is between the steady state energy equilibrium of those who are overweight and the means by which they became obese originally, when consumption must have exceeded expenditure. Overeating and weight gain may be harmful, but big eaters who stay lean appear to be at reduced risk. This may explain an observation from Czechoslovakia 10 years ago that those who had five meals a day seemed less prone to coronary heart disease than those who had only three (113); food energy consumption was not estimated, but it is possible that the big eaters eat more often.

Sucrose, Diabetes Mellitus, and Dietary Fiber

Linked in the popular mind to the hypothesis that overeating causes coronary heart disease is the suggestion made by Yudkin 20 years ago and vigorously prosecuted by him ever since that it is caused by eating sucrose (i.e., a sweet tooth) (12, 114–117). He claimed (12, 114) that international mortality trends for coronary heart disease correlated better with sucrose consumption over the previous decades than with fat. There is a high degree of correlation between fat and sugar consumption in the wealthy statistics-producing countries, so that they cannot easily be discriminated (4, 5, 13). However, there are indications that in some sugar cane–producing countries, such as those of South America, the Caribbean, and Mauritius, sugar is eaten with little fat, and coronary heart disease mortality rates are said to be low. If these countries are included in analyses, as some of them were in the International Atherosclerosis Project (17), there is a poorer correlation for sugar than for fat. Recent time trends in sugar consumption in different countries do not fit the mortality trends well either (although there are problems for the dietary fat theory here as well).

In the Seven Countries Study (20) the correlation coefficient between coronary heart disease incidence and dietary constituents in different groups was 0.86 for saturated fatty acids and 0.78 for sucrose with Japan included, and 0.84 and 0.75, respectively, with Japan excluded. Sucrose and saturated fatty acid consumption were highly correlated with each other ($r = 0.88$), so that the study failed to dissociate them, although statistical analysis was said to show that sucrose made no contribution to risk independent of its association with saturated fatty acids.

Yudkin has also published the results of case control studies alleging that patients with atherosclerosis habitually consume more sucrose than controls (115). Unlike other dietary constituents, sucrose consumption is fairly consistent from day to day and shows large differences between individuals, which can be estimated from questionnaires. High consumption of sucrose usually implies eating sweets, drinking soft drinks, or, particularly, drinking lots of tea or coffee with sugar added.

There have been a number of attempts to repeat Yudkin's work because his choice of controls was unsatisfactory and the reported levels of consumption rather surprising. The results are negative, either because coronary heart disease patients consume no more sucrose than controls, or because the difference is trivial and statistically insignificant, or because there is a difference that is explained away by an association between sucrose consumption and cigarette smoking, a known coronary risk factor, so that there is no excess of sucrose in cases when this has been corrected for (118–122). In a long-term prospective study in Chicago in which a dietary questionnaire was completed at the start (reducing possibilities of biased ascertainment) sucrose consumption was not significantly elevated in those who subsequently developed coronary heart disease as compared with those who did not (123).

The sugar story is not really supported by dietary experiments, either (20, 124). In animals dietary sucrose does produce atheromatous lesions when given in large quantities, but not in the absence of dietary fat and cholesterol, whereas the latter does it alone. In man sucrose feeding may lead to an acute, although temporary, rise in triglycerides, but there is a negligible effect on serum cholesterol. Trials on prevention of coronary heart disease by avoidance of sucrose have not been attempted. Yudkin produces a number of arguments from intermediary metabolism to explain why sucrose might cause arterial disease (insulin and lipid levels, etc.) but little convincing evidence that it does (117).

Although eating sugar may not predispose to atherosclerosis, diabetes mellitus as seen in Western countries undoubtedly does (70). Different studies have shown different independent contributions of glucose intolerance to risk when other risk factors have been taken into account. In a study of British civil servants the risk appears not to rise until the 98th percentile is reached (72). However, there is a correlation between diabetes, obesity, hypertriglyceridemia, and, in treated diabetics, even hypertension (125). That diabetes mellitus may not be a sufficient cause for atherosclerosis is suggested by Japanese diabetics, in whom it is rare. Not only might diabetics have a tendency to accelerated atherogenesis on Western diets, but the traditional low carbohydrate/high saturated fat diet used in its treatment may exaggerate this tendency.

The obverse of the sucrose story is the dietary fiber hypothesis. If many of the diseases of civilization are caused by consumption of refined carbohydrate (126), what has been extracted by refining is the fiber. The evidence that fiber is beneficial is that primitive communities subsisting largely on cereals appear to be free of many Western diseases and that these diseases became prominent in the West sometime after a change in the milling of wheat for bread (127, 128). However, it is not clear how any effect in preventing coronary heart disease might be mediated. Although it is claimed that dietary fiber reduces cholesterol levels, this has not been demonstrated even with considerable quantities of bran (129, 130); however, an effect has been observed with pectin and guar gum given in larger doses than would be consumed in primitive diets (131). It has been suggested that fiber may be related to silicon intake (132). There is a considerable degree of ignorance about the functions of dietary fiber (133, 134) that has not been aided by difficulties in definition. Originally defined as remnants of the plant cell wall (which excluded storage polysaccharides such as guar gum), dietary fiber has now been redefined as "plant polysaccharides and lignin which are resistant to hydrolysis by the digestive enzymes of man" (135).

With the difficulties of definition of dietary fiber have come inevitable problems of measurement and standardization for food tables, into which it is only just being introduced. However, the fiber hypothesis has received some support from a retrospective analysis for fiber in some of Morris's early dietary studies and correlation of these with coronary heart disease mortality (25). Men consuming more cereal fiber than their peers ran a lower risk of subsequent coronary heart disease. This effect appeared to be independent of other possible associations such as total food energy, fat intake, or serum cholesterol level.

Coffee and Alcohol and Vitamin C

The suggestion that coffee drinking was associated with coronary heart disease was first reported from the Boston Collaborative Drug Surveillance Program (136, 137) and Chicago (138), where it did not appear to be explained away by known risk factors such as cigarette smoking. However, other studies have failed to confirm these findings either because the association was not found or because it was explained away by the effect of cigarette smoking (110, 139–142).

Alcohol has created even greater interest because of its effects on intermediary metabolism. It raises serum triglycerides markedly (143, 144), but it is also associated with raised high density lipoprotein cholesterol (142) so that those interested in the former claim that it must increase coronary risk, and those concerned with the latter claim that it should be beneficial. The epidemiological evidence is in conflict. In Gothenburg, Sweden, there is an excess of coronary victims who have previously been registered with the Temperance Board for drink-related offences (75, 110). In New York in the Kaiser-Permanente study there was an excess of teetotalers among those with attacks (145) and the Japanese in Hawaii also seemed to be protected by beer (142). In Chicago, alcohol appears to be a risk factor, but not in Framingham (142) or in London busmen, suggesting either than alcohol has no effect or that different sorts of alcohol have different effects according to the quality or the quantity of what is consumed.

Ascorbic acid (vitamin C) has been found to lower serum cholesterol levels. There is no suggestion, however, that coronary-prone communities are deficient in their diet in this respect.

Minerals

In a number of countries an inverse correlation has been observed between the hardness of water supplies and coronary heart disease mortality rates, and in some cases mortality from other diseases as well (146, 147). The reports are not all consistent (148) and it is not clear whether the effects are mediated mainly by water calcium (which correlates best in Britain) or through some other mineral or trace element that is positively or negatively associated with it in water supplies, soil, and vegetables. It is difficult to think of water as a critical source of dietary calcium. In some British towns a change of water hardness was associated with a relative change of coronary heart disease mortality in the expected direction, some evidence that the association might be causal (149). However, a field study in Britain suggested that some of the mortality differences in towns with hard and soft water were mediated by traditional risk factors (150). These field studies are being repeated. The water story remains as a puzzling series of correlations without, at present, a plausible hypothesis as to the mechanism by which this could come about.

CONCLUSION

The evidence from coronary heart disease epidemiology is that the disease is culturally rather than genetically determined. The Seven Countries Study (19) and others suggest that diet shows greater differences between high and low incidence cultures than other known or postulated coronary risk factors. This chapter has covered a number of dietary hypotheses and demonstrated how many of the dietary factors are closely correlated, positively or negatively. Of all the conflicting hypotheses, that for dietary fat stands out as being supported not only from experiments in the animal laboratory but from demonstrable effects in intermediary metabolism, i.e., the serum cholesterol level, which is 1.5 times higher on average in eastern Finland than in rural Japan (19).

The dietary fat theory explains a large number of observations, but not all of them, and some of the loose ends have recently been given considerable publicity (151, 152). It is not well known, for example, that individual cholesterol levels are poor predictors in some communities of all-causes mortality (Table 8). In prospective studies subjects with below average cholesterol levels have been found to die more frequently from colon cancer, canceling out some of their advantage with respect to coronary disease (153). However, colon cancer is also associated with a high fat diet (see Table 4) in international studies, so that this is perhaps less an argument against reduction in

Table 8.   Serum cholesterol in the prediction of coronary heart disease, fatal cardio-vascular events, and death from all causes[a]

Age (yrs)	Serum cholesterol level		Men (rates/1000/yr)			Women (rates/1000/yr)		
	(mg/100 ml)	(mmol/l) (approx)	CHD[b]	CVD[c]	Death[d]	CHD	CVD	Death
45–54	96–204	2.7–5.6	5.5	3.7	10.1	1.5	0.3	4.7
	205–234	5.7–6.5	8.8	3.4	6.1	2.0	0.9	3.8
	235–264	6.6–7.4	8.9	4.5	8.2	2.8	1.7	5.7
	265–1,124	7.5–31.5	16.1	6.6	11.0	3.6	2.1	4.6
55–64	96–204	2.7–5.6	12.5	10.0	20.4	9.6	3.7	8.1
	205–234	5.7–6.5	21.7	12.9	18.6	6.5	3.7	8.5
	235–264	6.6–7.4	19.3	11.9	15.1	6.1	3.8	8.8
	265–1,124	7.5–31.5	26.9	11.8	18.1	13.2	4.6	7.9
65–74	96–204	2.7–5.6	16.5	26.4	47.8	5.6	26.7	42.2
	205–234	5.7–6.5	27.2	16.5	28.4	11.4	12.0	22.5
	235–264	6.6–7.4	13.8	15.0	31.2	10.5	7.2	12.3
	265–1,124	7.5–31.5	20.3	17.2	28.7	19.1	12.4	17.2

[a]Based on Framingham data (63).

[b]CHD, new coronary heart disease in those previously unaffected.

[c]CVD, death from any disease of the heart or blood vessels.

[d]Death, death from any cause.

fat intake than against concentrating this advice on those with high cholesterol levels. Results have recently been reported from a large trial of the cholesterol-lowering drug clofibrate in the primary prevention of coronary heart disease (155). The incidence of myocardial infarction was substantially reduced and the degree of reduction in risk correlated with the fall in cholesterol level. Unfortunately the drug proved to have serious side effects, which made its further use unacceptable. Nevertheless, this result gives strong support to the causal association of myocardial infarction with blood lipids.

Certain aspects of the dietary fat theory are theoretically unsatisfactory and suggest the need for further investigation. In practice, atherosclerosis is now a major disease and good reasons must be found for postponing action. Is present research likely to produce an answer for which it will have been worth waiting? Multifactorial trials now in progress are unlikely to produce good evidence for or against the dietary fat theory. If the results are positive, then diet change will be mixed up with control of other risk factors. If the outcome is negative, it may be because risk factors have been insufficiently changed or because the changes produced are too late in the natural history of the disease (i.e., in middle-aged men) to influence outcome. Trials of cholesterol-lowering drugs have been rather disappointing in secondary prevention (154, 155). This may be because cholesterol has been lowered too late or because coronary risk is mediated through other routes as well, as is suggested by dietary correlations with thrombogenesis and fibrinolysis (156, 157).

Table 9.   Average daily diet in Great Britain in 1976[a]

Energy source	Grams	Percent of total energy[b]
Protein	72.0	12.7
Animal protein	46.0	
Fat	105	41.7
Fatty acids		
Saturated	50.1	
Monounsaturated	39.7	
Polyunsaturated	10.5	
Carbohydrate	277	45.7
All Sources	100.0	

[a]Adapted from Ministry of Agriculture, Fisheries, and Food (160).
[b]Total is 2.280 kcals or 9.6 MJ.

What, then, should be done now? There is no shortage of advice from national bodies, recently reviewed by Shaper and Marr (158). Although these bodies disagreed in detail, their major recommendation was unanimous: there should be a reduction in food energy obtained from saturated fat. Although this can be done by interfering with the hydrogenation of fats in the ruminant stomach (159), this is less effective than substitution of cereals and vegetables for fat and, where fats have to be used, use of polyunsaturated oils. Tables 9 and 10 (160) show the breakdown of the present British diet, a culmination of 20 years of increase in fat consumption. There is little

Table 10.   Sources of saturated fatty acids in average diet in Great Britain in 1976[a]

Foodstuff	Percent of total saturated fat
Milk	18.5
Cheese	5.9
Dried milk and cream	1.7
Butter	21.2
Margarine	7.2
Other fats	7.7
Meat and meat products	24.0
Fish	0.6
Eggs	2.3
Vegetables	0.7
Fruit	0.4
Cereals	8.7
Other foods	1.1
Total	100.0

[a]Adapted from Ministry of Agriculture, Fisheries, and Food (160).

evidence that a decline from this peak would be harmful and some evidence that it would be beneficial (161).

REFERENCES

1. Morris, J. N., and Crawford, M. D. (1961). Lancet 1:47.
2. Ou, W. (1973). Br. Med. J. 4:1198.
3. Strong, J. P. (1972). Atherosclerosis 16:193.
4. Masironi, R. (1970). Bull. W. H. O. 42:103.
5. Knox, E. G. (1977). Br. J. Prev. Soc. Med. 31:71.
6. Stamler, J. (1967). Lectures on Preventive Cardiology, p. 60. Grune and Stratton, New York.
7. Keys, A. (1967). J. Am. Diet. Assoc. 51:508.
8. Malmros, H. (1969). Lancet 2:479.
9. Gresham, G. A. (1976). Triangle 15:39.
10. Armstrong, M. L. (1976). Postgrad. Med. J. 52:456.
11. Segall, J. J. (1977). Br. J. Prev. Soc. Med. 31:81.
12. Yudkin, J. (1964). Lancet 2:4.
13. Armstrong, B. K., Mann, J. I., Adelstein, A. M., and Eskin, F. (1975). J. Chronic Dis. 28:455.
14. Hollingsworth, D. (1974). Nutr. Rev. 32:353.
15. Clayton, D. G., Taylor, D., and Shaper, A. G. (1977). Health Trends 9:1.
16. Marr, J. W. (1973). Health Trends 5:37.
17. Scrimshaw, N. S., and Guzman, M. A. (1968). Lab. Invest. 18:623.
18. Keys, A., Aravanis, C., Blackburn, H. W., van Buchem, F. S. P., Buzina, R., Djordjevic, B. S., Dontas, A. S., Fidanza, F., Karvonen, M. J., Kimura, N., Lekos, D., Monti, M., Puddu, V., and Taylor, H. L. (1966). Acta Med. Scand. 179(suppl.):460.
19. Keys, A. (ed.). (1970). Circulation 41 (suppl. I):1.
20. Keys, A. (1971). Atherosclerosis 14:193.
21. Malhotra, S. L. (1967). Br. Heart J. 29:337.
22. Malhotra, S. L. (1967). Br. Heart J. 29:895.
23. Malhotra, S. L. (1971). Am. J. Clin. Nutr. 24:1195.
24. Mann, G. V., and Spoerry, A. (1974). Am. J. Clin. Nutr. 27:464.
25. Morris, J. N., Marr, J. W., and Clayton, D. G. (1977). Br. Med. J. 2:1307.
26. Groen, J., Tjiong, B. K., Kamminga, C. E., and Willebrands, A. F. (1952). Voeding 13:556.
27. Feldman, E. B. (1976). Nutrition and Cardiovascular Disease. Appleton-Century-Crofts, New York.
28. Vergroesen, A. J., and Gottenbos, J. J. (1975). In A. J. Vergroesen (ed.), The Role of Fats in Human Nutrition, pp. 1–41. Academic Press, Inc., New York.
29. Widdowson, E. M., Dauncey, M. J., Gairdner, D. M. T., Jonxis, J. H. P., and Pelikan-Filipkova, M. (1975). Br. Med. J. 1:653.
30. Garton, G. A. (1977). In T. W. Goodwin (ed.), MTP International Review of Biochemistry, Vol. 14, Biochemistry of Lipids II, p. 337. University Park Press, Baltimore.
31. Green, C. (1977). In T. W. Goodwin (ed.), MTP International Review of Biochemistry, Vol. 14, Biochemistry of Lipids II, p. 101. University Park Press, Baltimore.
32. Bronte-Stewart, B., Antonis, A., Eales, L., and Brock, J. F. (1956). Lancet 1:521.

33. Ahrens, E. H., Jr., Insull, W., Jr., Blomstrand, R., Hirsch, J., Tsaltas, T. T., and Peterson, M. L. (1957). Lancet 1:943.
34. Keys, A., Anderson, J. T., and Grande, F. (1965). Metabolism 14:747.
35. Keys, A., Anderson, J. T., and Grande, F. (1965). Metabolism 14:759.
36. Keys, A., Anderson, J. T., and Grande, F. (1965). Metabolism 14:766.
37. Kinsell, L. W., Friskey, R. W., Michaels, G. D., and Splitter, S. (1958). Lancet 1:334.
38. Sinclair, H. M. (1956). Lancet 1:381.
39. K. Diem and C. Lentner (eds.). (1970). Documenta Geigy, Scientific Tables, Ed. 7. Geigy, Basle.
40. Keys, A., Anderson, J. T., and Grande, F. (1965). Metabolism 14:776.
41. Grande, F., Anderson, J. T., and Keys, A. (1970). Am. J. Clin. Nutr. 23:1184.
42. Grande, F., Anderson, J. T., and Keys, A. (1972). Am. J. Clin. Nutr. 25:53.
43. Wells, V. M., and Bronte-Stewart, B. (1963). Br. Med. J. 1:577.
44. Rhomberg, H. P., and Braunsteiner, H. (1976). Br. Med. J. 1:1188.
45. Sirtori, C. R., Conti, F., Agradi, E., Mantero, O., and Gatti, E. (1977). Lancet 1:275.
46. Howard, A. N., and Marks, J. (1977). Lancet 2:255.
47. Reiser, R. (1973). Am. J. Clin. Nutr. 26:524.
48. Keys, A., Grande, F., and Anderson, J. T. (1974). Am. J. Clin. Nutr. 27:188.
49. Blackburn, H. (1974). In P. N. Yu and J. F. Goodwin (eds.), Progress in Cardiology, Vol. 3, p. 1. Lea and Febiger, Philadelphia.
50. Grande, F. (1975). Proceedings of the 9th International Congress of Nutrition, Mexico, 1972, Vol. 1, p. 346. Karger, Basel.
51. Shaper, A. G., and Jones, K. W. (1959). Lancet 2:534.
52. Truswell, A. S., and Mann, J. I. (1972). Atherosclerosis 16:15.
53. Morris, J. N., Marr, J. W., Heady, J. A., and Mills, G. L. (1963). Br. Med. J. 1:571.
54. Kahn, H. A., Medalie, J. H., Neufeld, H.N., Riss, E., Balogh, M., and Groen, J. J. (1969). Isr. J. Med. Sci. 5:1117.
55. Kannel, W. B., and Gordon, T. (1970). The Framingham Diet Study: diet and the regulation of serum cholesterol, Section 24. Department of Health Education and Welfare, Washington, D. C.
56. Truswell, A. S. (1976). Postgrad. Med. J. 52:425.
57. Truswell, A. S. (1977). Lancet 2:1173.
58. Gardner, M. J., and Heady, J. A. (1973). J. Chron. Dis. 26:781.
59. Mann, G. V., Pearson, G., Gordon, T., and Dawber, T. R. (1962). Am. J. Clin. Nutr. 11:200.
60. Dawber, T. R., Pearson, G., Anderson, P., Mann, G. V., Kannel, W. B., Shurtleff, D., and McNamara, P. (1962). Am. J. Clin. Nutr. 11:226.
61. Marr, J. W. (1973). Proc. R. Soc. Med. 66:639.
62. Marr, J. W. (1973). Nutrition 27:239.
63. Feinleib, M., Garrison, R. J., Fabsitz, R., Christian, J. C., Hrubec, Z., Borhani, N. O., Kannel, W. B., Rosenman, R., Schwartz, J. T., and Wagner, J. O. (1977). Am. J. Epidemiol. 106:284.
64. Kirkeby, K. (1966). Acta Med. Scand. 179(suppl.):443.
65. Sacks, F. M., Castelli, W. P., Donner, A., and Kass, E. H. (1975). N. Engl. J. Med. 292:1148.
66. Ruys, J., and Hickie, J. B. (1977). Br. Med. J. 2:87.
67. Easty, D. L. (1970). Br. J. Nutr. 24:307.
68. Blackburn, H. (1976). Postgrad. Med. J. 52:417.
69. Castelli, W. P., Cooper, G. R., Doyle, J. T., Garcia-Palmieri, M., Gordon, T., Hames, C., Hulley, S. B., Kagan, A., Kuchmak, M., McGee, D., and Vicic, W. J. (1977). J. Chronic Dis. 30:147.

70. Shurtleff, D. (1974). *In* W. B. Kannel and T. Gordon (eds.), The Framingham Study. 18-Year Follow-up, Section 30. Department of Health, Education, and Welfare, Washington, D. C.
71. Report of the Inter-Society Commission for Heart Disease Resources. (1970). Circulation 42:A39.
72. Reid, D. D., McCartney, P., Jarrett, R. J., Hamilton, P. J. S., Rose, G., and Keen, H. (1976). Lancet 2:979.
73. Carlson, L. A., and Böttiger, L. E. (1972). Lancet 1:865.
74. Kannel, W. B., Castelli, W. P., Gordon, T., and McNamara, P. M. (1971). Ann. Intern. Med. 74:1.
75. Wilhelmsen, L., Wedel, H., and Tibblin, G. (1973). Circulation 48:950.
76. Miller, G. J., and Miller, N. E. (1975). Lancet 1:16.
77. Berg, K., Bǿrresen, A.-L., and Dahlen, G. (1976). Lancet 1:499.
78. Hsia, S. L., Briese, F., and Hoffman, J. (1976). Lancet 1:799.
79. Miller, N. E., Thelle, D. S., Fǿrde, O. H., and Mjǿs, O. D. (1977). Lancet 1:965.
80. Gordon, T., Castelli, W. P., Hjortland, M. C., Kannel, W. B., and Dawber, T. R. (1977). Am. J. Med. 62:707.
81. Rose, G. A., and Blackburn, H. (1968). Cardiovascular Survey Methods, p. 117. World Health Organization, Geneva.
82. Shaper, A. G. (1976). Postgrad. Med. J. 52:464.
83. Research Committee. (1965). Lancet 2:501.
84. Research Committee to the Medical Research Council (1968). Lancet 2:693.
85. Leren, P. (1966). Acta Med. Scand. 179(suppl.)466.
86. Dayton, S., Pearce, M. L., Hashimoto, S., Dixon, W. J., and Tomiyasu, U. (1969). Circulation 40(suppl. II):1.
87. Miettinen, M., Karvonen, M. J., Turpeinen, O., Elusou, R., and Paavilainen, E. (1972). Lancet 2:835.
88. Rinzler, S. H. (1968). Bull. N. Y. Acad. Med. 44:936.
89. Halperin, M., Cornfield, J., and Mitchell, S. C. (1973). Lancet 2:438.
90. Ederer, F., Leren, P., Turpeinen, O., and Frantz, I. D., Jr. (1971). Lancet 2:203.
91. National Diet-Heart Study. (1968). Circulation 37(suppl. 1).
92. Whyte, H. M. (1975). Lancet 1:906.
93. Pinckney, E. R. (1973). Med. Counterpoint Feb., 1973.
94. Pinckney, E. R. (1973). Am. Heart J. 85:723.
95. World Health Organization European Collaborative Group. (1974). Int. J. Epidemiol. 3:219.
96. World Health Organization. (1977). The Prevention of Coronary Heart Disease. Report on a Working Group, Berlin 6-9, April, 1976. World Health Organization Regional Office for Europe, Copenhagen.
97. Farquhar, J. W., Maccoby, N., Wood, P. D., Alexander, J., Breitrose, H., Brown, B. W., Haskell, W. L., McAlister, A. L., Meyer, A. J., Nash, J., and Stern, M. P. (1977). Lancet 1:1192.
98. Thomas, L. H. (1975). Br. J. Prev. Soc. Med. 29:82.
99. Linden, V. (1974). Br. Med. J. 3:647.
100. Seelig, M. S. (1975). Br. Med. J. 3:648.
101. Crawford, M. A. (1968). Lancet 1:1329.
102. Davies, D. F., Davies, J. R., and Richards, M. A. (1969). J. Atherosclerosis Res. 9:103.
103. Davies, D. F., Rees, B. W. G., Johnson, A. P., Elwood, P. C., and Abernethy, M. (1974). Lancet 2:1012.
104. Mathews, J. D., Whittingham, S., and Mackay, I. R. (1974). Lancet 2:1423.
105. Toivanen, A., Viljanen, M. K., and Savilahti, E. (1975). Lancet 2:205.

106. Gaussett, P., Delespesse, G., Bastenie, P. A., Punsar, S., and Karvonen, M. J. (1977). Lancet 1:1006.
107. Kannel, W. B., Le Bauer, E. J., Dawber, J. R., and McNamara, P. M. (1967). Circulation 35:734.
108. Keys, A., Aravanis, C., Blackburn, H., van Buchem, F. S. P., Buzina, R., Djordjevic, B. S., Fidanza, F., Karvonen, M. J., Menotti, A., Puddu, V., and Taylor, H. L. (1972). Ann. Intern. Med. 77:15.
109. Keys, A. (1973). In G. A. Bray (ed.), Obesity in Perspective, Proceedings of a Conference, National Institutes of Health, Bethesda, Maryland, October 1-3, 1973. J. E. Fogarty International Centre for Advanced Study in the Health Sciences, Series on Preventive Medicine, Vol. 2, Part 2. Department of Health, Education, and Welfare, Washington.
110. Tibblin, G., Wilhelmsen, L., and Werko, L. (1975). Am. J. Cardiol. 35:514.
111. Ashley, F. W., and Kannel, W. B. (1974). J. Chron. Dis. 27:103.
112. Morris, J. N., Adam, C., Chave, S. P. W., Sirey, C., Epstein, L., and Sheehan, D. J. (1973). Lancet 1:333.
113. Fabry, P., Fodor, J., Geizerova, H., Hejl, Z., Balcarova, O., and Zvolankova, K. (1968). Lancet 2:190.
114. Yudkin, J. (1957). Lancet 2:155.
115. Yudkin, J., and Roddy, J. (1964). Lancet 2:6.
116. Yudkin, J. (1969). Nutr. News 9:32.
117. Yudkin, J. (1972). Proc. Nutr. Soc. 31:331.
118. Finnegan, A., Hickey, N., Maurer, B., and Mulcahy, R. (1968). Am. J. Clin. Nutr. 21:143.
119. Howell, R. W., and Wilson, D. G. (1969). Br. Med. J. 3:145.
120. Bennett, A. E., Doll, R., and Howell, R. W. (1970). Lancet 1:1011.
121. Elwood, P. C., Waters, W. E., Moore, S., and Sweetman, P. (1970). Lancet 1:1014.
122. Working Party on the Relationship between Dietary Sugar Intake and Arterial Disease. (1970). Lancet 2:1265.
123. Paul, O., MacMillan, A., McKean, H., and Park, H. (1968). Lancet 2:1049.
124. Grande, F. (1975). World Rev. Nutr. Diet. 22:237.
125. Keen, H. (1976). Postgrad. Med. J. 52:413.
126. Cleave, T. L., and Campbell, G. D. (1966). Diabetes, Coronary Thrombosis and the Saccharine Disease. John Wright, Bristol.
127. Trowell, H. (1972). Am. J. Clin. Nutr. 25:926.
128. Trowell, H. C. (1976). Dietary Fibre: Metabolic and Vascular Diseases. Norgine, Ltd., London.
129. Connell, A. M., Smith, C. L., and Somsel, M. (1975). Lancet 1:496.
130. Truswell, A. S., and Kay, R. M. (1975). Lancet 1:922.
131. Jenkins, D. J. A., Newton, C., Leeds, A. R., and Cummings, J. H. (1975). Lancet 1:1116.
132. Schwartz, K. (1977). Lancet 1:454.
133. Eastwood, M. A., Fisher, N., Greenwood, C. T., and Hutchinson, J. B. (1974). Lancet 1:1029.
134. Mendeloff, A. I. (1977). N. Engl. J. Med. 297:811.
135. Trowell, H., Southgate, D. A. T., Wolever, T. M. S., Leeds, A. R., Gassull, M. A., and Jenkins, D. J. A. (1976). Lancet 1:967.
136. Boston Collaborative Drug Surveillance Program. (1972). Lancet 2:1278.
137. Jick, H., Miettinen, O. S., Neff, R. K., Shapiro, S., Heinonen, O. P., and Slone, D. (1973). N. Engl. J. Med. 289:63.
138. Paul, O., Lepper, M. H., Phelan, W. H., Dupertuis, G. W., MacMillan, A., McKean, H., and Parks, H. (1963). Circulation 28:20.

139. Hrubec, Z. (1973). Lancet 1:548.
140. Klatsky, A. L., Friedman, G. D., and Siegelaub, A. B. (1973). JAMA 226:540.
141. Dawber, T. R., Kannel, W. B., and Gordon, T. (1974). N. Engl. J. Med. 291:871.
142. Yano, K., Rhoads, G. G., and Kagan, A. (1977). N. Engl. J. Med. 297:405.
143. Ginsberg, H., Olefsky, J., Farquhar, J. W., and Reaven, G. M. (1974). Ann. Intern. Med. 80:143.
144. Ostrander, L. D., Lamphiear, D. E., Block, W. D., Johnson, B. C., Ravenscroft, C., and Epstein, F. H. (1974). Arch. Intern. Med. 134:451.
145. Klatsky, A. L., Friedman, G. D., and Siegelaub, A. B. (1974). Ann. Intern. Med. 81:294.
146. Masironi, R. (1970). Bull. W. H. O. 43:687.
147. Crawford, M. D. (1972). Proc. Nutr. Soc. 31:347.
148. Bierenbaum, M. L., Dunn, J., Fleischman, A. I., and Arnold, J. (1975). Lancet 1:1008.
149. Crawford, M. D., Gardner, M. J., and Morris, J. N. (1971) . Lancet 2:327.
150. Stitt, F. W., Crawford, M. D., Clayton, D. G., and Morris, J. N. (1973). Lancet 1:122.
151. Oliver, M. F. (1976). Br. Heart J. 38:214.
152. Mann, G. V. (1977). N. Engl. J. Med. 297:644.
153. Rose, G., Blackburn, H., Keys, A., Taylor, H. L., Kannel, W. B., Paul, O., Reid, D. D., and Stamler, J. (1974). Lancet 1:181.
154. Coronary Drug Project Research Group. (1975). JAMA 231:360.
155. Committee of Principal Investigators. (1978). Br. Heart J. 40:1069.
156. Hornstra, G., Lewis, B., Chait, A., Turpeinen, O., Karvonen, M. J., and Vergroesen, A. J. (1973). Lancet 1:1155.
157. O'Brien, J. R., Etherington, M. D., and Jamieson, S. (1976). Lancet 1:878.
158. Shaper, A. G., and Marr, J. W. (1977). Br. Med. J. 1:867.
159. Nestel, P. J., Havenstein, N., Whyte, H. M., Scott, T. J., and Cook, L. J. (1973). N. Engl. J. Med. 288:379.
160. Ministry of Agriculture, Fisheries and Food. (1976). Household Food Consumption and Expenditure: 1976. Annual Report of the National Food Survey Committee. Her Majesty's Stationery Office, London.
161. Joossens, J. V., Vuylsteek, K., Brems-Heyns, E., Carlier, J., Claes, J. H., De Backer, G., Graffar, M., Kesteloot, H., Kornitzer, M., Lequime, J., Pannier, R., Raes, A., Van Houte, O., Vastesaeger, M., and Verdonk, G. (1977). Lancet 1:1069.

International Review of Biochemistry
Biochemistry of Nutrition IA, Volume 27
Edited by A. Neuberger and T. H. Jukes
Copyright 1979   University Park Press   Baltimore

10
Dietary Allowances of Energy and Nutrients

R. G. WHITEHEAD

University of Cambridge and Medical Research Council, Cambridge, England

---

This chapter is not intended as a review of the recommendations contained in various expert committee reports. Rather, it looks at the principal ways of studying requirements and examines the physiological problems that are involved.

Perhaps the major difficulty is defining the critical health parameters for each nutrient against which the adequacy of dietary intakes can be judged. Even when this has been done, interpretation is complicated by factors such as nutrient interaction, physiological variation among individuals, age, social and economic constraints, differing environmental conditions (including climate and pattern of infection), and the ability of individuals to adjust their metabolic efficiency to changed nutritional circumstances.

The first section deals with these basic principles and is followed by more detailed sections on energy and specific nutrients that illustrate the various physiological complexities that have been identified.

GENERAL PRINCIPLES

Planning and Surveillance

An accurate knowledge of nutrient requirements is important for a variety of reasons, but the main practical values of such information are that it enables food and nutrition planners to estimate food requirements, and that it forms a basis around which nutrition surveillance teams can interpret dietary intake data. Although these two functions are closely interrelated, there are more important differences in the way that nutrient requirement data need to be interpreted in order to be used in these ways.

When one is proposing nutrient requirements with planning in mind, one must clearly try to ensure that no one in that community, except the most extreme case, is ever likely to be undernourished or malnourished. The natural tendency is to err on the side of caution by introducing generous safety margins into recommended dietary allowances to cover every possible contingency. For the great majority of people, therefore, the recommended allowances are in excess of physiological needs and hence, for those individuals, wasteful; but since it is frequently impossible to know exactly which person has high needs and which has low ones, there is no option but to base one's calculations on the requirements of the most needful.

If, however, the same allowances are used uncritically to interpret dietary intake data, an unrealistic impression of the nutritional status of a community can emerge. Individuals will frequently be found who are not consuming as much as the recommended allowance, but by no means can one conclude they are necessarily malnourished. They may still be consuming well within their needs. This is an important point, because many investigators have mistakenly assumed that nutrient allowance tables can by themselves be used to *diagnose* the presence of malnutrition. This is not the case; the diagnosis of malnutrition is only possible by direct examination of the individual using the appropriate clinical, anthropometric, or biochemical techniques. Interpretation of dietary intake data on the basis of allowance values only provides a clue to the possible presence of malnutrition; it does not prove its existence.

Even for nutritional planning, tables of nutrient allowances should never be looked on as anything more than a guide. Usually these allowances have been derived from physiological or clinical considerations: they have rarely taken into account factors such as social acceptability, palatability, and economic feasibility. An exception is the 1969 report of the Department of Health and Social Security (DHSS) of Great Britain (1) in which, in its section on protein, the authors pointed out that, although physiologically it may appear unnecessary to have a protein-derived energy content greater than 6–7% for most age groups in Great Britain, a diet formulated around such a value would be quite unacceptable since British people have become accustomed to a diet of which 10–15% consists of protein. Consequently, recommended dietary intakes were based not on physiological data but on the minimum practical dietary protein content of 10%.

This decision was rational from a planning viewpoint, but its introduction has not been without attendant problems for those primarily concerned with surveillance. The National Food Survey Committee of the Ministry of Agriculture, Fisheries and Food (MAFF) initially used the 10% value to interpret their household purchase data, but the improbable conclusion that marginal protein deficiency might exist in some sectors of the UK population caused them to switch to interpretational criteria based on physiological considerations.

Basic Methods for the Estimation of Nutrient Requirements

Customary Intake Method   The original method used to define nutrient requirements involved measuring the nutrient intake of typical healthy people on the assumption that, when there is a free and open choice, intakes will roughly match requirement. This might have some validity with dietary energy intake, but there is little or no reason to believe that it is the case with protein and other nutrients; no specific "hunger" for most individual nutrients has been identified. Nevertheless, it is still occasionally necessary to fall back on this approach with some nutrients, such as trace elements, and it remains the principal means of defining the needs of the young infant on the basis that "breast must be best."

Clinical and Epidemiological Approach   It is easier to characterize improvement in morbidity than deterioration in health, and it is not surprising, therefore, that clinical assays for nutrient requirements have largely been based on the former approach. It has been reasoned that the minimum amount of a nutrient that can cure frank clinical signs of deficiency must surely also be adequate for the maintenance of health. A number of examples of this type of study will be described, but it will be seen that the interpretation is by no means so simple as just indicated.

A similar system that employs an epidemiological approach involves trying to define the minimum intake of a nutrient that is never associated with signs of clinical deficiency within the community being surveyed.

Physiological Evaluation   The main snag with techniques dependent on frank morbidity is that they ignore the possibility of deficiencies that impair overall metabolic efficiency, and hence health, but are not severe enough to give rise to clinical signs. If a metabolic sequence can be identified that is rate-limited by a specific nutrient, theoretically one has the basis for measuring the requirement for that nutrient. In principle, the metabolic process measured should be part of an essential pathway linking deficiency with health and disease. Unfortunately, for many nutrients — especially the vitamins and trace elements — our knowledge of intermediary metabolism in relation to pathogenesis is inadequate for this criterion to be completely satisfied. Nevertheless, data of this type have been used by various expert committees on nutrient requirements.

One of the most widely used physiological approaches to nutrient requirements involves the balance procedure, in which the excretion of a product via feces, urine, sweat, etc., is measured at graded levels of intake. Balance is considered to be the point at which intake equals output. A related approach measures obligatory body losses on zero intake of that nutrient from urine, feces, and skin. The amount of the nutrient required to replace these losses is then calculated, after taking into account factors such as the efficiency of utilization of the nutrient. To the balance or obligatory loss values, which are essentially estimates of maintenance requirements, are added the needs for other functions such as growth, pregnancy, and lactation. Protein requirements have been extensively studied using both these approaches and are dealt with in greater detail below.

Another physiological approach is of primary significance to the vitamins. It has been observed that for many vitamins there appears to be a maximum tissue concentration and levels of intake that would exceed this concentration are promptly excreted. Tissue saturation is usually identified by feeding graded levels of a vitamin until there is a sudden rise in urinary excretion of the vitamin or one of its degradation products. The precise meaning of tissue saturation is not clear, since levels of intake for its achievement invariably need to be far higher than for the prevention of signs of vitamin deficiency, but, until nutritional scientists define with greater certainty optimum intake values for health under all naturally prevailing circumstances, it is likely that tissue saturation will remain one of the major criteria for vitamin requirements.

In discussing the individual nutrients (see below) these different approaches — customary intake, clinical and epidemiological evaluation, and the various physiological assays — can be seen to give widely differing values. Deciding how to balance these conflicting impressions is one of the major tasks of expert committees.

Factors Complicating the Estimation of Nutrient Requirements

Nutrient Interaction   It is not possible to look at each nutrient as though it were in a separate packet. People eat food, not nutrients, and the nature of their food can influence the efficiency with which the constituent nutrients are utilized. Different nutrients interact for reasons that are not always clear, and it is important that nutritional studies be conducted in such a way that they take an adequate account of all the natural complexities involved.

For example, as protein intake increases, the excretion of calcium — and hence the amount required for calcium balance — increases. United States authorities (2) made a recommendation of 800 mg of calcium/day for adults, as opposed to the 500 mg/day recommended by the 1967 FAO/WHO committee (3), after acknowledging the fact that the protein intake of most Americans is considerably higher than their physiological requirement. A lower allowance for calcium would probably be quite adequate for people with more moderate protein intakes. Trace element requirements are probably higher in diets containing a large proportion of cereal because of cation binding to phytic acid and to certain of the unavailable carbohydrate fractions.

Clearly, traditional dietary patterns must be taken into consideration when nutrient allowances are being defined for one's own country. The deliberations of the expert committees of the international agencies provide excellent guidance, but their conclusions should not be copied uncritically; there may well be special circumstances arising from traditional dietary habits that must be accommodated.

Physiological Variation Among Individuals   A major difficulty in defining nutrient requirements is the fact that there is a considerable variation in the needs of individuals. Safe levels or recommended dietary intakes and allowances are usually quoted as only being sufficient to meet the needs of *practically* all healthy persons in a population.

For many nutrients scientists have little factual knowledge about ranges of needs, and they can only produce safety margins that in their judgment should cover almost everyone. Inevitably there is a tendency to err on the side of caution in such circumstances. Ideally, however, safety margins should be defined on a mathematical basis. Conventionally, the upper limit of requirement within a community has been set at the mean + 2 SD. Obviously the shape of the distribution curve must be established and the appropriate mathematical procedures applied, for it is by no means certain that the data will conform to a simple Gaussian pattern. With the exception of protein and possibly calcium, however, there are really insufficient physiological data for this type of analysis to be carried out with any real validity. The data should also be truly representative of the population under consideration, taking age, sex, and genetic factors fully into account. It is perhaps not surprising, considering the low level of financial support given to nutritional science, that so few of these important criteria have been sufficiently satisfied for unequivocal recommendations to be made.

A safety margin added to average requirements assumes that what is an excess nutrient intake for the great majority of people will produce no harmful effects. This procedure cannot be applied to dietary energy, however, and this is why only mean requirements are quoted for this component. This must always be borne in mind when energy intake data are being interpreted. One should find that around 50% of the population are receiving less than the recommended dietary allowance, but it does not mean that they are undernourished, even though this has been concluded on more than one occasion!

There are numerous reasons for these differences in nutrient requirements. Variations in digestive and absorptive capacity represent one important factor. Nutrient interaction, as already mentioned, can modify the availability of nutrients for absorption from the gut.

Once the nutrients have become absorbed, endocrine balance determines to what extent nutrients are used for anabolic processes or are catabolized and the products excreted. Insulin that is secreted following a meal stimulates a transient uptake of amino acids by muscle, making them less available to the liver and thus reducing the risk of a temporary excess being wastefully catabolized and excreted. This metabolic process is related to the protein-sparing effect of carbohydrate. It is well known, however, that the insulin response is not identical in all people and this must lead to differences in ability to conserve amino acids following a meal.

Differences among individuals in the way that they cope with moderately high energy intakes are well established. Some people respond primarily by synthesizing fat, while others are able to dissipate, to a greater or lesser extent, some of this excess energy as heat. Likewise, with low energy intakes some are able to maintain a particular weight while others become excessively thin. The ways by which individuals effect these different responses to the same energy intake are the subject of much research.

Social Habits   Metabolic efficiency, and thus nutrient requirements, can be affected in a number of other ways. The amount of dietary vitamin C required to maintain an adequate plasma or leucocyte ascorbic acid level, for example, is greater in people who smoke than in nonsmokers. A minor cold, a sudden change of environment such as occurs in South African laborers who leave a rural way of life to work in the gold mines, or the use of oral contraceptives all have the same apparent effect on vitamin C requirements. Steroid therapy and oral contraceptives affect apparent nutritional status as measured biochemically with a range of vitamins. Whether or not there is any need to correct for these metabolic abnormalities by recommending an extra intake of vitamin is not clear, but it does illustrate the large number of considerations that must be taken into account when one is interpreting dietary intake measurements.

Abnormal Environmental Conditions   Most tables of recommended dietary allowances are prefaced by a statement to the effect that they are only intended to cover the needs of healthy people. The allowances are sufficient to cover routine minor trauma such as the occasional upper respiratory tract infection, but not more serious or chronic conditions. This is a rational provision, because it is impossible to make general recommendations to cover an infinite number of unspecified conditions.

Things become less clear, however, when one is primarily concerned with recommendations for some developing countries, where infections such as infantile diarrhea and malaria are so prevalent as to be almost part of the normal scene. There is no simple answer to the question of whether or not one should make an allowance for high levels of endemic infection. Earlier WHO/FAO expert committees did so for protein, but this decision was reversed by the 1973 FAO/WHO committee (4). Obviously the real solution is to remove the causes of these infections, but this is easier said than done. There is no doubt, however, that nutrient requirements are quite different when people are frequently affected by infection.

Apart from the anorexic effect that most diseases produce, gut parasites and pathogenic bacteria also result in a reduced proportion of ingested nutrients being available for adsorption. Worm infestations, such as roundworms and tapeworms, affect the nutritional status of the host because the products of digestion are also used to support the growth and well-being of the parasite. Other worms, such as the hookworm, may damage the gut wall and result in the loss of blood constituents, which have to be replenished from the host's diet. Measles also affects the gut wall and results in a leakage of substances such as albumin into the lumen, causing a marked drop in plasma albumin concentrations. Gardia can affect nutrient absorption by "coating" the gut villi and thus reducing the absorptive area. Once nutrients are absorbed, infection may affect the efficiency with which they are used for anabolic purposes. A raised plasma cortisol concentration, which often accompanies infection, particularly when there is pyrexia, can greatly impede the utilization of amino acids for protein synthesis.

The interaction between infection and nutrient requirements is not just confined to the acute phase of illness. Recovery involves replenishment of tissues and, in children, catch-up growth. If these are to be efficiently achieved, raised intakes of some nutrients may be necessary.

These few examples illustrate the complexity of allowing for infection in dietary allowance tables. This does not usually create a practical problem when one is dealing with socially privileged people, but it is something that must be taken into account in many poor countries. It is usually not possible to make any effective blanket allowance in such circumstances, but specific needs of the individual must be borne in mind and extra allowances *prescribed* when this is justified clinically.

Metabolic Adaptation to Altered Nutrient Intakes   The possibility of metabolic adaptation to altered nutrient intakes must be taken into account when one is defining requirements. Physiological studies performed on subjects who have lived in circumstances of dietary excess may be misleading for communities with different dietary patterns. Adaptation to temporary increased requirements is also possible. For example, when an individual's iron status is maximal, only about 10% of the dietary iron ingested is likely to be absorbed. However, if that individual should develop a special need for extra iron, such as during pregnancy, up to 20% may be absorbed from the same diet. Thus it is not necessary to increase iron recommendations by the same amount. As will be described, there is similar evidence for adaptation to customary calcium intakes.

One should be equally wary about relating experiences observed in people living in extreme environmental conditions to those of people who have been born and bred in communities offering more hospitable circumstances. One can envisage a situation in which a wide range of nutritional requirements originally existed but the traditional diet was only capable of satisfying a portion of these needs. Natural selection would have tended to favor the survival of those persons having lower individual requirements, and thus, with time, there might have evolved a much narrower and lower range of requirements in that community. One can speculate that this could have occurred with calcium and perhaps also protein and energy in the developing countries. It would be dangerous to assume that levels of dietary intake that are perfectly compatible with health in a community that has been subject to this type of selection would necessarily be adequate for all the world.

Age　There is much more direct nutritional information available on healthy young men and women of 20–22 years of age (mainly students) than for all other age groups, with the debatable exception of early infancy, where breast milk composition and output data form valuable guides to requirements. For most other age groups allowances are determined either by extrapolation, or on differences in energy intake, body size, or basal metabolic rate (BMR). Clearly, more direct information is desirable, particularly in the elderly, growing children, and adolescents. The balance between requirements for maintenance and growth has an important bearing on overall nutrient needs, but the interrelationships for the different nutrients are complex.

Sex　Differences in allowances for males and females are also made by taking into account their separate energy requirements, body size, basal metabolic rate (BMR), and, to a lesser extent, their pattern of growth. Generally speaking, work and physical activity tend to be greater in males than females and this creates an extra need for dietary energy. Pregnancy and lactation create special needs, but dietary allowances often have to be adjusted for these functions on a rather arbitrary basis (see below). Thiamin is also required for the metabolism of energy metabolites and recommended daily intakes for very active men are considerably greater than for the average woman. For most other nutrients, however, there is no evidence that extra energy expenditure by itself confers special needs, and for these the main consideration is body size and metabolic mass.

Climate　There are less firm data concerning the relationship between requirements and climate. Theoretically, cold conditions should increase energy requirements for the maintenance of body temperature, but in practice extra clothing and warm housing minimize these needs. Likewise, the effects of hot conditions are also lessened by adjustments of the microenvironment, and it is difficult to justify separate allowances for tropical and temperate climates.

Apart from energy, there is little reason to believe that climate will affect requirements for most nutrients. Sweating can increase obligatory losses of nitrogen, but since this represents only a small fraction of the total nitrogen excretion it is unlikely to be of great importance. In practical nutrition the most important consideration connected with a hot climate may be in its differential effect on energy and nutrient intakes. Prolonged exposure to such conditions can reduce overall body activity and this will be mirrored in a lower dietary energy and food consumption. With customary diets of only marginal quality it is possible that an individual's requirements for specific nutrients may not be met at these lower intake levels.

Of all the nutrients, water and salt requirements show the greatest variation with climatic conditions. When individuals are engaged in heavy manual work in hot conditions, water loss through the skin can be very great, and if it is not replaced regularly an acute need can develop very rapidly, as can a concomitant need for salt replacement.

General   These brief remarks indicate some of the complexities that are involved in the definition of nutrient requirements. It is not surprising that with such a range of potential variables few, if any, of the nutrients have been studied in sufficient depth to produce data that can be used without reservation for the determination of recommended allowances. The next sections dealing with specific energy and nutrient requirements, do not aim to criticize, but to point out some of the crucial gaps in our knowledge about a subject of such vital importance to man's health, efficiency, and progress.

ENERGY REQUIREMENTS

It is almost impossible to produce tables of recommended daily allowances for energy that can be applied uncritically. The problem is the considerable variation in requirement that exists among different individuals. At practically any age the customary energy intake spans a range in which maximum values are at least twice minimum values, and this is still true when the data are selected to exclude those individuals with obvious obesity or undernutrition.

Activity

The most obvious factor complicating the estimation of energy requirements is the level of activity. Durnin and Passmore (5) have demonstrated, for example, that the energy required for light activities such as working in a laboratory, typing, sewing, and ironing may be no greater than 2.0 kcal/min

Table 1. Energy requirements throughout the day of young adult men with differing work and leisure activities[a]

Occupation	Sedentary	Moderately active	Very active
Energy expenditure			
In bed (kcal/8 h)	500	500	500
At work (kcal/8 h)	900	1200	1800
Nonoccupational			
(kcal/8h)	800–1800	800–1800	800–1800
Energy requirement			
from food			
(kcal/24 h)	2200–3200	2500–3500	3100–4100
Recommended intake			
for a group			
(kcal/24 h)	2700	3000	3600

[a]From the DHSS (1).

for the average woman or 2.5 kcal/min for a man, whereas scrubbing floors, shopping with a heavy load, or working in the garden may use up to 7.5 kcal/min. Likewise, leisure activity can vary considerably; watching television requires little more than 1 kcal/min, but playing squash can consume 12 kcal/min. It is easy, however, to overestimate the contribution of sport to overall daily energy requirements, since usually these activities last for only a short time and their effect is often canceled by a much longer period of relative inactivity after the game is over!

A range of estimated energy requirements depending on different levels of activity during the day for a standard 65-kg man is given in Table 1. The range is wide — 2200–4100 kcal/day — and in an attempt to simplify the situation there has been a tendency to assume that the "average" man requires the "average" energy intake of this range, i.e., around 3000 kcal/day. This is not the case, however. In most countries, including Great Britain, the 50th percentile man requires considerably less. In industrialized countries many jobs, even those conventionally thought of as being quite active, are in reality not so energy demanding because of the long periods of standing around and sitting they involve. For example, the 1969 DHSS report (1) placed into the "sedentary" category shop workers, doctors, and journalists; even the jobs of farm workers and builders' laborers were considered to be only moderately active. In poor countries a lack of opportunity to work is compounded by a minimal social stimulation to be involved in other high energy activities. It is also very unusual for a man with a moderate or very active job to take part in very active nonoccupational activities. All these factors bias toward lower energy requirements within the population and thus it is not surprising that even in rich countries, where food is abundant, it is rare for the average adult male energy consumption to be as high as the 1973 FAO/WHO requirement value of 3000 kcal/day.

One could argue about the desirability of this situation and claim that the recommended allowance is correct for the level of activity that *should* be occurring, but a social change toward increased activity is unlikely to be achieved by recommending an increase in energy consumption. If complied with, such a recommendation would more likely lead to an increase in the incidence of obesity. Except where there is actual primary undernutrition or malnutrition, the nutritionist can only match his recommendations to satisfy the existing social norm.

In England, at practically all age groups, mean measured intakes are some 15% below 1969 DHSS recommended daily intakes, even after different levels of work activity have been taken into account, and the Household Food Consumption and Expenditure Report (6) provided evidence for a progressive decline in energy consumption during the years 1970–1975, and this trend is known to be continuing.

Body Size

Body size constitutes another component of variability in energy requirements. Tables of daily allowances quote values for only one body size for adults, usually 65 kg for men and 55 kg for women. When dealing with people who deviate markedly from this weight, theroretically it would seem desirable to make an allowance; but how this can be done is not easy to determine. The relationship between body weight and energy expenditure is not particularly close, and correlation coefficients are 0.4 at best. One reason could be that heavy people tend to be less active than light ones, and this negative relationship partly cancels the positive one between size and basal metabolic rate (2). Although care has to be exercised in correcting recommended daily energy allowances for body size, WHO/FAO (4) has suggested how this can be done, and its corrections for men who are moderately active are shown in Table 2.

Age

Apart from the obvious considerations of childhood and adolescence, age also affects energy requirements, but again the relationship is a complex one because of its multifactorial nature. Basal metabolic rate declines throughout adulthood at a rate of approximately 2% per 10 years (5). At the same time, people usually become heavier with age, which tends to cancel any consequent reduction in energy requirements.

Although people become less active as they grow older, there is no fixed pattern of change — change depends to a large extent on the social environment. In general it may be assumed, however, that the degree of change is likely to be more marked in individuals who have been engaged in heavy work and leisure activities in their youth.

It is not surprising that individual expert committees have made different allowances for age. Table 3 records the 1973 FAO/WHO conclusions for

Table 2. Adjustment of energy requirement for men with different body weights, assuming moderate activity[a]

Body weight (kg)	Energy (kcal)
50	2300
55	2530
60	2760
65	3000
70	3220
75	3450
80	3680

[a]From the FAO/WHO (4).

moderately active men and women, assuming weight is constant. It is concluded that there is no change before 30 but that a steady decline occurs thereafter until, by 70 years, requirement is calculated to be only 70% of the young man or woman. On the other hand, the NRC (2) only reduced energy allowances for people over 50 years of age by 10%, and even then warned that this was inappropriate if the individual remains active. ·

Ambient Temperature

To some extent the need to adjust energy intakes for different ambient temperatures is eased by our control of the microenvironment. In industrial countries temperature control in the home, at work, and in the car are routine, and we vary the amount of clothes we wear when out-of-doors. The early FAO Committees on Calorie Requirements (7, 8) were conscious, however, that they had to consider the problems of people who might not be able to compensate for the environment in this way.

The 1950 FAO committee (7) based all of their energy recommendations on an annual *mean* temperature of 10°C and suggested, for planning purposes, that energy requirements should be increased by 5% for every 10°C of mean annual external temperature below this reference temperature; this was amended by a second committee in 1957 (8) to only 3%. Both the 1950 and 1957 committees recommended that energy allowances should be decreased by 5% for every 10°C above the reference temperature.

Table 3. Energy requirements and age[a]

Age (years)	65-kg man (kcal)	55-kg woman (kcal)	% of reference
20–39	3000	2200	100
40–49	2850	2090	95
50–59	2700	1980	90
60–69	2400	1760	80
70–79	2100	1540	70

[a]From the FAO/WHO (4).

Extra energy is thought to be necessary in cold conditions in order to support an increased thermogenesis. The thermogenesis is of two types: "shivering," which results in increased muscular heat production, and "nonshivering," which involves a substantially altered metabolism and is the response to more long-term exposure to cold. In moderately hot conditions it has been suggested there might be a reduction in basal metabolic rate, but this notion comes from studies in developing countries, and the possibility of dietary energy deficiency in the subjects cannot be ruled out; not all investigators have confirmed this response of BMR to temperature.

For men who have to work continuously at very high temperatures, energy requirements may actually become increased due to a rise in metabolic rate, since extra energy has to be expended to maintain thermal balance.

It was apparent to the 1973 FAO/WHO expert committee that the situation was much more complicated than had been appreciated by the two earlier committees, and they concluded that there was no quantifiable basis for either introducing a temperature correction factor to BMR or increasing energy requirements in general. They suggested, very reasonably, that the biggest energy response to prolonged excessively high temperatures would be a restriction of activity, which could best be allowed for by careful selection of the appropriate activity category.

Most individual countries do not have a wide enough temperature range to make this an important problem, but the 1974 NRC report stated that, although it was not necessary to adjust requirements for temperatures up to 30°C, above this, wherever people were required to be *physically active* (i.e., to expend over 3000 kcal/day), energy allowances should be increased by 0.5% for every degree of temperature above 30°C. They also pointed out that in cold conditions (9) the energy cost of work was approximately 5% greater when mean temperature was below 14°C than when it was between 20 and 30°C. The actual wearing of extra cold weather clothing could also increase energy expenditure by 2–5% by its "hobbling effect."

It is obvious that a considerable degree of judgment needs to be exercised in whether or not to allow for different ambient temperatures, but it seems that any allowance is likely to be small in comparison with overall requirements and adjustments on the basis of changes in activity.

Metabolic Differences Among Individuals

Even when energy expenditure has been standardized for size, activity, age, and temperature, it is quite apparent that a considerable degree of variation remains. Durnin (10) has concluded that the standard deviation of energy expenditure between adults after these corrections is of the order of 20% and thus, assuming a normal distribution, requirements may cover an 80% range between −2 SD and +2 SD of the mean. These differences in metabolic efficiency are apparent in both resting and activity expenditures, but it has not been established whether or not the same individuals who have efficient BMRs are equally efficient in their other activity expenditures.

The reasons behind this biological variability in BMR are by no means fully understood. One possible factor is the proportion of the different organs within the body. In the young child heart, brain, kidneys, liver, lungs, and diaphragm account for most of the resting oxygen consumed (about 85%) and skeletal and smooth muscle take only 15% (11). As the individual grows older, the BMR/kg falls, reflecting a decreasing ratio of the former group of organs to body weight. Clearly, not all people are identical, and there is some degree of variation in this development.

It is unlikely, however, that body compositional differences provide more than a partial explanation, and it seems probable that there are additional metabolic differences among individuals. These are largely speculative, but there is considerable current interest in the so-called futile metabolic cycles, in which energy metabolites circulate in an energy-consuming sequence of metabolic reactions for no apparent rational purpose. A frequently quoted example is that involving the fructose 6-phosphate/fructose 1,6-diphosphate cycle (12):

$$
\begin{array}{ccc}
& \text{Glucose} & \\
& \downarrow & \\
& \text{F-6-P} & \\
\text{Fructose diphosphatase} & \big(\quad \big) \quad \text{Phosphofructokinase} \quad \big(\begin{array}{l} \text{ATP} \\ \text{ADP} \end{array} \\
& \text{F-1,6-diP} & \\
& \downarrow & \\
& \text{Pyruvate} &
\end{array}
$$

One molecule of ATP is used up in each cycle and gives rise to a considerable waste of energy within individuals for whom this metabolic process is an active one. Whatever the nature of biochemical individuality in energy efficiency, it is of considerable practical significance. It is important in the pathogenesis of obesity, and also explains why some people remain excessively thin on an apparently adequate energy intake. It could also be linked with the processes of metabolic adaptation, which people possess to different degrees, when they are switched from high to low energy intakes, and vice versa. It is also of important to planners, particularly those who have to plan for emergency rationing. There will always be people with requirements considerably in excess of the mean and who possess little ability to adapt to reduced circumstances; too rigid an approach would inevitably lead to difficulties.

Childhood and Growth

Most of the complexities detailed above for adults apply equally or even more so to children. The NRC (2) stated that its recommended energy allowances were proposed only as averages and for feeding *groups*. There are considerable variations in the energy expenditures of children and due con-

Table 4. Energy requirements for maintenance, growth, and activity in children of differing ages[a]

		Energy cost per day		Energy for activity (kcal)
Age	Weight (kg)	Maintenance (kcal)	Growth (kcal)	
3 months	4.6	365	128	57
9–12 months	9.6	800	60	150
2–3 years	13.6	1020	30	310
4–5 years	17.4	1200	35	485
9–10 years	31.3	1750	30	640
16–17 years	60.3	2500	60	540

[a]From the FAO/WHO (4).

sideration must be taken of this fact. It should also be appreciated, particularly in modern industrialized societies, that relatively inactive children can become obese even on an apparently low energy intake. On the other hand, a deficiency of dietary energy is the major cause of most protein-energy malnutrition in children of the developing world.

In general, energy requirements fall with age, from an estimated 120 kcal/kg in early infancy to 100 kcal/kg between 1 and 3 years of age and to around 40 kcal/kg in the adult. Changes in growth rate in fact constitute only a small proportion of the energy requirements of a child and of the variations among individuals. The FAO/WHO (4) considered a series of different estimates for the energy cost of growth and concluded that the amount was approximately 5 kcal (21 kJ) per g of tissue, assuming it consisted of 16% fat and 18% protein. Table 4 provides relative energy estimates for growth, maintenance, and activity, using this value at different ages. The table shows that, although growth represents 23% of total energy needs in the first trimester of life, by age 4–5 this has fallen to 2%. The major reason for the drop in energy requirements per unit of body weight is the fall in BMR per units of body weight.

A comparison of the 1974 NRC recommended dietary allowances and the 1973 FAO/WHO international standards for children reveals that the American values are lower. The 1969 DHSS guidelines are nearer the international ones, but recent field studies in England have revealed that in practice average intakes are lower, up to 15% lower, than recommended intakes, and it is probable that the British recommendations will also be lowered.

The reason for the differences between the FAO/WHO and NRC recommendations is partly that the international committee was very much aware that a substantial proportion of the world's population is undersize, underweight, and underactive, all possibly because of a deficiency in dietary energy. The opposite is true for the United States, where obesity is the major nutritional health problem. It is not surprising that these two contrasting situations biased the committees to somewhat different conclusions.

Pregnancy and Lactation

Extra energy to support growing tissues is also needed during pregnancy. It has been calculated that the energy cost of pregnancy is of the order of 80,000 kcal (13). A large proportion of this energy is accounted for by fat storage, which begins early during pregnancy. This fat has two functions: it protects the fetus against dietary energy deficit during the phase of rapid growth toward the end of pregnancy, and it greatly aids the synthesis of milk during lactation. Sufficient energy to lay down fat during pregnancy is thus of major health significance.

Determination of how much extra dietary energy must be provided during pregnancy is complicated by social factors. The amount of work a woman does while pregnant in contrast to that done during her prepregnancy state varies. In some societies pregnancy is not allowed to make a difference, and women continue even with hard manual work. In other countries women are "protected" at this time and assume a more or less sedentary existence. For international purposes it had to be assumed that a woman carries on working as previously and thus the whole 80,000 kcal is allowed for. The FAO/WHO (4) increased allowances by 150 kcal/day during the first trimester and 350 kcal/day for the remainder of pregnancy. The DHSS (1), on the other hand, decided that only 200 kcal/day for the second and third trimesters (36,000 kcal per pregnancy) was a sufficient supplement because of the predominance of reduced activity during pregnancy for British women.

It is well known, however, that many women do not increase their dietary energy intake during pregnancy. In Gambia (14), for example, 1500 kcal/day is the average energy intake during both pregnancy and nonpregnancy. The baby at birth does tend to be small (2.8 kg), but not excessively so, and the women are then able to breastfeed for very long periods. One can only assume that pregnancy may be accompanied by a considerable increase in efficiency of energy utilization.

The extra dietary energy needed to support adequate lactation is also difficult to define precisely. Breast milk provides on average 70 kcal/100 ml. If a child were to exist on breast milk alone until 6 months (and many authorities recommend this), he would theoretically need to receive up to 1160 ml of milk (15), since at 6 months the average male infant has a recommended energy intake of 814 kcal (4). Most expert committees have based their estimates on the assumption that a woman will be producing 850 ml of milk per day, and thus an extra 600 kcal has to be accounted for. The validity of only allowing for 850 ml must be looked at more critically, however, since in practice it is quite possible that 110–120 kcal/kg of body weight is an overestimate of energy needs and, furthermore, efficiency of energy utilization might vary also according to supply.

It is now agreed that maternal dietary energy is converted to milk energy with an 80% efficiency (16) and thus approximately 90 kcal is required for the production of 100 ml of milk; for 850 ml an extra 765 kcal of energy would thus be required. However, a woman should have stored up to 4 kg of fat (36,000 kcal) and the 1973 FAO/WHO committee reasoned that only 550 kcal/day in addition to normal needs is required to support lactation. It warned, however, that women who had not laid down fat, or who breastfed in excess of 6 months (common in developing countries), would require more dietary energy because by this time any fat stores would have been used up.

The above arguments have assumed that it is a normal practice to breastfeed up to 6 months but, of course, in many urbanized communities this is not the case, although there is evidence that this situation may be altering. This is another example of the interaction between nutritional requirements and social practice. Once again it is important that the nutritionist adopt a flexible approach in defining recommended intakes and ensure that these keep pace with changing attitudes and practices.

It must be pointed out that theory and practice about nutrient requirements for successful, long-term lactation do not always coincide. It is rare for a Gambian woman (14), for example, to have anything like a dietary intake of 2500–3000 kcal/day during lactation; the average intake in fact is of the order of 1500 kcal/day. Despite this, a breastmilk output of 500–600 ml/day is common, and the energy content of this milk is maintained at 70 kcal/100 ml (lactation is continued up to 18 months). After allowing for the 400 kcal this milk contains, the lactating woman seems to be able to carry out a considerable degree of heavy manual work on the remaining 1100 kcal, a figure near her theoretical resting metabolic rate. Clearly a more detailed understanding of the mechanisms of energy utilization during pregnancy and lactation is required before recommended daily energy allowances can be made for all prevailing environmental circumstances.

NUTRIENT REQUIREMENTS

Protein

With the exception of dietary energy, recommended dietary allowances for protein have received more detailed consideration than any other component of dietary allowance tables. This was to be expected, since protein is the traditional body-building food and for many years it was thought by everyone that primary protein malnutrition was widespread in many parts of the world. Furthermore, protein is an expensive commodity to produce and it was necessary to find out what was the smallest protein intake that was compatible with a healthy nation.

Typical trends in recommended dietary allowances for protein for a 2-year-old child are given in Table 5. It will be seen that, in general, estimated requirements for protein have been falling and this means that some dietary patterns that were originally considered to provide an inadequate balance between protein and energy would now be thought acceptable.

Table 5.   Trends in recommended dietary allowances for a two-year-old child during recent years[a]

Year	Energy [g/kg body weight (kcal)]	Protein (g/kg body weight)	Protein/ energy ratio (%)	References
1941, 1945, 1948	418(100)	3.3	13.2	NRC(1948)
1963	418(100)	2.5	10.0	NRC(1964)
1965	—	1.5	—	FAO/WHO(1965)
1968	385 (92)	2.1	9.1	NRC(1968)
1969	439(105)	1.7	6.5	DHSS(1969)
1973	424(101)	1.5	5.9	FAO/WHO(1973)

[a]From Whitehead (27).

Obligatory Nitrogen Loss and Nitrogen Balance   Two main procedures have been used to define adult protein requirements: one is based on estimates of obligatory nitrogen losses, and the other on nitrogen balance. The 1973 FAO/WHO report provides many excellent examples of how to estimate protein requirements by both these methods, and the following is a brief summary to outline the principal features of its approach (see also Table 6).

The obligatory nitrogen loss method estimates the nitrogen needed to replace losses in the feces and urine and from the skin. These have only been studied to any significant extent in young adult men. Nitrogen intake is reduced to zero and obligatory nitrogen loss is taken to be that nitrogen that continues to be lost after the body has returned to a steady state again, which usually takes about 1 week.

Table 6.   Example of calculation for the protein requirements of a young child[a]

Nitrogen to cover obligatory losses: nitrogen per basal kcal × BMR/body weight (2 × 800/17.42)	= 92 mg/kg/day
Nitrogen for growth	= 8.5 mg/kg/day
Total nitrogen	= 100 mg/kg/day
Adjustment for utilization efficiency of milk protein (× 1.3)	= 130 mg of nitrogen/kg/day
Provision for individual variation (× 1.3)	= 160 mg of nitrogen/kg/day
Protein requirement (× 6.25)	= 1.06 g of protein/kg/day
Provision for efficiency of utilization of British-type diet relative to egg/milk (100/80)	= 1.325 g of protein/kg/day
Minimal intake for average 4-year-old child, 17.42 kg	= 23.1 g of protein/day

[a]Based on the 1973 FAO/WHO report (4).

In order that obligatory losses can be defined for age groups other than young adult men, these have been related to metabolic body size as measured by the basal metabolic rate. It has been assumed, although not proved, that total obligatory losses per basal energy unit are constant regardless of age, sex, or physiological status. This value has been calculated to be approximately 2 mg of nitrogen/basal kcal. About 70% of the nitrogen is lost via the urine, 20% from the feces, and 10% from the skin and other miscellaneous sources.

The 2 mg/basal kcal is first multiplied by the relevant BMR value for that age and sex to obtain a nitrogen value for the whole body. To this is added, when necessary, the nitrogen requirement for growth. This is calculated from the amount of new tissue that is deposited and is based on average weight gain data at different ages and published values for the nitrogen content of that new tissue. During pregnancy and lactation, appropriate additions are made for these functions, too. The product represents the total nitrogen needs for the average individual, assuming 100% efficiency of conversion from dietary nitrogen to tissue nitrogen.

It was observed, however, that when the calculated requirement based on obligatory losses was compared against known requirements for nitrogen balance in young adults, there was a discrepancy of about 30% even with the best-utilized dietary proteins, such as egg and milk. This was assumed to reflect the degree of efficiency with which nitrogen is utilized around the balance point.

It was assumed that efficiency of nitrogen utilization should be the same for all ages and thus, where no nitrogen balance data were available, the 1973 FAO/WHO committee multiplied estimated nitrogen requirements to replace obligatory losses by 1.3 to obtain an estimate of balance needs. It was recognized that not all individuals of the same size, age, and physiological status would have identical obligatory losses, nor possess the same efficiency in dealing with dietary protein. An estimate of individual variation was obtained from experimental data on obligatory nitrogen losses in young adults, and the coefficient of variation was set at 15% for all ages. Consequently, an additional 30% (+ 2 SD) was added to the nitrogen balance data to cover the needs of the conventional 97% of the population.

This final nitrogen value was then multiplied by 6.25 to convert it to the reference protein for nitrogen balance studies — milk or egg protein. An adjustment then had to be made for the quality of different dietary proteins relative to milk and egg. There are various ways by which this can be determined, but the most widely used is the net protein utilization method (NPU), usually with the rat as the test animal. The previously calculated protein value is then multiplied by the ratio NPU egg:NPU test food to give the theoretical safe level for protein with the diet being tested. In practice, one can generally assume that the mixed diet normally eaten in European countries has a protein value of 80% relative to that of egg or milk, a mixed cereal-based diet, 70%, and a starchy root- or plantain-based diet, around 60%.

Appraisal of the 1973 FAO/WHO Approach   Recommendations based on the above type of physiological considerations have received wide acceptance. There has, however, in the past year or two been criticism of some of the assumptions made. The most vociferous objections came from Dr. Nevin Scrimshaw of the Massachusetts Institute of Technology (18). Although his criticisms perhaps represent a minority opinion, they are sufficiently important to be considered in some detail. It is obvious that more experimentally derived data are urgently required from centers representative of the conditions existing in other parts of the world.

One of the trickiest factors complicating the estimation of protein requirements is the amount of dietary energy consumed along with the protein. An excess of dietary energy over needs apparently improves the efficiency of dietary nitrogen utilization. Garza, Scrimshaw, and Young (17) have criticized the applicability of much of the nitrogen balance data used by the FAO/WHO (4) because, they claimed, most were carried out under conditions in which there was an over-generous supply of dietary energy to make absolutely certain that a lack of energy was not adversely affecting the efficiency of nitrogen utilization. They showed that when the "safe level" for protein was fed to young United States male students, together with an intake of energy relevant to their requirement but no more, the majority went into negative nitrogen balance. This could be reversed by increasing the energy intake, but in doing so all the subjects gained weight, indicating they were laying down fat. This clearly needs to be studied in greater detail, as most people in the world certainly do not have an excessive energy intake — rather the opposite is true.

Considerable controversy (18) has also been generated by the validity of the 30% factor adopted to adjust calculated obligatory nitrogen values to the amounts of egg or milk nitrogen needed for balance. From the data that were available it was obvious to the 1973 FAO/WHO committee that this was variable, and it now seems possible that the magnitude of the nitrogen efficiency factor depends on the long-term dietary background of an individual. If he has been used to a relatively low protein intake, a person may be able to utilize nitrogen more efficiently, and the 1.3 factor will over-estimate needs (19, 20). For the exact opposite reason, it is apparently too low a value for the meat eating, socially privileged people studied by Scrimshaw and his colleagues (18).

Differences in efficiency of nitrogen utilization have also been demonstrated when people are switched from their customary diet containing proteins of high quality to ones of low biological value. American students fed the type of cereal-based diet customarily consumed in many developing countries apparently needed considerably higher quantities for balance than would have been predicted from the relative NPUs of the two diets (18). It was obvious that Nigerian adults fed a very similar diet were utilizing the nitrogen with a much greater efficiency (19, 20).

Other investigators have been concerned about the allowance made to cover individual variation, but it is obvious that these worries will not be resolved until more knowledge is made available. Sukhatme (21) has suggested that much of the overall variation was *within* individuals rather than *among* individuals, and thus there was no need to make anything like such a high safety margin allowance as +30% (2 standard deviations). On the other hand, Scrimshaw and his colleagues (22) have reasoned that in the same way that efficiency of nitrogen retention becomes less as intakes approach the balance point, the difference between individual efficiencies will become more scattered. If this proved to be true, then a standard deviation of 15% may prove inadequate.

The nitrogen balance method assumes that when the body as a whole is in balance each organ is receiving sufficient nitrogen for optimum function. Scrimshaw (23) and his colleagues cast doubt on this assumption, too. They have produced enzyme evidence that could be interpreted as a sign of liver malfunction, even though nitrogen balance data appeared satisfactory. Subsequent work on balance studies in rats has also demonstrated that nitrogen balance differs between organs, with the liver and heart needing considerably more dietary nitrogen than muscle before balance is achieved (24).

A clarification of the best way of defining recommended dietary allowances is of more than academic interest. Although it is clearly desirable to protect each and every member of society under as wide a range of environmental and physiological circumstances as possible, such an aim can lead to impossible and even undesirable goals, particularly in the developing countries. Increases in total food production are still inadequate to match population increases. If protein requirements are set sufficiently high to ensure a blanket coverage of those with exceptional needs, and agricultural planners use these requirements as the basis of their food production policies, this could give rise to an inefficient use of resources. An exclusive concentration on protein-rich crops and on the production of animal protein reduces the food energy yield per acre. In most developing countries the deficiency is more of energy than of protein, and consequently such a policy might well do more harm than good. This is a matter of considerable importance and is a danger that must be emphasized. An alternative approach to blanket coverage is to ensure that the health services are adequate to detect persons with exceptional requirements and to treat them as special dietary cases.

Requirements for Growth   The extra nitrogen increment needed for average rates of growth makes very little difference to overall protein requirements, except in the first year of life. During infancy and childhood, the average rate of growth falls off rapidly and nitrogen requirements for maintenance represent an increasing proportion of total needs (Table 7).

Table 7. Nitrogen requirements (mg/kg/day) for maintenance and growth at different ages[a]

Age	Obligatory loss	Growth	Total
6–8 months	112	42	154
9–11 months	110	26	136
1 year	104	16	120
2 years	100	12	112
3 years	96	10	106
4 years	92	8.5	100

[a]From the FAO/WHO (4).

Calculations of protein requirements for growth at different ages have usually been based on Boston 50th percentile data (25). Doubt has been expressed, however, as to whether diets containing protein and energy only in the proportions necessary to support *average* rates of growth are really adequate to cover growth as it occurs in practice (26, 27). Even perfectly healthy children exhibit marked variations in rates of growth; Figure 1 illustrates an example of a young female child. For weeks children may, for no apparent reason, grow relatively little, and this is followed by an episode of catch-up growth in which velocity of weight gain is considerably in excess of the 50th percentile. In circumstances where there are periodic infections, variations in rate of growth become exaggerated. Any growth faltering or loss of weight becomes the stimulus for catch-up after the illness is finished.

Waterlow and Payne (28) and Whitehead (27) have attempted to estimate protein relative to energy requirements for different rates of growth, and from both their calculations it would appear that for an individual to show rapid catch-up he needs a diet with a relatively higher protein content than would be necessary if he were only growing at the Boston 50th percentile rate. This fits in with common biological experience. The greater the rate of growth of a species (g/kg of body weight) the higher must be the protein content of the diet, relative to energy. The importance of this balance between protein and energy (the P:E ratio) for catch-up growth is greater the younger and smaller the child is. The example in Table 8 is for a 7-kg child, a frequently encountered weight among children in the developing countries between 6 and 24 months, who clearly have a need for catch-up growth.

An analysis of growth rate data in Table 9 shows that monthly weight gain increments do vary widely between individual children, much more so than the ± 30% safety margin allowed for in the calculation of the safe level.

It is not yet known how much this really matters in practice, but if a child's catch-up growth is limited by the P:E ratio of his diet he will take longer to catch up after an episode of illness. In situations in which infection is a frequent occurrence, as in many developing countries, this would give rise to permanent faltering, a not uncommon finding.

Pregnancy During pregnancy, about 950 g of protein are synthesized by the mother as fetus and maternal reproductive tissues. This protein is not

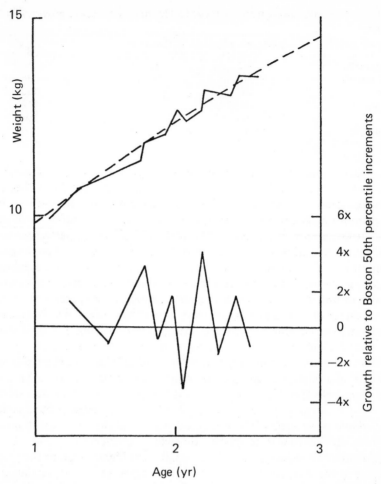

Figure 1.   The growth and growth velocities of a European child during the second two years of life, relative to Boston 50th percentile weight increments.

laid down uniformly throughout pregnancy, however: Hytten and Leech estimated from an analysis of fetuses, stillborn children, and placental tissues that the rates of protein accretion during the successive ten-week quarters of pregnancy were 0.6, 1.8, 4.8, and 6.1 g/day. Some expert committees have made no allowance for these differences, mainly because there is some evidence (29) that nitrogen can be stored during the early phases of gestation and then released when protein needs become particularly high. The DHSS (1) assumed that an average increase of 5 g of protein/day during the second and third trimesters was an adequate extra allowance. On the other hand, FAO/WHO (4) recommended only an extra 1 g of protein/day for the first quarter of pregnancy, but 4, 8, and 9 g/day during the final three

Table 8. Protein and energy requirements for different rates of growth in a 7-kg child[a]

Growth rate (maintenance plus normal growth)	Protein (g/kg/day)	Energy (kJ/kg/d)	P:E ratio (%)
× 1	1.25	465	4.55
× 2	1.40	490	4.80
× 3	1.55	515	5.05
× 4	1.70	540	5.30
× 5	1.85	565	5.50

[a]Data are based on requirements for milk or egg protein. Protein increment for normal growth was taken as 0.15 g/kg/d. From Waterlow and Payne (28).

quarters. There is evidence from balance experiments, however, that nitrogen retention is about twice that, which can thus be accounted for by nitrogen increments in the fetus and reproductive tissues (13). Furthermore, and rather surprisingly, there is evidence that the efficiency of protein utilization may be lower in pregnant than in nonpregnant women. Because of these unexplained findings, the NRC (2) decided to act cautiously and recommended an extra 30 g of protein/day throughout pregnancy.

Exactly what is the significance of these high nitrogen retentions during pregnancy remains to be seen, but it is widely recognized that many facets of

Table 9. Variations in monthly growth increments in preschool children in three different communities[a]

Age (months)	Number	Percentiles of weight change		
		3rd	50th	97th
Uganda				
10–12	92	−724	217	977
13–15	99	−579	174	869
16–18	83	−805	145	1086
19–24	179	−521	174	869
25–30	126	−553	217	869
Gambia				
10–12	193	−819	95	760
13–15	159	−652	108	760
16–18	144	−819	117	984
19–24	346	−869	109	936
25–30	241	−811	117	1014
Jamaica				
10–12	616	−189	227	642
13–15	401	−189	189	605
16–18	579	−340	189	680
19–24	700	−302	151	718
25–30	700	−378	151	718

[a]Increments at the Boston 50th percentile used by WHO/FAO (1973) were: 9–11 months, 330 g/month; 1–2 years, 208 g/month; and 2–3 years, 170 g/month.

growth and health are fixed early during development, and where the economy and traditional dietary habits conform to a high protein intake it would be unwise to dissuade pregnant women from the practice. At the same time, poor people living in the developing countries consume nothing like this amount of protein, and a better understanding of nitrogen retention is required before such an expensive change could be recommended.

Lactation Fortunately, calculating allowances for lactation is not as complicated as for pregnancy, with the exception of defining a realistic milk output. On the basis of an 850-ml output, assuming it contains 1.2 g of protein/liter and that dietary nitrogen utilization is operating with normal efficiency, an extra 17 g/day of milk or egg protein was recommended for lactating women by the FAO/WHO (4). The NRC (2) recommended 20 g/day because milk yield might range between 850 ml and 1200 ml. The DHSS (1) only allowed an extra 13 g/day, but its baseline recommendations for nonlactating women were higher.

It is apparent that, although protein requirement has been subject to much greater scrutiny than that of any other nutrient, much more work needs to be done before we have a really sound basis for our recommendations. Nevertheless, protein has set an example for the degree of objectivity and thought that needs to be adopted for the whole range of nutrients.

Fat Soluble Vitamins

Vitamin A Vitamin A is necessary for a variety of body functions. It is derived either from food as the preformed vitamin retinol, or from related carotenoids, the most plentiful of which is β-carotene. One way of expressing vitamin A requirements is in "μg retinol equivalents."

One of the earliest attempts to define vitamin A requirements was the war-time study of Hume and Krebs (30), who found that 390 μg of retinol were necessary to achieve optimum night vision, but more than this amount was needed to raise plasma vitamin A concentrations up to conventionally accepted normal values. The DHSS (1) adopted a recommendation of 750 μg for adults, which it assumed would not only produce desirable plasma concentrations but would also cover individual variability. There was no measure of individual variability as such available, and it was impossible to provide a safety margin on the basis of mean + SD, as was the case with protein.

More recently, Hodges and Kolder (31) in the United States looked not only at plasma levels and dark adaptation, but at a whole range of vitamin A–dependent functions, including balance, taste and smell thresholds, skin lesions, and electroretinogram performance. It was found that these functions reached their maximum performance on widely different levels of vitamin intake. The most easily attained was dark adaptation (a 150-μg intake), whereas skin lesions were only controlled with a 600-μg intake. The US adult male recommendation was therefore made 1000 μg retinol equivalents, and that for a female, 800 μg. The safety margin was included to cover individual requirements. This is higher, however, than the 1967 FAO/WHO value (3) and those for all European countries, which tend to be similar to those in the British guidelines.

Retinol is required for pregnancy and lactation. The DHSS (1), however, decided not to make an extra addition during pregnancy, in contrast to the NCR (2), which recommended a further 200 μg. The British committee did not consider that the somewhat lower plasma vitamin A concentrations found in pregnancy were of any physiological significance.

Breast milk contains about 50 μg of retinol/100 ml, and, on the assumption that the mother will secrete 850 ml, an extra dietary allowance of around 450 μg/day is made by most authorities for lactation, but clearly a mother producing more milk may need great supplementation. It is also assumed that the retinol content of 850 ml of human milk represents the approximate need of a young infant, but this has not been confirmed either experimentally, which would be difficult ethically, or by epidemiological survey. Intermediate values between those recommended for infancy and young adults have been adopted for other ages during childhood.

One of the difficulties in defining retinol requirements is that the body contains substantial stores, which take many months, or even years, to deplete. Vitamin A deficiency is, however, relatively common and in some developing countries it is as big a problem as protein-energy malnutrition, with which it frequently coexists. In such people intakes are considerably lower than the above recommended values.

One finding of fundamental importance to all nutrients has emerged from studies on vitamin A requirements. Different physiological functions may need different dietary levels of a nutrient to achieve optimum performance. This should be borne in mind when other vitamins are considered. With vitamin A we are fortunate to have identified various functions of pathological relevance, and thus have had the opportunity to investigate their individual requirements. With most vitamins we have only a rather vague and imprecise knowledge of their range of functions.

Vitamin D   Vitamin D is necessary for calcium absorption from the gut and for the deposition of calcium in bone. It is probably also necessary for calcium metabolism in many other tissues, including muscle and nervous tissue.

It is very difficult to quote any really meaningful requirements because, except during early infancy, it would seem that needs can be synthesized by sunlight from steroid precursors in the skin. Recent studies in the UK on children, young adults, and old age pensioners, have demonstrated that in healthy subjects diet makes very little contribution to plasma 25-hydroxycholecalciferol concentrations, but the latter correlate closely with variations in sunlight exposure among individuals (32).

It seems probable that in infancy the natural source of the vitamin is the water soluble sulfate. Human breast milk contains a plentiful supply of the vitamin in this form.

Vitamin D is not distributed widely in foods. Natural sources are fatty fish, eggs, liver, and butter. Margarine is fortified in most countries with vitamin D_2. In some countries cow's milk is also fortified, but in others this fortification is limited to certain brands of tinned milk. Infant milks are similarly fortified. In countries such as England, which has clinical rickets once again (mainly in Asian immigrants), the right type of food to fortify represents a problem. The possibility of fortifying flour with encapsulated vitamin D has been tested experimentally, but its general introduction would require fresh legislation and there is doubt that it would be really effective. Some authorities believe that taking vitamin D capsules prophylactically as a medicine, rather than providing a dietary source of D, is the more rational way of dealing with a deficiency that is limited to relatively few people. One of the potential dangers of fortification is hypervitaminosis D. Amounts of vitamin D only five times the United States recommended dietary allowance have resulted in hypercalcaemia in infants and kidney stones in both children and adults.

Vitamin D is another vitamin for which different requirements have been proven for its individual metabolic functions. In infancy, for example, 2.5 μg of vitamin D/day seems adequate to prevent rickets, improve calcium absorption from the gut, and allow normal mineralization of bone, but it would appear that 10μg/day promotes better growth. It is this level, 10 μg/-day, that was recommended for infancy by both the DHSS (1) and the NRC (2). The latter maintained this recommendation for all stages of childhood and adolescence, and during pregnancy and lactation, but they made no recommendation for adults over 22 years of age on the assumption they could synthesize all their needs from sunlight. The DHSS (1) adopted a different approach, dropping recommendations to 2.5 μg/day for all ages and sexes from 5 years, except during pregnancy, where it was again 10 μg/day. Clearly these different recommendations represent judgment rather than a reflection of firm fact.

Vitamin E   Primary vitamin E deficiency is unknown as a public health problem in man and has only been demonstrated after prolonged impairment of fat absorption. Plasma concentrations are also correlated with plasma lipid levels. Low plasma vitamin E levels have been reported in low birth weight infants fed milk formulas with only a low vitamin E content. The deficiency was accompanied by edema and anemia. Low blood vitamin E levels increase susceptibility to hemolysis; erythrocyte survival time is also reduced.

The DHSS (1) made no specific recommendation for vitamin E, but it pointed out that the vitamin occurred widely in many plants and in milk and eggs; British diets provided 10 mg/day or more and there was little evidence of E deficiency.

The NRC (2), on the other hand, was clearly concerned about vitamin E requirements in infancy and the nutritional adequacy of infant formulas. It recognized that plasma vitamin E levels varied with the amount of fat fed, because there was an apparently greater requirement with the type of fat contained in artificial formulas than with that in human milk. A milk concentration of 3 mg of α-tocopherol/liter containing 3.5% fat was recommended; 3-4 mg/day was the recommended intake for the first year of life. For older children it was assumed that requirement increased with body size, but not proportionately, and thus for a 40-kg individual around 10 mg was recommended (12 IU). The committee was also conscious of reports indicating a link between polyunsaturated fat intake and vitamin E requirements, and their recommendation assumed a linoleic acid consumption of no greater than 7% of total dietary energy.

The view has been expressed that, physiologically speaking, vitamin E requirements should be defined as that level of intake that maintains an adequate cellular concentration, relative to polyunsaturated fatty acid content, to permit satisfactory functioning during stress, as well as in normal situations. Unfortunately, there are few data on these parameters in man, and the NRC (2) recommendations for adults are based on an argument that is typical of the type of reasoning that expert committees are forced to adopt for many nutrients. The NRC assumed that in the adult a total blood tocopherol concentration of 0.5 mg/100 ml *should* ensure adequate tissue levels. Secondly, it stated that blood levels less than this were rare in the United States; therefore the dietary intake of between 10-20 IU/day (about 9-18 mg) must be sufficient to maintain these levels. It was assumed that somewhat more vitamin E would be needed during pregnancy and lactation.

Vitamin E raises an important quandary: it is clear that many more data are required for a truly accurate assessment of needs at all ages, but, in the absence of signs of deficiency at the public health level, would all the effort and expense of obtaining the necessary physiological information be worthwhile? Inevitably, the scientific community must consider the cost/benefit factor in the research they do. With vitamin E perhaps only the infant and young child need to be given immediate attention.

Vitamin K   Vitamin K deficiency results in defective blood coagulation. There is a range of chemical compounds with vitamin K activity; all are derivatives of naphthoquinone. K_1 is found primarily in plants, and K_2 is synthesized by intestinal bacteria, although the significance of the contribution of the latter source to overall human needs is doubtful.

There is no real basis of knowledge on which vitamin K requirements can be based. Vitamin K deficiency has only been reported by one author (33), in young infants prior to the development of their gut flora. On the basis of this finding, the NRC (2) recommended that 0.5-1 mg of vitamin K should be administered intramuscularly immediately after birth to assist adequate blood clotting, but this procedure is not widely adopted in other parts of the world. It is also possible that vitamin K deficiency might occur following prolonged antibiotic therapy, which could alter the intestinal flora; supplementation by chemotherapy in such circumstances would be advisable.

Water Soluble Vitamins

Vitamin C   Scurvy among deep water sailors was one of the first recognized dietary disorders, but in spite of this the actual amount of vitamin C required for health is still a controversial issue. The difficulty, as with so many of the vitamins, is that we do not know exactly what all of its functions are, and it is always possible that some physiological processes might need more vitamin C than others.

Most recommendations are based on the amounts of vitamin C necessary to alleviate and cure the clinical signs of scurvy (34); this was shown to be about 10 mg/day. The DHSS (1) added to this value a generous safety margin and said that it was highly unlikely that 30 mg/day for an adult would not cover every possible eventuality.

Such an amount would, however, not maintain tissue levels at or near saturation levels (35, 36, 37, 38); and vitamin C concentrations have been shown to be saturated in all healthy animals capable of synthesizing their own. Although saturated tissue levels have not been proved to confer any particular advantage to man, concern has been expressed by some scientists as to whether levels of intake incapable of achieving near saturation would be capable of sustaining optimal health under adverse conditions. Thus, the NRC (2) recommended a higher allowance than the British — 45 mg/day, sufficient to maintain a total body pool of 1500 mg.

It is obviously undesirable, however, to base vitamin allowances solely on either the size of body stores or the correction of extreme pathological signs, such as those seen in scurvy. Theoretically, it would be better if one could define the pathophysiological events leading up to scurvy and to base requirements on the optimum functioning of these metabolic processes. Vitamin C is known to be involved in the synthesis of collagen through the hydroxylation of proline to hydroxyproline, but so far it has not proved possible to use this knowledge for defining requirements. It would be unwise, however, to confine studies just to collagen metabolism. Vitamin C is known to play a role in many other oxidation-reduction reactions, including the synthesis of adrenalin and of anti-inflammatory steroids. Plasma and leukocyte vitamin C content has also been shown to fall during episodes of infection (39) and with emotional stress, such as when rural Africans begin work down in the mines (40). Smoking also has the same effect (41). All these metabolic processes need to be evaluated before vitamin C requirements can be defined unequivocally.

The benefits that have been claimed for pharmacological doses of vitamin C (0.5–5 g/day), particularly with respect to their relieving the symptoms of the common cold, are a totally different issue. Such levels of intake lie quite outside those capable of being supplied by normal diets and, even if the various claims that have been made were substantiated, they could hardly be viewed as dietary requirements (see also Schrauzer, this volume).

Requirements at different ages have not been subjected to careful experimental scrutiny. Plasma and leukocyte vitamin C levels do tend to be substantially lower in older people. Whether this indicates a lower degree of efficiency in utilization or just lower intakes remains to be seen.

Artificially fed infants do not develop signs of scurvy at levels of intake of about 7 mg/day, and thus the DHSS (1) made 15 mg/day its recommended intake for infancy. The intake of breastfed infants is considerably greater than this, however. Breast milk contains on average 40–55 mg ascorbic acid/liter and thus if a child receives 850 ml his intake will be around 30–40 mg. The NRC (2) followed the time-honored assumption that until more is known it would be judicious to assume that the breast knows best, and recommended 35 mg/day for infancy. Since there is no evidence to suggest that infants need more vitamin C than older children, the NRC graded its allowances with age from 35 mg up to the adult value of 45 mg. Likewise, British recommended intakes following infancy were graded from 15 to 30 mg.

Considerable extra allowances have been made for lactation in order to allow for the vitamin C content of breast milk. In England the recommended intake was raised from 30 to 60 mg/day, and in the United States from 45 to 80 mg/day. Extra vitamin C requirements for pregnancy are more difficult to define and both countries increased their recommended intakes to 60 mg/day.

Thiamin The major clinical feature of severe thiamin deficiency is beri-beri, and it is also known that thiamin is important in the metabolism of carbohydrates and their catabolic derivatives, with the most extensively studied reaction being the oxidative decarboxylation of pyruvic acid.

Estimations of requirements have been based either on the amount of thiamin needed to prevent clinical signs of beri-beri, on intakes necessary for tissue saturation, or on intakes needed to maintain normal red cell transketolase levels, the conventional parameter measured in assays of thiamin status. As in so many cases, the lowest requirements are those needed to prevent the appearance of clinical signs. Much clinical evidence came from studies in prisoner-of-war camps, from which it was concluded that the range of protective intakes was 0.2–0.4 mg/1000 kcal (42). As would be anticipated, thiamin requirements are closely linked with the amount of carbohydrate to be metabolized; thus it is customary to quote requirements on the basis of total energy intake.

Other investigators have measured the amount of the vitamin and its metabolites excreted in urine following an oral dose, but the results have been variable. Some studies have indicated that tissue saturation was achieved at an intake of 0.35 mg/1000 kcal, and the FAO/WHO (3) suggested an average thiamin requirement of 0.33 mg/1000 kcal. On the other hand, other studies have been interpreted as showing that tissue saturation was only attained at 0.5 mg/1000 kcal (43, 44).

In transketolase studies dietary intakes of 0.5 and 0.6–0.8 mg/1000 kcal have been shown to be necessary for accepted erythrocyte enzyme levels. Older people seemed to need more because of inefficient utilization (45, 46, 47). It must be admitted, however, that the physiological significance of enzyme studies based on erythrocytes is not understood.

In the light of these differences it is not surprising that recommended allowances for young adults vary considerably. The DHSS (1) value for men consuming 3000 kcal is 1.2 mg/day, similar to that of the FAO/WHO (3), but the NRC (2) opted for 1.5 mg.

Thiamin requirements for infants have generally been based on the composition of human breast milk, which contains around 0.3 mg/1000 kcal. Children and adolescents have been allotted intermediate allowances dependent on their energy intake.

Because human milk contains around 0.2 mg of thiamin in a day's typical secretion, and because extra dietary energy is recommended for lactation, the allowances for women are also raised at these times by an average of 0.3 mg/day. The pregnancy allowance is similar.

Riboflavin   Riboflavin is needed for the flavoprotein group of coenzymes. Clinical signs of riboflavin deficiency, lesions in the mucous membranes, apparently disappear when adult consumption levels rise above 0.3 mg/1000 kcal energy intake (48, 49). A marked rise in riboflavin excretion takes place when intake exceeds 0.4–0.5 mg/1000 kcal, which probably indicates the saturation level. Although most bodies relate their requirements to energy intake, physiologically this is misleading since riboflavin, unlike thiamin, is not directly involved in energy expenditure.

The FAO/WHO (3) accepted 0.44 mg riboflavin/1000 kcal as representing average requirements, and, after adding an apparently arbitrary allowance of 25% for individual variation, made its recommendation 0.55 mg/1000 kcal. The NRC (2) based its calculations on 0.60 mg/1000 kcal, but because of the link with energy intake lower requirements were quoted for older people (1.5 mg/day) as compared with 19–22-year-old-men (1.8 mg/day). There is little factual basis for believing that metabolic need truly falls away in this manner.

Another example of how linking nutrient requirements to energy can give rise to dubious reasoning is the DHSS (1) adjustment for requirements at different ages. At 0.55 mg/1000 kcal, they calculated that a 65-kg man consuming 3000 kcal would receive around 1.7 mg/day, which is equivalent to an intake of 0.07 $mg/kg^{0.75}$, which in turn is equivalent to 1 mg/1000 resting kcal. On the basis of this latter value and standard BMR tables, requirements for the two sexes at different ages were calculated. Although this scheme is not without its logic, it is clearly undesirable that roundabout calculations of this type should be necessary.

About 0.3 to 0.5 mg of riboflavin are secreted in breast milk each day, depending on concentration and output. The DHSS (1) allowed an extra 0.5 mg/day to cover this amount during lactation (50).

Nicotinic Acid and Its Derivatives   This group of nutrients is named niacin in the United States and consists of nicotinic acid and nicotinamide. Tryptophan is also a source of these two compounds, but only a small portion appears to be convertible and it has become customary to assume that, for every 60 mg of tryptophan consumed, about 1 mg of nicotinic acid and its derivatives are made available to supplement vitamin requirements. An examination of the original data (51, 52, 53) reveals a considerable variation between individuals — it appears that no fixed proportion of tryptophan is converted to nicotinic acid, and thus the 60:1 figure should only be used for guidance.

A further difficulty in defining nicotinic acid requirements is availability. Much of the nicotinic acid in cereal foods is in a bound form, and the extent to which it is metabolically available is not known for certain, but it may be limited. For practical purposes it may be wiser to assume that cereal products, unless fortified, are not a good source of nicotinic acid.

Nicotinic acid requirements have largely been investigated by studies in adults (54, 55, 56), which have looked either at tissue saturation levels or dietary intakes necessary for the prevention of pellagra. As would be expected, the former provides a larger value than the latter, and it is the saturation level that has usually been adopted to establish requirements. After allowing for individual variation, the FAO/WHO (3) reasoned that 6.6 mg of nicotinic acid/1000 kcal, or its equivalent, was a reasonable basis for the calculation of requirements. This was fixed on the assumption that a large proportion of the dietary intake would be in the form of cereal products. The same value was adopted, with minor modifications, by both the DHSS (1) and the NRC (2).

There is no direct information on the needs of children from infancy to adulthood, but nicotinic acid requirements for infants up to 6 months have been based on the breast milk content of nicotinic acid and tryptophan.

Likewise, there is a dearth of data for pregnancy and lactation. As with many nutrients, the efficiency of dietary utilization, particularly the conversion of tryptophan to nicotinic acid, may be greater at this time; but this is by no means certain. In the light of this lack of knowledge, most expert committees have assumed that extra vitamin allowances should be increased proportionately with energy at these times. As with riboflavin, however, there is no physiological justification for linking vitamin requirements to energy in this way.

Vitamin B_6   The metabolism of this vitamin is closely linked with that of nicotinic acid. Vitamin B_6, too, is not a single compound but a collective term for various pyridoxine derivatives. Metabolism and deficiency are particularly difficult to establish because of the variety of apparently unrelated clinical symptoms that seem to be linked with vitamin B_6: convulsions in children, microcytic anemia, depression and confusion, vomiting, and electro-encephalographic abnormalities.

Requirements have been variously based on the usual range of clinical, tissue saturation, and specific enzyme function tests, but the establishment of allowances is greatly complicated by the fact that requirements seem to rise with the level of protein in the diet (57). Requirements may also be greater in high fat diets (59). There may be an age factor, with young men being able to utilize B_6 more efficiently than older men (58). The use of oral contraceptives also results in an excess excretion of tryptophan metabolites (2), and affects the activity of B_6-dependent enzymes so much that it is unlikely that these could be corrected by the amount of B_6 normally present in a diet.

For all these reasons, recommended dietary allowances for B_6 must be regarded with circumspection, particularly when dietary intake data are being interpreted; an intake that is below the allowance might be perfectly safe because the substantial safety factor that has been included to cover the above contingencies could be uncalled for in that particular situation. Although the recommended adult allowance of 2 mg/day is speculative, it would almost certainly be absolutely safe for all except for some women taking oral contraceptives.

There are no satisfactory data on B_6 requirements in children. At birth the infant has a store of B_6 and the concentration in breast milk is initially low (0.01 mg/liter) but later rises to 0.1 mg/liter. Infants are perhaps a group in which deficiency can occur; convulsions have been detected in children receiving 0.1 mg/day, and 0.3 mg/day are necessary to protect against abnormal excretion of tryptophan metabolites after a test dose. In the United States it has been suggested that infant milk formulas should provide 0.04 mg/100 kcal (60); thus a 6-kg infant would receive 0.26 mg/day.

Likewise, there is little or no information for pregnant women or lactating mothers. Only an arbitrary addition can therefore be made, and the NRC (2) allowed an extra 0.5 mg/day for both conditions.

Folic Acid   Folic acid deficiency is one of the more common vitamin deficiencies because of the greatly increased requirements of pregnant women. Indeed, in most industrialized countries medicinal folic acid is provided as a routine during pregnancy.

Defining requirements is complicated by a number of different factors. First, there is the complex chemical nature of folic acid derivatives in food, which are chiefly in the form of formyl or methyl derivatives of tetrahydrofolic acid conjugated with additional glutamic acid residues. The digestion and efficiency of absorption of these derivatives are variable and incompletely understood. Once absorbed they exhibit different degrees of efficiency in their capacity to be converted to the coenzyme form of the vitamin.

Nutrient composition data are now obtained by a standardized microbiological assay procedure, using *Lactobacillus casei* after incubation with chick pancreas deconjugase, but it is recognized that pure folic acid may be required in amounts only one-quarter of this assay value.

Functionally, folic acid is concerned with the metabolism of the "active one-carton units" so important in the synthesis of nucleic acids. Thus deficiency would be expected to have widespread consequences in cellular metabolism. Blood seems to be the tissue most susceptible, and recommended allowances have been greatly influenced by the levels needed for the remission of hematological signs. For the adult this would seem to be 50 μg of pure folic acid per day (61). This value must then be adjusted to food values ($\times$ 4) and an allowance made for digestibility ($\times$ 2). Thus NRC (2) adopted a requirement of 400 μg/day as being appropriate to the American diet.

For infants there is no option but to assume that breast milk composition provides adequate guidance about requirements. Breast milk contains 5 μg/100 ml (or 5 μg/70 kcal); thus 40 μg/day of the type of folic acid in milk would probably represent a safe level for a young infant. Obviously more would be required if it were present in forms found in other foods. Needs of older children and adolescents have been predicted by interpolation.

For pregnancy, the NRC (2) allowed an extra 400 μg of *total* folate, assuming it existed in the customary dietary form of the United States. It was acutely conscious of the need to protect not only the developing fetus but the mother as well for subsequent pregnancies. Since breast milk contains 50 μg of folate per liter, and assuming a 25% efficiency of digestion, absorption, and conversion to milk folate, an extra 200 μg/day was recommended for lactating women.

With a vitamin as closely linked with human health status as folic acid, it would clearly be desirable to identify needs at different ages and physiological states with greater factual exactitude.

Vitamin B$_{12}$ Vitamin B$_{12}$ is closely linked functionally with folic acid. Requirements are difficult to define by physiological experiment because healthy people have substantial liver stores, the contents of which are readily available to the body as a whole. Proven deficiency is rare and is usually associated with poor digestion and absorption from the intestine, although low dietary levels can make a contribution if prolonged over many months. It is generally recognized that old people are among those most likely to be at risk, and it is important to ensure that they have available sufficient food of animal origin. Vegans are also potentially in a similar position, but can be protected by prophylactic B$_{12}$.

Requirements are not known with certainty, but it is usually considered that 3–4 μg/day is adequate. Needs of infants are based on breast milk composition and have been estimated as 0.3 μg/day. Children and adolescent recommendations have been suggested by interpolation. Pregnancy appears not to create special problems and is probably well allowed for by the 3–4 μg/day allowance for nonpregnant women. Breast milk, too, does not contain large amounts of B$_{12}$, and 3–4 μg/day would probably be satisfactory here also. These latter comments and reasoning are clearly not completely satisfactory, and once again there is need for more information.

Pantothenic Acid and Biotin   There are even less data than usual on which to base recommendations for these two nutrients. This is probably because clinical deficiencies are virtually unknown in man and thus defining requirements is largely an academic exercise. Biotin is widely distributed in food, but it can also be synthesized by the gut flora and it is doubtful if there is any dietary need at all in man for this substance. Pantothenic acid is widely distributed, too. It is doubtful that a good scientific case can be made for extensive new work on these vitamins, even though our knowledge about their dietary and health significance is so rudimentary.

Minerals

Calcium   Calcium is the mineral for which man has the highest daily requirement. Most of the body's calcium is present in the bones, but about 1% is in the soft tissues, where it plays an essential role in a variety of physiological processes, including the control of excitability in nerves and muscle, blood coagulation, and cardiac and voluntary muscle function. The maintenance of blood calcium is one of the most precisely controlled homoeostatic mechanisms in the body.

Physiological measures of calcium requirements have mainly been based on the amount needed to replace body losses, with the two principal approaches being, as with nitrogen, the balance technique and the estimation of obligatory losses. Both methods are troubled by a number of interpretational complexities. If a person has become accustomed to a relatively large calcium intake, he apparently becomes relatively inefficient in his ability to absorb calcium. Adaptation does occur (62), but this can be slow, and considerable differences have been noted in the ability of individuals to accommodate new circumstances (63). This means that if measurements are carried out in people from "westernized" countries, apparent requirements are much higher than if the same studies are performed in subjects from one of the developing countries, where customary intake has been relatively low.

Nordin (64) and colleagues have analyzed all available balance data from Europe and North America and have concluded that mean intake for balance in adult males is around 600 mg/day, and if one plans to cover the mean + SD of the population to define a "safe level" one would come up with a value of around 900 mg/day. Likewise, in the United States it has been found (65) that up to 320 mg of calcium are lost daily in urine, and if absorption is working at 40% efficiency the recommended dietary allowance would need to be 800 mg/day.

Equally, however, it has been widely demonstrated that children and adults grow healthy bones in many countries on considerably less calcium, and the FAO/WHO (66) suggested what it called a "practical allowance" of 500 mg/day. It has been shown that individuals in such countries (67) achieve calcium balance on as little as 200–400 mg/day.

Although the average calcium intake of adults in England is considerably higher (around 1 g/day), the DHSS (1) also adopted 500 mg/day for its recommended intake. The NRC (2), although it accepted the fundamental argument that people consuming low levels of calcium can be of adequate calcium status, still felt it was possible that higher calcium intakes might afford some protection against progressive calcium loss after 40 years of age (68). Furthermore, there is a known association between protein intake and calcium absorption: the higher the dietary protein, the lower the efficiency of calcium maintenance (69). The need for higher calcium intakes may become more pressing with the move in many countries to diets with a higher whole meal cereal content. These have been shown to increase calcium requirements for balance (70).

Efficiency of calcium absorption is also important in infant feeding. With breast milk about 70% of the ingested calcium is retained, whereas with cow's milk this figure is only 25–30%. Thus, although the latter contains considerably more calcium, overall retention is about the same.

Defining requirements for children and adolescents creates as great a quandary as for adults. Although apparently healthy growth is possible with less calcium, it has been suggested (71) that calcium laid down within the bone crystal lattice during early life may be a reservoir that mitigates against the worst effects of calcium loss in later life. Therefore, the NRC (2) recommended allowances of 800 mg/day for most of childhood and raised this up to 1200 mg for the ages of 10 to 18. In contrast, the 1969 DHSS recommended intakes were never higher than 700 mg.

The FAO/WHO (66) reasoned that, since the breast milk secreted each day during lactation contained about 250–300 mg of calcium, intake should be raised from 500 up to 1200 mg/day. This assumed an efficiency of absorption of 30–40%. The recommendation in Britain and the United States was also 1200 mg of calcium/day but the NRC (2) warned that some women secreted over 1 g of calcium/day in their milk and thus intakes must be considered on the basis of individual need.

Calcium needs for pregnancy have been calculated from changes found with age in fetal calcium content. At birth a baby contains on average 25 g of calcium and, although calcium absorption is probably increased in efficiency during pregnancy, recommended intakes have been raised considerably, and 1200 mg/day is virtually universal. While this intake is achievable for women in Western countries, this recommendation must be seen as an unattainable, and perhaps unnecessary, target in many developing countries. It is undesirable to have this type of two-tiered recommendation unless there really is a justifiable physiological basis. This can only be determined by much more intensive research than is occurring at the moment. Comparative studies in the two types of dietary situation are essential.

Iron   Although required in considerably less quantity than calcium, iron is one of the most important minerals physiologically because of its central role in oxygen transport and cellular oxidation.

Iron is present in the body in two main forms: in "stored" forms as ferritin and hemosiderin (5–20 mg/kg of body weight), or in active forms, as hemoglobin, myoglobin, and, to a lesser extent, in association with a number of enzymes. During the initial stages of iron deficiency it is the stored forms that first become reduced in content and thus they provide the most sensitive index of dietary need. It is only when these are significantly depleted that blood hemoglobin concentrations begin to drop.

Losses of iron from the body, apart from unabsorbed nutrient, are not great and are confined to exfoliated cells or to bleeding, the latter being particularly important in menstruating women. Thus, in general, daily requirements are relatively small. The intestine is the main organ of homeostatic control. Normal efficiency of iron absorption is about 10%, but when this becomes insufficient to meet needs, such as during pregnancy, lactation, after bleeding, or in low intakes, its efficiency can increase by up to 20–30% (72).

Calculations to take account of dietary iron absorption are also complicated by the different chemical forms found in food. Heme iron in meat has the highest absorption of natural iron compounds. Absorption of the iron in egg or vegetables can be influenced considerably by other dietary components (73). For example, phytate or dietary fiber can bind such iron, making it much less available. Not all dietary interactions are disadvantageous. Ascorbic acid, for example, enhances the absorption of nonheme iron, and there are reports that the presence of heme iron can enhance the absorption of nonheme iron (74).

For an adult man or a nonmenstruating woman who is not iron deficient, and who is receiving a well-balanced diet, requirements have been estimated to be around 1 mg/day; thus (assuming a 10% efficiency of absorption) the requirement becomes 10 mg/day, and this is the value recommended by most expert committees.

Infancy is one of the critical periods of life when iron deficiency may occur. The iron content of breast milk is not high enough to enable the child to build up stores and those laid down during pregnancy are usually depleted by 6 months. This means that even the well-fed infant is very sensitive to the iron content of weaning foods. At 3 months the "artificially" fed child probably needs around 1 mg/kg/day of dietary iron, but low birth weight children may need double this (2).

Another group potentially at risk are women during menstruation (75). Menstrual losses are very variable, and to take account of the full range the NRC (2) recommended 18 mg/day for women during the ages of menstruation, in contrast to 10 mg for men and nonmenstruating women. In practical *family* diets, however, this level is difficult to achieve and the British approach (1) was to raise *dietary* recommendations only to 12 mg/day and to assume that the health services would detect women with exceptionally high needs, who could then be provided with the necessary iron in *medicinal* form.

Pregnancy is a further "at risk" time because of the demands of the fetus, and losses at childbirth. It is considered by many that these needs, too, should be met from nondietary iron sources.

The fortification of foods with iron is a controversial matter (76). It can be argued that a well-balanced diet provides sufficient iron for all normal needs and that medicinal iron should be used to cover exceptional requirements. This counsel is not necessarily applicable to all communities, however, and it seems that food supplementation with readily absorbable iron chelates will become more common. This will mean, of course, that some sectors of the community will receive considerably more than their needs, but it does not seem likely that this will create a health hazard.

Zinc Zinc is one of the minerals that has been of increased interest to nutritionists in recent years. Frank zinc deficiency has been reported from Egypt (77), and the growth of infants fed milk formulas has been shown to be affected by the zinc content of the diet (78). Biochemical evidence of zinc deficiency, based on hair or plasma zinc concentrations, has also been detected in communities living in the United States (79), but the physiological significance of these findings has not really been established.

The greatest effort to define zinc requirements has been in the United States (2). Estimates have largely been based on balance studies carried out in infancy and in young adults. Zinc is predominantly found in animal foods; it is also present in cereal products, but availability is probably low. As a result, the adequacy of a person's diet as judged by 1974 NRC criteria is very dependent on the proportion of animal foods consumed. Data from many countries, particularly during infancy, early childhood, and pregnancy, would indicate the possibility of widespread deficiency. As with calcium, however, it seems likely that need and efficiency of utilization will depend greatly on the dietary level to which the individual has become accustomed, and uncritical extrapolation from American experiences to the developing countries may not be fully justified.

Sodium and Potassium Dietary requirements of sodium and potassium in adults living in Western countries are more than met by the diet, and the main concern is *overconsumption*. Occasional exceptions are the elderly, with low total food intakes, who may become potassium deficient, especially if they are taking purgatives or diuretics in an uncontrolled manner. Excessive sweating can also create salt deficiencies, and this is a problem for those doing heavy manual work in hot climates or, alternatively, in excessively hot factory conditions, such as in old-fashioned boiler houses or iron foundries.

Worries about salt intake as an important factor in the development of hypertension in man are contentious. Many authorities would claim that in spite of the evidence from animal experiments there is little practical evidence in man that salt intake is a primary etiological factor. Salt can, however, exacerbate existing hypertension, and people with this condition certainly need a lower salt diet. It must be pointed out, however, that a general reduction in salt intake in the United States was one of the dietary goals of the McGovern Senate Committee (80), and others (81) have recommended that children should be dissuaded from eating salty preparations like beef concentrates, (for example, Marmite) so that they do not develop a taste for other salty foods in later life.

It is not customary for sodium and potassium requirements to appear in tables of nutrient requirements, but they have been considered here because of growing interest in their dietary importance for health.

Other Cations   There are a whole range of other cations, including copper, chromium, cobalt, manganese, molybdenum, and selenium, that are known to be essential for growth and well-being, but their public health significance for man is by no means understood. Most of the practical nutritional experience concerning these minerals comes from agricultural and veterinary studies. It is well established in farm animals that a variety of mineral deficiencies in the soil result in physiological defects in grazing animals. Modern animal husbandry methods, which result in particularly rapid growth in the young animal, have also forced the farmer to take special note of a wide range of trace element requirements.

In the industrial countries, man is to a large extent protected from trace element deficiency because, if at all possible, he eats meat and the animal has, in effect, concentrated essential elements even sparsely available in the soil. The situation is not the same, however, for communities who live predominantly on vegetable crops, since they face the same primary difficulty as the farm animal. The nutritional advantage of the customary high animal protein diet of the Western world lies, perhaps, not in its protein per se, but in the high mineral and trace element content of animal products.

It would clearly be desirable, although perhaps not immediately essential, for work to be begun or expanded on mineral requirements in order to cover a wider range than has hitherto been the case. It is to be hoped that when this work is started it will be designed to adequately investigate practical physiological complexities such as nutrient interaction, efficiency of digestion, absorption, tissue utilization, critical metabolic role in health, and variation in requirements between individuals at different stages of development.

Anions   The human body needs specific anions as well as cations. Chloride is, of course, the principal anion in extracellular fluid, but usually if sodium requirements are satisfied so are those for chloride. However, in some clinical conditions in which dietary sodium needs to be severely restricted, such as cases of heart or kidney disease, alternative sources of chloride may be needed.

Iodine is a dietary anion that is of practical concern for nutritionists concerned with public health. Endemic goiter resulting from iodine deficiency is a problem in many countries. Females are more affected than males, particularly during child-bearing age. Although goiter does predominate in countries with generally low intakes of iodine, it is not always possible to achieve a significant correlation between biochemical indices of iodine status, such as urinary iodine secretion, and the severity of the clinical condition (82). This indicates, as is the case with so many nutritionally related diseases, that goiter is multifactorial in origin.

Iodine requirements in adults have been roughly defined by the NRC (2) on the basis of the clinical evidence that goiter can be prevented by an intake of 1 μg/kg of body weight. Infant requirements were based, as is becoming the custom for most nutrients, on the composition of breast milk from healthy mothers. Extra allowances were made for pregnancy and lactation.

It is perfectly possible to meet dietary iodine requirements from a well-balanced diet, but if there is an overall shortage of animal and dairy products there is potential trouble. In many industrialized countries the risk of iodine deficiency is overcome by the addition of iodine to table salt. Iodine is not customarily added to other salts in order to minimize the risk of excessive levels of dietary iodine.

Fluorine is also essential for growth in animals, although growth failure due to fluorine deficiency is not a known public health problem for man. The main health interest in dietary fluorine concerns the incorporation of this element into the lattice of dental enamel, which has the effect of hardening the structure, thus conferring some protection against dental caries (83). Fluorine is present in animal products, in tea, and in many samples of drinking water (and hence in many cooked foods as well), but the fluorine content of water is variable and many public health authorities now supplement drinking water with fluorine as a public health measure. There is little need to point out that for some people this is a highly contentious procedure (84). Mottling of teeth or more serious toxic effects are never seen at the levels of public health fortification, however, and it is the opinion of most that the benefits of this procedure outweigh any identified risk.

NUTRIENTS AS EATEN

This chapter has largely been concerned with the physiological background to dietary allowances, and as such has been confined mainly to those topics usually considered by expert committees given the task of defining allowances for their country. However carefully worked out, most present recommendations should be viewed only as the best that can be done with the scientific knowledge available. A plea has been made throughout for more knowledge, and for the recognition of this need by authorities responsible for funding medical and scientific research.

In the future, tables of recommended dietary allowances for optimum health will inevitably become more complex. This chapter has only dealt with major classifications of nutrients. The differences between various energy sources have, for example, not been mentioned, but some metabolizable carbohydrates, such as sucrose, may be linked to health hazards, whereas starches are not. Likewise, some "unavailable" carbohydrates confer health advantages that other chemically similar unavailable carbohydrates do not. There is also intense current interest in the biological significance of the percentage of fat in the diet, and the importance of different saturated and unsaturated fats in relation to the etiology of heart disease.

It is not inconceivable that such considerations will ultimately also be incorporated into tables of dietary allowances, but before this can be done with any degree of scientific confidence we must develop a better understanding of what we mean by health. Only then will we have a baseline for nutritional considerations of such complexity.

REFERENCES

1. DHSS. (1969). Recommended Intakes of Nutrients for the United Kingdom. Reports on Public Health and Medical Subjects, No. 120. Her Majesty's Stationery Office, London.
2. Food and Nutrition Board, National Research Council. (1974). Recommended Dietary Allowances, 8th ed. National Academy of Sciences, Washington, D. C.
3. Joint FAO/WHO Expert Group on Requirements of Vitamin A, Thiamine, Riboflavine and Niacin. (1967). FAO Nutrition Meetings Report Series, No. 41; WHO Technical Reports Series, No. 362. United Nations, New York.
4. FAO/WHO. (1973). Energy and protein requirements. Report of a joint FAO/WHO ad hoc Expert Committee. WHO Technical Reports Series, No. 522; FAO Nutrition Meetings Report Series, No. 52. WHO, Geneva.
5. Durnin, J. V. G. A., and Passmore, R. (1967). Energy, Work and Leisure. Heinemann, London.
6. Household Food Consumption and Expenditure. (1975). Annual Report of the National Food Survey Committee, Ministry of Agriculture, Fisheries and Food. Her Majesty's Stationery Office, London.
7. FAO Committee on Calorie Requirements. (1950). [Report.] FAO Nutritional Studies, No. 5. United Nations, New York.
8. FAO Second Committee on Calorie Requirements. (1957). [Report.] FAO Nutritional Studies, No. 15. United Nations, New York.
9. Johnson, R. E. (1963). Fed. Proc. 22:1439.
10. Durnin, J. V. G. A. (1977). Personal communication.
11. Alleyne, G. A. O., Hay, R. W., Picou, D. I., Stanfield, J. P., and Whitehead, R. G. (1977). Protein-Energy Malnutrition. Edward Arnold, London.
12. James, W. P. T., and Trayhurn, P. (1976). Lancet 2:770.
13. Hytten, F. E., and Leitch, I. (1971). The Physiology of Human Pregnancy, 2nd ed. Blackwell Scientific Publications, Oxford.
14. Whitehead, R. G., Paul, A. A., Prentice, A. M., Rutishauser, I. H. E., and Hutton, M. A. (1978). Br. J. Nutr. (in press).
15. Whitehead, R. G. (1976). Lancet 2:1192.
16. Thomson, A. M., Hytten, F. E., and Billewicz, W. Z. (1970). Br. J. Nutr. 24:565.
17. Garza, C., Scrimshaw, N. W., and Young, V. R. (1977). Br. J. Nutr. 37:403.
18. Scrimshaw, N. S. (1976). N. Engl. J. Med. 294:198.
19. Nicol, B. M., and Phillips, P. G. (1976). Br. J. Nutr. 36:337.
20. Nicol, B. M., and Phillips, P. G. (1976). Br. J. Nutr. 36:337.
21. Sukhatme, P. V. (1974). J. R. Stat. Soc. A. 137:166.

22. Scrimshaw, N. S. (1977). Personal communication.
23. Garza, C., Scrimshaw, N. S., and Young, V. R. (1976). Am. J. Clin. Nutr. 29:280.
24. Whitehead, R. G., Coward, W. D., Lunn, P. G., and Sawyer, M. (1978). Br. J. Nutr. (in press).
25. Stuart, H. C., and Stevenson, S. (1959). In W. E. Nelson (ed.), Textbook of Pediatrics. Saunders, Philadelphia.
26. Whitehead, R. G. (1977). Am. J. Clin. Nutr. 30:1545.
27. Whitehead, R. G. (1973). In J. W. G. Porter and B. A. Rolls (eds.), Protein in Human Nutrition. Academic Press, New York.
28. Waterlow, J. C., and Payne, P. R. (1975). Nature 258:113.
29. Naismith, D. J. (1969). Proc. Nutr. Soc. 28:25.
30. Hume, E. M., and Krebs, H. A. (eds.). 1949. Vitamin A requirement of human adults. Report of the Vitamin A Sub-committee of the Accessory Food Factors Committee. Medical Research Council Special Report Series, No. 264. Her Majesty's Stationery Office, London.
31. Hodges, R. E., and Kolder, H. (1971). In J. G. Bieri (ed.), Summary of Proceedings, Workshop on Biochemical and Clinical Criteria for Determining Human Vitamin A Nutriture. National Academy of Sciences, Washington, D. C.
32. Lawson, D. E. M., Cole, T. J., and Poskitt, E. M. E. (1978). Manuscript in preparation.
33. Sutherland, J. M., Glueck, H. I., and Gleser, G. (1967). Am. J. Dis. Child. 113:524.
34. Medical Research Council, Accessory Food Factors Committee. (1953). Vitamin C Requirements of Human Adults. Medical Research Council Special Report Series, No. 280. Her Majesty's Stationery Office, London.
35. Baker, E. M., Saari, J. C., and Tolbert, B. M. (1966). Am. J. Clin. Nutr. 19:371.
36. Baker, E. M., Hodges, R. E., Hood, J., Sauberlich, H. E., and March, S. C. (1969). Am. J. Clin. Nutr. 22:549.
37. Baker, E. M., Hodges, R. E., Hood, J., Sauberlich, H. E., March, S. C., and Canham, J. E. (1971). Am. J. Clin. Nutr. 24:444.
38. Levenson, S. M., Manner, G., and Seifter, E. (1971). In S. Margen (ed.), Progress in Human Nutrition, Vol. I. AVI Publishing Co. Inc., Westport, Conn.
39. Hume, R., and Wayers, E. (1973). Scot. Med. J. 18:3.
40. Kotze, H. F., Van der Walt, W. H., Rogers, G. C., and Strydom, N. B. (1977). J. Appl. Physiol. 42:711.
41. Pelletier, O. (1975). Ann. N. Y. Acad. Sci. 258:156.
42. Burgess, R. C. (1946). Lancet 2:411.
43. Williams, R. D., Mason, H. L., Smith, B. F., and Wilder, R. M. (1942). Arch. Intern. Med. 69:721.
44. Williams, R. D., Mason, H. L. and Wilder, R. M. (1943). J. Nutr. 25:71.
45. Haro, E. N., Brin, M. and Faloon, W. W. (1966). Arch. Intern. Med. 117:175.
46. Horwitt, M. K., Liebert, E., Kreisler, O., and Wittman, P. (1948). Investigations of Human Requirements for B-Complex Vitamins. NRC Bulletin. National Academy of Sciences, Washington, D. C.
47. Oldham, H. G., Davis, M. V., and Roberts, L. J. (1946). J. Nutr. 32:163.
48. Sebrell, W. H., Jr., Butler, R. E., Wooley, J. G., and Isbell, H. (1941). Public Health Rep. 56:510.
49. Horwitt, M. K., Harvey, C. C., Hills, O. W., and Liebert, E. (1950). J. Nutr. 41:247.

50. Bro-Rasmussen, F. (1958). Nutr. Abstr. Rev. 28:1, 369.
51. Horwitt, M. K., Harvey, C. C., Rothwell, W. S., Cutler, J. L., and Haffron, D. (1956). J. Nutr. (suppl. 1) 60:1.
52. Goldsmith, G. A., Miller, O. N., and Unglaub, W. G. (1961). J. Nutr. 73:172.
53. Vivian, V. M. (1964). J. Nutr. 82:395.
54. Goldsmith, G. A., Sarett, H. P., Register, U. D., and Gibbens, J. (1952). J. Clin. Invest. 31:533.
55. Goldsmith, G. A., Hosenthal, H. L., Gibbens, J., and Unglaub, W. G. (1955). J. Nutr. 56:371.
56. Goldsmith, G. A., Gibbens, J., Unglaub, W. G., and Miller, O. N. (1956). Am. J. Clin. Nutr. 4:151.
57. Baker, E. M., Canham, J. E., Nunes, W. T., Sauberlich, H. E., and McDowell, M. E. (1964). Am. J. Clin. Nutr. 15:59.
58. Ranke, E., Tauber, S. A., Horonick, A., Ranke, B., Goodhart, R. S., and Chow, B. F. (1960). J. Gerontol. 15:41.
59. Emerson, G. A., Walker, J. B., and Ganapathy, S. N. (1960). Am. J. Clin. Nutr. 8:242.
60. Food and Nutrition Board, National Research Council. (1968). Recommended Dietary Allowances, 7th ed. National Academy of Sciences, Washington, D. C.
61. Herbert, V. (1968). Am. J. Clin. Nutr. 21:743.
62. Malm, O. J. (1958). Calcium Requirement and Adaptation in Adult Man. Oslo University Press, Oslo.
63. Lawson, D. E. M., Cole, T. C., and Whitehead, R. G. (1977). Unpublished data.
64. Marshall, D. H., Nordin, B. E. C., and Speed, R. (1976). Proc. Nutr. Soc. 35:163.
65. Goldsmith, G. A. (1966). *In* Food and Civilization. A Symposium, Chap. 4, Charles C Thomas, Springfield, Ill.
66. FAO/WHO. (1962). Calcium requirements. Report of a FAO/WHO Expert Committee on Calcium Requirements. WHO Technical Reports Series, No. 230. FAO, Rome.
67. Hegsted, D. M., Mosioso, I., and Collazos, C. (1952). J. Nutr. 46:181.
68. Nordin, B. E. C. (1962). Am. J. Clin. Nutr. 10:384.
69. Margen, S., and Calloway, D. H. (1968). Fed. Proc. 27:726(A).
70. Branch, W. J., Southgate, D. A. T., and James, W. P. T. (1975). Proc. Nutr. Soc. 36:120A.
71. Newton-John, H. W., and Morgan, D. B. (1968). Lancet 1:232.
72. U. S. Department of Health, Education, and Welfare. 1972. Ten-State Nutrition Survey, 1968–70. IV. Biochemical. DHEW Publication No. (HSM) 72-8132. U. S. Dept. Health, Education, and Welfare, Washington, D. C.
73. Layrisse, M., Martinez-Torres, C., and Roche, M. (1968). Am. J. Clin. Nutr. 21:1175.
74. Cook, J. D., Layrisse, M., Martinez-Torres, C., Walker, R., Monsen, E., and Finch, C. A. (1972). J. Clin. Invest. 51:805.
75. Monsen, E. R., Kuhn, I. N., and Finch, C. A. (1967). Am. J. Clin. Nutr. 20:842.
76. Finch, C. A., and Monsen, E. R. (1972). JAMA 219:1462.
77. Prasad, A. S. (1966). *In* A. S. Prasad (ed.), Zinc Metabolism. Charles C Thomas, Springfield, Ill.
78. Walravens, P. A., and Hambidge, K. M. (1976). Am. J. Clin. Nutr. 29:1114.
79. Hambidge, K. M., Hambidge, C., Jacobs, M., and Baum, J. D., (1972). Pediatr. Res. 6:868.

80. McGovern, G. (1977). Dietary Goals for the United States. Select Committee on Nutrition and Human Needs, United States Senate. U. S. Government Printing Office, Washington, D. C.

81. Turner, R. (1977). Personal communication.

82. McGanity, W. (1970). *In* Food and Nutrition Board, National Research Council. Iodine Nutrition in the United States. National Academy of Sciences, Washington, D. C.

83. British Ministry of Health (1962). R. Soc. Health J. 82:173.

84. Food and Nutrition Board, National Research Council. 1953. The Problem of Providing Optimum Fluoride Intake for Prevention of Dental Caries. Publication 294. National Academy of Sciences, Washington, D. C.

Index

DATE DUE			
Chemistry Dept			
5/6/80			

Biochemistry   169637